Pediatric Heart
Disease

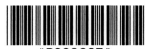

Pediatric Heart Disease
A Practical Guide

Edited by

Piers E. F. Daubeney MA, DM, FRCP, FRCPCH
Consultant Paediatric and Fetal Cardiologist
Royal Brompton Hospital;
Reader in Paediatric Cardiology
National Heart and Lung Institute
Imperial College
London, UK

Michael L. Rigby MD, FRCP, FRCPCH
Consultant Paediatric Cardiologist
Royal Brompton Hospital
London
UK

Koichiro Niwa MD, PhD, FACC, FAHA
Director
Department of Cardiology
Cardiovascular Center
St Luke's International Hospital
Tokyo, Japan

Michael A. Gatzoulis MD, PhD, FACC, FESC
Professor of Cardiology, Congenital Heart Disease
Royal Brompton Hospital;
National Heart and Lung Institute
Imperial College
London, UK

WILEY-BLACKWELL
A John Wiley & Sons, Ltd., Publication

Library of Congress Cataloging-in-Publication Data
Pediatric heart disease : a practical guide / Piers E. Daubeney ... [et al.].
    p. ; cm.
  Includes bibliographical references and index.
  ISBN-13: 978-0-7279-1861-1 (hard cover : alk. paper)
  ISBN-10: 0-7279-1861-3
  I. Daubeney, Piers E. F.
  [DNLM: 1. Heart Defects, Congenital. 2. Child. 3. Infant. WS 290]
  LC-classification not assigned
  618.92′12043–dc23
                        2011030257

A catalogue record for this book is available from the British Library.

Wiley also publishes its books in a variety of electronic formats. Some content that appears in print may not be available in electronic books.

Cover designer: Nathan Harris

Set in 9.25/11.5 pt Minion by Toppan Best-set Premedia Limited
Printed and bound in Malaysia by Vivar Printing Sdn Bhd

1 2012

Contents

List of Contributors

Lee Beerman MD
Professor of Pediatrics
University of Pittsburgh School of Medicine;
Children's Hospital of Pittsburgh of UPMC
Pittsburgh, PA, USA

Sian Bentley BPharm, MRPharmS
Specialist Pharmacist, Paediatrics
Royal Brompton Hospital
London, UK

Margarita Burmester MBBS, MRCP, FRCPCH
Consultant Paediatric Intensivist
Royal Brompton Hospital;
Imperial College
London, UK

Jamie Cheong BPharm (Hons), Cert Pharmacy Practice, MSc
Specialist Pharmacist, Antimicrobial
Royal Brompton Hospital
London, UK

Michael Cheung BSc (Hons), MB ChB, MRCP (UK), MD
Director, Department of Cardiology
Heart Research Group Leader
Murdoch Childrens Research Institute;
Principal Fellow
University of Melbourne
The Royal Children's Hospital
Melbourne, VIC, Australia

Piers E. F. Daubeney MA, DM, FRCP, FRCPCH
Consultant Paediatric and Fetal Cardiologist
Royal Brompton Hospital;
Reader in Paediatric Cardiology
National Heart and Lung Institute
Imperial College
London, UK

Brian Feingold, MD
Assistant Professor of Pediatrics,
University of Pittsburgh School of Medicine;
Children's Hospital of Pittsburgh of UPMC
Pittsburgh, PA, USA

Helena M. Gardiner PhD, MD, FRCP, FRCPCH, DCH
Reader in Perinatal Cardiology
Imperial College;
Honorary Consultant
Queen Charlotte's & Chelsea Hospital
London, UK

Michael A. Gatzoulis MD, PhD, FACC, FESC
Professor of Cardiology, Congenital Heart Disease
Royal Brompton Hospital;
National Heart and Lung Institute
Imperial College
London, UK

Georgios Giannakoulas MD, PhD
Consultant Cardiologist
Ahepa Hospital
Aristotle University
Thessaloniki, Greece;
Royal Brompton Hospital
London, UK

Alex Gooi FRACP, FCSANZ, MBBS, BSc (Med)
Paediatric and Fetal Cardiologist
Mater Children's Hospital
Brisbane, QLD, Australia

Nick Hayes BSc, MBChB, MRCPCH
Paediatric Cardiology Specialist Registrar
Royal Brompton Hospital
London, UK

Michael Y. Henein MD, MSc, PHD, FESC, FACC, FECP
Professor of Cardiology
Heart Centre and Department of Public Health and Clinical Medicine
Umea University
Umea, Sweden

S. Yen Ho PhD, FRCPath, FESC
Professor of Cardiac Morphology
Royal Brompton Hospital
London, UK

Victoria Jowett MD
Paediatric and Fetal Cardiologist
Royal Brompton Hospital
London, UK

Bradley B. Keller MD
Professor of Pediatrics, Pharmacology and Toxicology, and Bioengineering
Kosair Charities Chair and Chief, Division of Pediatric Heart Research
Cardiovascular Innovation Institute
Vice Chair for Research, Department of Pediatrics
University of Louisville
Louisville, KY, USA

Alan G. Magee BSc, MRCP, MB, BCh (Hons), FRCP
Consultant Paediatric Cardiologist
Royal Brompton Hospital
London, UK

William H. Neches MD
Emeritus Professor of Pediatrics
Cardiology Division
Children's Hospital of Pittsburgh of UPMC
Pittsburgh, PA, USA

Koichiro Niwa MD, PhD, FACC, FAHA
Director
Department of Cardiology
Cardiovascular Center
St Luke's International Hospital
Tokyo, Japan

Alan W. Nugent MBBS, FRACP
Associate Professor Pediatrics
University of Texas Southwestern Medical Center;
Director Cardiac Catheterization
Children's Medical Center
Dallas, TX, USA

Eric Quivers MD
Medical Director
Dean Health System
Middleton, WI, USA

Michael L. Rigby MD, FRCP, FRCPCH
Consultant Paediatric Cardiologist
Royal Brompton Hospital
London, UK

Phil Roberts MBChB, DCH, MRCPCH, FRACP
Interventional Cardiologist Heart Centre
for Children
Children's Hospital at Westmead
Sydney, NSW, Australia

Maria Virginia Tavares Santana PhD
Director
Department of Pediatric Cardiology
Instituto Dante Pazzanese
São Paulo, Brazil

Cleusa Cavalcanti Lapa Santos MD
Paediatric Cardiologist
Department of Pediatric Cardiology
Instituto Dante Pazzanese
São Paulo, Brazil

Anna Seale MBBChir, MRCP
Consultant Paediatric and Fetal Cardiologist
Royal Brompton Hospital
London, UK

Zdenek Slavik MD, FRCPCH
Consultant Paediatric Cardiologist/Intensivist
Royal Brompton Hospital
London, UK;
Associate Professor of Paediatrics
Charles University
Prague, Czech Republic

Mark S. Spence MD, MB, BCh, BAO (Hons), FRCP
Consultant Cardiologist
Royal Victoria Hospital
Belfast Trust;
Honorary Senior Lecturer
Queen's University
Belfast, UK

Shigeru Tateno MD
Director
Pediatric and Adult Congenital Heart
Disease Unit
Chiba Cardiovascular Center
Chiba, Japan

Gregory H. Tatum MD
Assistant Professor
Pediatric Cardiology
Duke University Medical Center
Durham, NC, USA

Jan Till MD
Consultant Paediatric Cardiologist
Department of Cardiology
Royal Brompton Hospital
London, UK

Anselm Uebing MD
Consultant Congenital Cardiologist
Adult Congenital Heart Centre and Centre
for Pulmonary Hypertension
Royal Brompton Hospital
London, UK;
Department of Congenital Heart Disease
and Pediatric Cardiology
University Hospital of Schleswig-Holstein
Kiel, Germany

Hideki Uemura MD, FRCS
Consultant Cardiac Surgeon
Department of Cardiothoracic Surgery
Royal Brompton Hospital
London, UK

Steven A. Webber MBChB, MRCP
Professor of Pediatrics and Clinical and
Translational Science
University of Pittsburgh School of
Medicine;
Chief, Division of Cardiology
Children's Hospital of Pittsburgh of UPMC
Pittsburgh, PA, USA

Preface

Pediatric cardiology is a niche specialty when compared to most others and international collaboration has been an essential part of the amazing progress in diagnosis and treatment achieved during the past 25 years. The frequency and range of congenital heart malformations, with few exceptions, is the same worldwide, whereas the incidence of acquired heart disease is subject to extreme variability. We have assembled experts from all over the world, who have combined their talents and knowledge in the production of this new textbook. This is a true manifestation of international friendship and collaboration and a reflection of the global family of pediatric cardiologists and cardiac surgeons caring for what is a common and global disease.

Nevertheless, many major congenital heart malformations are relatively rare; consequently, limited numbers of cases are seen in an individual institution or even in a single country. National and international research and audit must continue to develop, if further advances in management are to take place. Despite the emphasis on fetal, neonatal, and infant cardiology in modern practice, pediatric cardiology should merge seamlessly with adolescent and adult congenital heart disease; the involvement of Michael Gatzoulis in the editorial team has certainly assisted in this goal. An additional challenge to us all is the lack of availability of comprehensive cardiology services for children and young adults born with congenital heart disease in many countries around the world, including some with thriving economies. There must be a continuing stimulus to international collaboration in teaching and sharing expertise, research, and treatment.

It is therefore timely and appropriate that the editors have brought together experts from all continents, including Australasia, Asia, Europe, Africa, and North and South America, to produce this focused and much needed textbook, which will be an invaluable resource to physicians – senior and junior – and other disciplines involved with the care of the young patient with congenital heart disease. The list of contributors is impressive, which is not surprising, considering the international training and expertise of all four editors. We also count many of the contributors as personal friends and know they all accepted their invitations without hesitation and delivered excellent chapters. It is relatively unusual for a small textbook to have such an array of authors, but this reflects a major strength of the specialty of pediatric cardiology and long may it continue.

Piers E. F. Daubeney
Michael L. Rigby
Koichiro Niwa
Michael A. Gatzoulis

1   Epidemiology and genetics

Bradley B. Keller

University of Louisville, Louisville, KY, USA

Understanding the causes of congenital cardiovascular malformations

This is usually the third question asked by new parents of a child with congenital heart disease. The first four questions are:

1. What is wrong with our child's heart?
2. Will our child be alright?
3. Why does our child have a heart defect?
4. What did I do or not do during my pregnancy that caused my child's problem? (particularly asked by mothers)

Over the past 50 years dramatic progress in the diagnosis and management of congenital cardiovascular malformations now allows almost all newborns with congenital heart disease to survive with either palliative or complete "repairs." There has been comparable progress over the past 25 years in identifying the developmental mechanisms that regulate cardiovascular morphogenesis and that alter this complex process to generate malformations. This now provides the molecular and genetic insights that allow physicians to begin to answer parents when they ask, "Why did this happen?" With a more complete understanding of the mechanisms for congenital heart disease, physicians can also begin to answer more accurately the fifth question asked by some parents and patients:

5. Will our next child also have a heart problem?

Developmental mechanisms of congenital heart disease

While truly fascinating, a discussion of the developmental mechanism that produce "altered trajectories" in developing cardiovascular systems, trigger adaptive mechanisms, and result in the congenital heart disease detected at birth are beyond the scope of this handbook. However, for the purposes of understanding the specific malformations discussed in later chapters, it is important to recognize that normal cardiovascular development requires:

- A complex and dynamic sequence of temporally- and spatially-restricted gene expression (and suppression);
- The proliferation, migration, differentiation, and death of multiple cell subpopulations;
- A dynamic process of tissue remodeling throughout the developing heart and vasculature;
- A geometric increase in the biomechanical performance of the heart and vasculature;
- Multiple adaptive mechanisms for altered developmental events;
- A supportive "environment."

For humans, this occurs within the uterine environment and thus also includes both maternal hemodynamic and metabolic influences, as well as the environmental influences of both biologic and inert teratogens. Numerous recent reviews of normal and altered cardiovascular development are available for further reading.

Incidence of congenital heart disease

Congenital heart disease is commonly described to occur in 1% of liveborn infants based on several cross-sectional epidemiologic surveys. However, several important concepts require discussion to understand the accuracy (and limitations) of epidemiologic data on the incidence of congenital heart disease.

First, the definition used for heart disease greatly impacts the estimated incidence. For example, cross-sectional

Pediatric Heart Disease: A Practical Guide, First Edition. Piers E. F. Daubeney, Michael L. Rigby, Koichiro Niwa, and Michael A. Gatzoulis.
© 2012 Blackwell Publishing Ltd. Published 2012 by Blackwell Publishing Ltd.

population studies suggest that approximately 1% of live-born infants have heart disease, yet this estimate does not include affected fetuses who die *in utero*. Almost 30% of human pregnancies end during the first trimester and a major cause is failure of the developing heart and vasculature. The 1% incidence of congenital heart disease also does not include relatively "silent" abnormalities, such as a bicuspid aortic valve, small atrial septal defects, or subtly abnormal mitral valves, which may present as heart disease in adults or may be noted as incidental findings on postmortem examination. Finally, few studies on the incidence of congenital heart disease include the truly silent variations in cardiac anatomy, such as mitral valve-to-aortic valve discontinuity or aortic arch malformations, which may reflect genetic risk for congenital heart disease.

Second, the methods used to detect heart disease influence the estimation of incidence. Early population studies depended on family history and physical examination, but not all family members underwent echocardiography. Echocardiography has become one "gold-standard" in identifying congenital heart disease and with the increasing resolution and accuracy of current systems, the detection rate of silent or clinically "non-significant" findings continues to increase. These subtle abnormalities may still represent genetic risk for congenital heart disease with phenotypic expression determined by other modifying genes.

Third, the population studied greatly influences the rate of heart disease detected. While an estimated incidence of 1% is reasonable for newborns with obvious congenital heart disease, it is often the recurrence risk that parents want to know after they have had a first child with congenital heart disease. Accurately answering this important question is much more difficult as the recurrence risk for an individual couple is directly related to the underlying genetic or non-genetic (environmental) mechanism for the specific malformation. The basic answer for a family with a first child with non-syndromic and isolated congenital heart disease is that the recurrence risk for a second affected sibling may be as low as 2–5%, but may be higher based on the mechanism for a specific defect. It is important to note that there are differences in recurrence risk based on the sex of the affected child as well as the sex of the subsequent child.

The remainder of this chapter presents the general categories of congenital cardiovascular malformations grouped by underlying genetic or environmental mechanisms, including the relative incidence and recurrence risks for each group.

Genetic associations and congenital heart disease (Table 1.1)

Chromosomal disorders

Most parents are aware that chromosomal disorders cause developmental defects. Autosomal disorders are due to a decreased or increased number of genes or to altered genes on chromosomes other than X or Y.

Down syndrome (trisomy 21; discovered in 1959) is the most commonly recognized disorder associated with congenital heart disease. Of children born with a heart defect, 1 in 20 has trisomy 21. Specific to cardiac malformations, at least 40% of patients with trisomy 21 have abnormal atrioventricular septal morphogenesis and 30% have multiple cardiac anomalies. In autopsy series, at least 50% of the hearts of patients with trisomy 21 are abnormal and if silent malformations are included the incidence is even higher. The association between trisomy 21 and atrioventricular septal defect has been shown to be due to abnormal remodeling of the endocardial cushions triggered by the overexpression of the cell adhesion molecule DSCAM.

Trisomy 18 (Edward syndrome) occurs in 1 in 3500 newborns and is often associated with dysplastic and thickened cardiac valves and a triangular-shaped large ventricular septal defect.

Trisomy 13 (Patau syndrome) occurs in 1 in 7000 newborns and has a high incidence of heart disease, including laterality defects and both atrial and ventricular septal defects.

There are numerous partial duplication or deletion disorders associated with multiple congenital anomalies, including congenital heart disease. The involvement of a clinical genetics team in identifying the pattern and underlying cytogenetic disorder in a patient with multiple congenital anomalies is required to provide the family with accurate information both on the mechanism and the recurrence risk.

Turner syndrome is a genetic disorder of aneuploidy of the X chromosome, resulting in 45 rather than 46 chromosomes. Often associated with congenital heart disease, Turner syndrome has an extremely high rate of intrauterine loss such that the liveborn incidence of 32 in 10 000 births may reflect only 8% of conceptions with 45 (X,O). Patients with Turner syndrome have a disorder of lymphatic drainage which may explain some of the phenotypic features of neck webbing, wide-spaced nipples, and puffy feet noted at delivery. The prevalence of heart disease in patients with Turner syndrome is approxi-

Table 1.1 Common congenital heart defects and genetic associations

Anatomic defect/syndrome	Genetic associations
Atrial septal defect (ASD)	*GATA4* (8p23–22), *NKX2.5* (5q34)
Holt Oram syndrome	*TBX5* (12q24.1)
ASD and cardiomyopathy	*CSX* 5Q34
Ellis–van Creveld syndrome	*EVC* (4p16.1)
Ventricular septal defect	
22q11 deletion syndrome	22q11
Atrioventricular septal defect	*CRELD1* (3p25)
Down syndrome	Trisomy 21
Pulmonary valve stenosis	
Noonan syndrome	*PTPN11* (12q22)
Patent ductus arteriosus	
Char syndrome	*TFAP2B* (6p12-p21)
Tetralogy of Fallot	*TBX1* (22q11), *GATA4*
DiGeorge syndrome	22q11 deletion
Alagille syndrome	*jagged 1* (20p12)
Aortic valve stenosis	
Turner syndrome	45 (X,0)
Williams syndrome	7q11 deletion including *elastin* gene
Transposition of the great arteries	*ZIC3, CFC1*
Heterotaxy syndromes	*ACVR2B, CRYPTIC, LEFTYA, PITX2, ZIC3*
Connective tissue sisorders	
Marfan syndrome	*FBN1* (fibrillin, 15q21)
Ehlers–Danlos syndrome	*col3A1* (2q31)
Cardiomyopathy	
Barth syndrome	*Tazaffin* (Xq28)
Duchenne muscular dystrophy	*Dystrophin* (Xp21)
Fabry disease	*α-gallactosidase* (Xq22)
Hunter syndrome	*Iduronate sulphatase* (Xq27-28)
Hurler syndrome	*IDUA* (4p16)
Pompe disease	*α-glucosidase* (17q23)
Long QT syndrome	*KCNE2*
Jervell–Lange–Nielson syndrome	*KCNQ1* (11p15), *KCNE1* (21q11)
Romano–Ward syndrome	*KCNH2 "HERG"* (7q3)
	SCN5A (3p2)

mately 10%, with the highest association to left heart structures, including the mitral and aortic valves, and aortic arch.

Microdeletions

The recognition that a microdeletion on the long arm of chromosome 22 (22q11) was the genetic cause of **DiGeorge syndrome** in the early 1980s has resulted in a dramatic increase in the interest of clinicians in identifying genetic causes of congenital heart disease. First, it is important to note that while the deletion of a contiguous region of a single chromosome during DNA replication can be associated with congenital heart disease, the absence of a "deletion" based on the use of fluorescent *in situ* hybridization (FISH) techniques in no way defines the region of interest to be normal.

The association between a deletion in the 22q11 region and DiGeorge syndrome became apparent with the identification of a family with a translocation between chromosomes 20 and 22 and features of DiGeorge syndrome. Additional cases led to the identification of the 22q11 deletion and to the search for the DiGeorge "critical region" required for the clinical features, and specifically required to produce congenital heart disease. Deletions in the 22q11 region are now known to cause defects in craniofacial development (producing both information processing disorders, unique facial features, and cleft lip and palate), pharyngeal arch development (producing hypoparathyroidism and thymic aplasia with immune deficiency), aortic arch malformations (aortic arch interruption type B and anomalous origin of the subclavian artery), and cardiac defects (truncus arteriosus, tetralogy of Fallot, ventricular septal defect, and others). It is important to note that there can be significant phenotypic variation within an individual family harboring a specific 22q11 deletion due to both genetic and epigenetic modifiers. For example, a parent may have only mildly dysmorphic facial features while three of four children may have structural heart disease; and the heart disease between siblings can vary in location and severity.

Developmental studies in mouse models continue to identify underlying mechanisms for cardiac malformations, including the abnormal migration and patterning by "neural crest cells" that are required for normal aortic arch and aortopulmonary septal formation. The role of neural crest cells in this developmental process was initially identified by Kirby and colleagues in a series of neural crest ablation experiments using chick embryos, and has been subsequently confirmed by mouse models targeting the genes and proteins that affect neural crest migration and fate. Elegant temporal and spatial mapping studies in animal models have identified genes within the 22q11 region as well as genes outside this region.

The incidence of a deletion in the 22q11 region is still under investigation in population studies, but it is estimated to be as common as 13 in 10 000 newborn infants. Since this deletion acts as an autosomal dominant disorder, the recurrence risk for subsequent first-degree relatives may be as high as 40% (10 times higher than the recurrence risk for the first-degree relatives of a patient with isolated and non-syndromic congenital heart disease).

Williams syndrome (microdeletion on chromosome 7q11 including the *elastin* gene) includes a developmental disorder of vasculogenesis that is associated with supravalvar aortic and pulmonary artery stenosis as well as stenosis at the origins of vessels, including the coronary ostia and aortic coarctation.

Alagille syndrome (microdeletion on chromosome 20p12) has been identified to be caused by a loss of function of the gene *jagged 1* which produces a ligand for the transcription factor Notch 1 required for early laterality pattern formation. This results in cardiac anomalies including segmental pulmonary arterial hypoplasia.

Singe gene disorders

At least 80% of newborn infants with congenital heart disease have "normal" karyotypes as defined by standard genetic analysis including FISH probes. However, due to the many genes and proteins involved in cardiovascular morphogenesis, errors in a single gene down to the level of a single base pair error can still result in clinically significant and even lethal congenital anomalies. For some genes, loss of a single copy of the gene (heterozygous condition) is sufficient to alter cardiovascular morphogenesis and generate structural malformations.

Examples of single gene, heterozygous conditions include:
• **Holt–Oram syndrome** (atrial septal defect, conduction disorders, and cardiomyopathy) is caused by a heterozygous error in the *TBX5* gene;
• **Marfan syndrome** (connective tissue disorder with mitral valve prolapse and aortic aneurysm and rupture) is caused by a heterozygous error in the *fibrillin* gene;
• **Noonan syndrome** (pulmonary valve stenosis, hypertrophic cardiomyopathy) can be caused by heterozygous errors in a protein phosphatase PTPN11, as well as errors in the *SOS1, RAF1, KRAS, NRAS,* and *BRAF* genes.

Many of these genetic diseases are lethal in the homozygous mutant state in mice, and likely also in humans. The severity of disease in individuals with the same single gene heterozygous error is influenced by both genetic and epigenetic modifying factors during development, and these can either increase or decrease in severity in subsequent generations. For the parents of a child with a heterozygous, single gene disorder the recurrence risk for subsequent children can be as high as 50%, though often this is not the case owing to variations in the phenotypic severity due to modifier genes that can impact fetal survival. For example, left heart defects that may be due to an autosomal dominant gene in a single family may represent a clinical spectrum from very mild (silent) variations in aortic valve structure to very severe (*in utero* lethal) left heart hyperplasia. These syndromes can also occur as new mutations and this is more likely when both parents are phenotypically normal or if the syndrome is associated with significantly reduced fertility (such as in Turner syndrome).

Abnormalities of metabolic and structural pathways

For genes that are required for metabolic pathways, often two copies of the abnormal gene are required for a clinically detectable syndrome. For example, **Pompe disease** (glycogen storage disease type IIa or acid maltase deficiency) occurs in 1 in 40 000 newborns as an autosomal recessive disorder and is associated with progressive and lethal hypertrophic cardiomyopathy.

Duchenne muscular dystrophy (skeletal and cardiac myopathy) is a good example of of a disorder caused by genes restricted to the sex (X,Y) chromosomes; clinical presentation is usually restricted to affected males with females acting as carriers. The affected *dystrophin* gene is on the X chromosome. Rarely, affected carrier females inactivate the "normal" X chromosome and display the disease.

Heart disease in twins

Twins represent unique biologic siblings that can have concordant or discordant cardiac findings. The risk of congenital heart disease in all twins remains close to the population average of 1% with a slightly increased risk of almost 2% in monozygotic twins. The absence of heart disease in many siblings of monozygotic twins was an early rationale for a polygenic or environmental mechanism for congenital heart disease. In fact, monozygotic twins are not "identical" as the process of cleaving the early developing embryo results in two embryos with unequal laterality cues. These patterning cues for the developing embryo cause differences in gene expression (or suppression) that can dramatically alter final phenotype.

Maternal disorders associated with congenital heart disease

For centuries, both mothers and physicians have suspected a maternal mechanism for congenital heart disease. Common maternal causes for congenital heart disease have included:
• **Maternal (and subsequently congenital) rubella infection**: 35% risk of patent ductus arteriosus, pulmonary arterial hypoplasia, septal defects;
• **Diabetes**: 3–5% risk of transposition of the great arteries, ventricular septal defect;
• **Alcohol abuse**: 25–30% risk of septal defects;
• **Phenylketonuria**: 25–50% risk of tetralogy of Fallot;
• **Systemic lupus erythematosus**: up to 40% risk of congenital heart block;
• **Lithium**: up to 20% risk of tricuspid valve anomalies;
• **Retinoic acid exposure**: associated with at least 50% risk of conotruncal defects.

The mechanisms by which these maternal diseases or exposures alter cardiovascular morphogenesis are varied, but reflect injury to vulnerable cells and tissues during unique developmental windows. The severity and lethality of these events can also be modified by both genetic and epigenetic factors.

Polygenic inheritance

A basic set of rules for determining polygenic inheritance is:
• Recurrence risk depends on the gene incidence in the population with the risk to first-degree relatives being the square root of the incidence;
• Risk is greater in first-degree relatives than in distant relatives;
• Risk is increased when there are multiple affected family members;
• Risk may be higher when the disorder is more severe;
• When the incidence varies by sex, the risk is greater in relatives of the more rarely affected sex.

Thus, one of the critical aspects of providing families with an accurate assessment of the possible causes and possible recurrence risk for congenital heart disease requires a detailed family history for congenital cardiac and non-cardiac malformations (with the greatest level of accuracy available).

Summary

Despite the complexity of cardiovascular morphogenesis, only 1% of children are born with obvious congenital heart disease. It is likely that many more affected fetuses with congenital heart disease die *in utero*, and there are many more individuals with subtle errors in cardiac structure and function who may present with heart disease later in life or who may carry a genetic risk for congenital heart disease with minimal phenotypic expression. The underlying genetic, molecular, and epigenetic mechanisms for congenital heart disease are becoming increasingly apparent, and together with the expanded availability of targeted and genome-wide genetic testing, this is aiding families in understanding both the underlying mechanism and the recurrence risk for these disorders. Most importantly, we need to be honest with families in stating that at the present time we simply do not know the underlying cause of congenital heart disease for most patients, but that for most families the risk of recurrence in subsequent children appears to be relatively low (<5%).

Further reading

Boldt T, Andersson S, Eronen M. Etiology and outcome of fetuses with structural heart disease. *Acta Obstet Gynecol Scand* 2004;83:531–535.

Bruneau BG. The developing heart and congenital heart defects: a make or break situation. *Clin Genet* 2003;63:252–261.

Burggren W, Keller BB. *Development of Cardiovascular Systems: Molecules to Organisms*. New York: Cambridge University Press, 1997.

Burn J. The aetiology of congenital heart disease In: Anderson RH, Baker EJ, Macartney FJ, Rigby ML, Shinebourne EA, Tynan M, eds. *Paediatric Cardiology*, 2nd edn., London: Churchill Livingstone, pp. 141–213.

Epstein JA, Parmacek MS. Recent advances in cardiac development with therapeutic implications for adult cardiovascular disease. *Circulation*. 2005;112:592–597.

Ferencz C, Rubin JD, Loffredo CA, Magee CA. Epidemiology of Congenital Heart Disease: The Baltimore-Washington Infant Study 1981–1989. In: Anderson RH, ed. *Perspectives in Pediatric Cardiology*, Volume 4. Mount Kisco: Futura Publishing Co, 1993.

Harvey RP, Rosenthal N. *Heart Development*. San Diego: Academic Press, 1999.

Lin AE, Pierpont ME. Special issue: Heart developments and the genetics aspects of cardiovascular malformation. *Am J Med Genet* 2001;97.

Pierpont MEM, Moller JH. *The Genetics of Cardiovascular Disease*. Boston: Martinus Nijhoff Publishing, 1987.

Srivastava D. Genetic assembly of the heart: implications for congenital heart disease. *Annu Rev Physiol* 2001;63:451–469.

2 Basic cardiac physiology

Michael Cheung

Murdoch Childrens Research Institute and The Royal Children's Hospital, Melbourne, VIC, Australia

The ability of the heart to alter contractile patterns and generate adequate cardiac output in response to demand is remarkable in terms of chronicity, rate of response, and also magnitude of change. Some of the governing factors in this process will be discussed in this chapter, and a brief account of the fetal circulation and postnatal changes will be presented.

Initiation of contraction

Much of our knowledge regarding cardiac muscle contraction is derived from the study of skeletal muscle. Although there are some important differences between cardiac and skeletal muscle, the general scheme of excitation–contraction coupling is similar.

Cardiac muscle consists of thick (myosin) and thin (actin) filaments, contractile components linked to these, and a major protein titin, which is important in the passive spring-like properties of the myocardium. Associated with these filaments are the contractile components, which consist of troponin subunits (I, C, and T) and tropomyosin. The troponin subunits function to bind calcium (TnC) and tropomyosin (TnT), and also inhibit this interaction (TnI). Essentially then, the cardiac action potential influences ion channels, resulting in a transient calcium ion influx. This entry of calcium into the cell causes release of a larger amount of calcium from the sarcoplasmic reticulum, so-called calcium-induced calcium release. In the absence of calcium the interaction between myosin and actin is blocked by the binding of TnI to actin. With the binding of calcium by TnC however, a change in configuration of tropomyosin permits interaction between myosin and actin and subsequent force generation. This process requires energy and appears to be driven by the activity of myosin ATPase. Once attached to actin, the power stroke of myosin head rotation causes myofilament shortening. The reuptake and release of calcium from TnC permits relaxation to occur.

There are multiple levels where this process can be affected. For example, alterations in the myosin heavy chain isoforms and ATPase activity have been shown in disease states such as hypothyroidism and diabetes. Furthermore, genetic mutations resulting in abnormal troponin development account for particular types of cardiomyopathy.

Properties of myocardium

Force–velocity relationship

Contractile performance of muscle, defined as its ability to do work, can be expressed in different ways. One of the fundamental properties of the myocardium is its force–velocity relationship. This relationship describes the ability of myofilaments to shorten more rapidly and to a greater degree when faced with a light load as compared to a heavy load. Conversely, in the face of a heavy load, a muscle shortens more slowly and also to a lesser degree. Using *in vitro* methods of measurement, such as the isovelocity release technique, plots of the load dependence of these shortening velocities yield hyperbolic force–velocity curves (Figure 2.1). It can be seen that maximal velocity of shortening (V_{max}) occurs at zero load. V_{max} is considered to reflect the intrinsic velocity of myosin cross-bridge turnover, which can be measured *in vitro* as myosin ATPase activity. The x-intercept of this curve, where generated force is maximal, is designated P_0. It is important to note therefore, that for the same contractile state, the changes in performance in the face of changing load are a reflection of the way in which work is performed in the face of a changing hemodynamic environment.

Pediatric Heart Disease: A Practical Guide, First Edition. Piers E. F. Daubeney, Michael L. Rigby, Koichiro Niwa, and Michael A. Gatzoulis.
© 2012 Blackwell Publishing Ltd. Published 2012 by Blackwell Publishing Ltd.

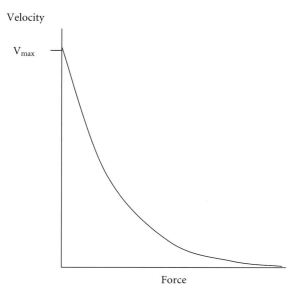

Figure 2.1 Force–velocity relationship.

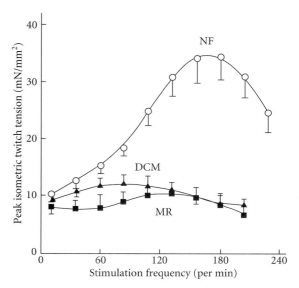

Figure 2.2 Plot of peak force versus rate of stimulation for normal non-failing myocardium (NF), and myocardium from patients with dilated cardiomyopathy (DCM) and chronic mitral regurgitation (MR). (Reproduced from Alpert NR, Leavitt BJ, Ittleman FP, *et al*. A mechanistic analysis of the force-frequency relation in non-failing and progressively failing human myocardium. *Basic Res Cardiol* 1998;93:23–32, with kind permission of Springer Science + Business Media.)

Length–tension relationship

This is another fundamental property of muscle which relates the maximum developed force to sarcomere length. It is thought that the generated force is dependent upon the degree of overlap of thick and thin myofilaments. As muscle length is gradually increased, developed force on contraction increases up to an optimal length. In skeletal muscle, it is possible to continue beyond this length to such a degree that the developed force decreases, to a point where there is no overlap of myofilaments and therefore force cannot be generated. Cardiac muscle differs significantly however, in that under physiologic conditions it does not appear possible to elicit this descending limb of the relationship. The heart therefore functions on the ascending limb of the length–tension curve. This relationship is thought to partly account for the Frank–Starling relationship (see below).

Force–frequency relationship

First described by Bowditch in 1871, the intrinsic property of the myocardium to alter contractile force with change in rate of stimulation is known as the force–frequency relationship (FFR) or "treppe" effect. The majority of data support rate-related fluctuations in calcium cycling as the underlying mechanism for this phenomenon.

In vitro studies have shown that the response of normal myocardium to an increasing stimulation rate is to increase the force of contractility (Figure 2.2), up to an optimal rate where generated force is maximal, after which there is a decline in force. The effect of increasing stimulation rate is thought to be an increase in activity of sarcoplasmic reticulum calcium ATPase. The rate-dependent intracellular flux of calcium can be demonstrated through the use of calcium dyes such as aequorin.

Using the same approach, dramatically differing responses may be observed in samples of diseased myocardium. In patients with dilated cardiomyopathy, for example, the FFR may become negative. Consequently, at relatively low heart rates the generated force decreases with increasing rate of stimulation.

The heart as a pump

The main function of the heart is to act as a pump and supply the body with blood, and in order to understand this, it is worthwhile considering the different phases of the cardiac cycle as described in the Wiggers diagram

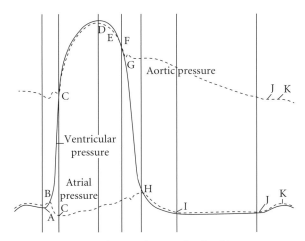

Figure 2.3 Wiggers diagram (see text for details).

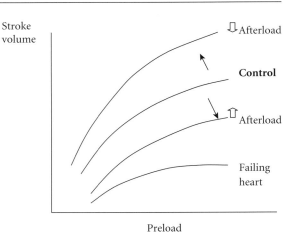

Figure 2.4 Ventricular function curve (see text for details).

(Figure 2.3). Wiggers divided the cardiac cycle for the left ventricle into separate phases. Systole begins with isovolumic contraction (A–C), followed by maximum ejection (C–D), and ending with a period of reduced ejection (D–F). In the first period of diastole, known as protodiastole (F–G), the first effect of relaxation is a drop in ventricular pressure leading to closure of the aortic valve. Ventricular pressure continues to fall as myocardial relaxation proceeds throughout this period of isovolumic relaxation (G–H). Once the ventricular pressure is lower than that of the atrium, the mitral valve opens and the period of early rapid filling begins (H–I). Ventricular pressure continues to fall during this phase, albeit at a slower rate. In the normal heart the majority of ventricular filling (approximately 70%) occurs during this period. A period of diastasis (I–J) may be observed when transmitral flow ceases, or occurs at a slow rate as pressure in the atrium and ventricle approximate prior to atrial contraction (J–K). It is important to consider blood flow in the heart as being driven by pressure gradients and that these changes in relative pressure in the connecting chambers and vessels explain the flow profiles demonstrated, for example, by echocardiography.

Ventricular function curves

Understanding the properties of isolated myocardium presented above is useful; however, control of pump function *in vivo* is a more complicated issue since there are additional reflexes involved. The major factors that influence ventricular pump function *in vivo* are preload, afterload, contractility, and heart rate. The relationship of

some of these factors can be described by examining the ventricular function curve (Figure 2.4). For the individual heart a whole family of curves is generated in response to the changing environment and demands of the patient. As can be seen in the control curve, the varying preload alters stoke volume or the amount of blood ejected per beat (Frank–Starling relationship). The most appropriate manner to assess preload (usually expressed as either end-diastolic pressure or end-diastolic volume) is debatable; however, essentially this is a reflection of the length–tension relationship mechanism (see above), which accounts partly for the Frank–Starling relationship. Note that the ventricular function curves do not have a downward or descending limb; indeed several studies have demonstrated no reduction in stroke volume despite elevation of preload to non-physiologic levels. In the control curve, the effect of increasing preload is to increase stoke volume. The effect of varying afterload is demonstrated by the other curves. Afterload reduction increases the amount of blood ejected and conversely an increase in afterload reduces stroke volume. Improved contractility causes a leftward shift to a different ventricular function curve.

Optimizing pump function

In the heart that is failing due to impaired contractility, it can be seen from the ventricular function curves that improvements in stroke volume could be brought about through either afterload reduction or by giving a positive inotrope to improve contractility, both of which should induce a leftward shift to a different curve. Further increases in preload will produce less improvement in stroke volume since the curve is relatively flatter in these patients with failing myocardium. Indeed, in these patients, although preload reduction in the form of diuretics may provide symptomatic improvement, stroke volume may not increase.

Diastolic function

It is of course obvious that if the heart does not fill properly, then output will be reduced. Referring to the Wiggers diagram (see Figure 2.3), there seem to be discrete phases of diastole which could potentially be assessed. The whole period of diastole is complex, however, with overlap of multiple processes affecting this part of the cardiac cycle. Following systolic contraction the ventricle has been deformed by shortening of myocardial fibers. The ventricle has passive elastic properties and as a consequence of this deformation there is stored potential energy which is released upon onset of relaxation. The process of relaxation is active and energy consuming. The fall in pressure during isovolumic relaxation therefore is influenced by a combination of active relaxation and also the release of the stored potential energy due to deformation of elastic material. Pressure cross-over with atrial pressure exceeding that of the ventricle opens the mitral valve and the generated pressure gradient across the valve induces flow into the ventricle during the so-called early rapid phase of ventricular filling. With equalization of ventricular and atrial pressures, a period of diastasis ensues during which time there may be no or only a small amount of low velocity flow. With atrial contraction an increase in the pressure gradient between the atrium and ventricle is developed, which drives blood into the ventricle. It can be seen therefore that during diastole there are two main phases of blood flow into the ventricle. These periods of blood flow during diastole can be routinely examined non-invasively using techniques such as echocardiography. Changes in diastolic filling may be due to abnormalities of relaxation, ventricular compliance, and timing, e.g. duration of diastole relative to the total duration of the cardiac cycle, atrioventricular delay, and rhythm. The common final mechanism, however, is the effect of these processes on the relative pressures within the atrium and ventricle and thus the impetus to blood flow.

Fetal circulation

The circulation in the fetus is different from that in postnatal life in that the systemic circulation is fed by the left and right ventricles in parallel. Shunting of blood occurs at three important levels (ductus venosus, foramen ovale, and ductus arteriosus) in this circulation. The placenta serves to oxygenate blood in addition to many other functions. Of the blood returning from the placenta via the umbilical vein, some goes to the hepatic veins, and the rest goes through the ductus venosus to enter the right atrium. Some of this highly oxygenated blood is diverted through the foramen ovale to the left atrium where it mixes with the small amount of pulmonary venous return. Blood supply to the coronaries and cerebral circulation is largely via the left ventricle and with relatively highly oxygenated blood (approx 65% saturated). Since the fluid-filled lungs are not inflated *in utero*, vascular resistance in this compartment is relatively high. The blood entering the pulmonary artery via the right ventricle therefore goes predominantly to the descending aorta via the ductus arteriosus, with a small proportion (approx 10%) of blood from the right ventricle being directed to the lungs. The left ventricle largely supplies the upper body, cerebral circulation, and coronaries, whilst the lower body is supplied by the right ventricle. The two vascular beds are connected by the aortic isthmus, the portion of the aorta between the left subclavian artery and the insertion of the ductus arteriosus.

The parallel nature of the fetal circulation means that changes in output can occur in one ventricle to compensate for derangements in the contralateral ventricle. These changes lead to the disproportionate growth of ventricles seen in many forms of congenital heart disease.

Fetal ventricular function

The contractile performance of the fetal myocardium has been shown to be reduced in comparison with adult myocardium *in vitro*. At similar muscle lengths, less active tension is developed by the fetal myocardium. This is perhaps not surprising considering the immaturity of structure and function of the fetal myocardium. The responses of the fetal ventricle to changes in loading conditions are also different. It appears that, although the stroke volume of the fetal ventricle increases in response to an increase in preload, the magnitude of response is limited and furthermore the right ventricle responds less than the left ventricle. The Frank–Starling mechanism is intact but within the fetus the ventricle is operating at the top, relatively flat part of the function curve. The fetal ventricular response to an increase in afterload created by balloon occlusion of the descending aorta in animal studies is a dramatic fall in right ventricular output. It appears therefore that changes in fetal heart rate are the major determinant of cardiac output.

Postnatal circulatory changes

With the first postnatal breath and inflation of the lungs, pulmonary vascular resistance falls and the amount of blood flow to the lungs increases. With increasing pulmonary venous return, left atrial pressure rises above that of the right atrium, leading to closure of the foramen ovale. Pulmonary vascular resistance continues to fall but may take several weeks to reach the lowest levels. Increasing levels of blood oxygenation stimulate the ductus arteriosus to close and this usually occurs in the first few days of life. Closure of the shunts present in fetal life creates a circulation in series, in contrast to the previous situation of a circulation with the ventricles supporting a parallel circulation.

In addition to the changes in the circulation, changes occur in myocardial function in postnatal life, albeit more slowly. Continued maturation of the myocardium occurs with alterations in systolic function with increased active tension development and altered responses to changes in loading conditions. Ventricular filling patterns change with a gradual improvement in early relaxation during childhood prior to a gradual decline in diastolic function during adulthood, both in terms of active relaxation and also passive properties of the myocardium. These normal age-related changes in ventricular function must be considered during assessment of ventricular performance.

Summary

Consideration of the factors involved in the control of ventricular function is important in the assessment and interpretation of clinical findings. Furthermore, understanding these factors is useful in instituting appropriate therapy.

Further reading

Alpert NR, Leavitt BJ, Ittleman FP, Hasenfuss G, Pieske B, Mulieri LA. A mechanistic analysis of the force–frequency relation in non-failing and progressively failing human myocardium. *Basic Res Cardiol* 1998;93:23–32.

Gwathmey JK, Slawsky MT, Hajjar RJ, Briggs GM, Morgan JP. Role of intracellular calcium handling in force–interval relationships of human ventricular myocardium. *J Clin Invest* 1990;85:1599–1613.

Pieske B, Kretschmann B, Meyer M, *et al.* Alterations in intracellular calcium handling associated with the inverse force–frequency relation in human dilated cardiomyopathy. *Circulation* 1995;92:1169–1178.

3 Cardiac morphology and nomenclature

S. Yen Ho

Royal Brompton Hospital, London, UK

To cope with the complexities of structural malformations of the heart and the myriad of variations that are observed, clinicians practicing in the field of congenital heart disease have developed ways of analyzing the heart in a systematic fashion. While the approaches used are similar, the terminologies employed differ widely. Some terminologies are in Latin, some relate to putative embryonic derivatives of cardiac structures or mechanisms of development, some are descriptive, and so on. Given the penchant of busy clinicians to use short-hand and acronyms, the nomenclature of congenital heart defects acquired an unwarranted reputation of being too complex and difficult for the novice in the field. This chapter summarizes an approach based entirely on morphology that is logical and simple.

The analysis of any congenitally malformed heart is simplified by first examining each segment of the heart:
• Atria;
• Ventricles;
• Great arteries (Figure 3.1).

By taking note of how each chamber relates and connects to another in a sequential fashion, even seemingly complex malformations can be described readily. This approach, **sequential segmental analysis**, provides the basic framework, but is not complete until account is taken of all associated malformations. Thus, most hearts have usual connections and relations of the chambers, but the associated lesions, such as a large ventricular septal defect or severe stenosis of the pulmonary valve, will dictate the clinical course. It is imperative, nevertheless, to analyze the heart sequentially before embarking on listing the associated defects.

Morphologic approach to segmental analysis

Based entirely upon recognition of the **morphology** of the cardiac chambers, this approach is **not** dependent on prior knowledge of embryology. Therefore, it has the advantage of not having to speculate on how the defect could have occurred during cardiac development. Instead, it is firmly based on descriptive anatomy. For segmental analysis, the morphologic distinction between right and left atria is as important as the distinction between right and left ventricles. The key is morphology rather than location. As is obvious in the human heart, right and left heart chambers are not strictly in the right and left positions. When the normal heart is viewed from the front, there is overlap of the right chambers over significant portions of the left chambers. Furthermore, the chambers in the malformed heart may also be abnormally located in relation to one another.

An in-depth description of the morphology of the cardiac chambers and great arteries is beyond the scope of this handbook and is well-described elsewhere. The salient morphologic features are summarized below. There are, undoubtedly, subtle differences from one patient to another, but one or more of the diagnostic features should be recognizable.

Briefly, the morphologic right atrium has a characteristic broad and triangular-shaped appendage that contains extensive pectinate muscles arising from the terminal crest, whereas the morphologic left atrium is smooth walled since the pectinate muscles are mainly confined to

Pediatric Heart Disease: A Practical Guide, First Edition. Piers E. F. Daubeney, Michael L. Rigby, Koichiro Niwa, and Michael A. Gatzoulis.
© 2012 Blackwell Publishing Ltd. Published 2012 by Blackwell Publishing Ltd.

Morphologic features of cardiac chambers

Atria

- Morphologic right:
  - Triangular, broad-based appendage
  - Extensive pectinate muscles
  - Terminal crest
  - Rim of oval fossa
- Morphologic left:
  - Tubular, narrow-based appendage
  - No terminal crest
  - Valve of oval fossa (no rim)

Ventricles

- Morphologic right:
  - Coarse apical trabeculations
  - Leaflet of atrioventricular valve attached directly to the septum (septal leaflet of tricuspid valve)
  - Moderator band
  - Septomarginal trabeculation
- Morphologic left:
  - Fine apical trabeculations
  - Smooth upper part of septum (without attachment of mitral valve)
- Morphologic indeterminate:
  - Very coarse trabeculations
  - No ventricular septum (solitary ventricle)

Great arteries

- Aorta:
  - Origin of coronary arteries
  - Aortic arch, usually with three arch arteries
- Pulmonary trunk:
  - Bifurcates into right and left pulmonary arteries
- Common arterial trunk (all three components mentioned below must be present):
  - Origin of coronary arteries
  - Origin of ascending aorta and aortic arch
  - Origin of pulmonary trunk or pulmonary arteries
- Solitary arterial trunk;
  - Origin of coronary arteries
  - Origin of ascending aorta and aortic arch
  - Collateral arteries supply lungs (no intrapericardial pulmonary arteries)

within its narrow, finger-like appendage that lacks a terminal crest. On the septal aspect of the morphologic right atrium, the valve of the oval fossa (septum primum) appears like a depression surrounded by a muscular rim (septum secundum). The fossa valve is the true interatrial septum and deficiencies in the valve are described as oval fossa defects (so-called secundum atrial septal defects). The septal aspect of the morphologic left atrium is the fossa valve itself but without a muscular rim.

Ventricles are described as having three components: inlet, apical trabecular, and outlet. The trabecular patterns, coarse in morphologic right and fine in morphologic left, are distinctive of the ventricles. The right ventricle has a muscle bundle known as the septomarginal trabeculation that is adherent to the septum. From it arises the moderator band that crosses the ventricular cavity to insert into the parietal wall of the right ventricle. In addition, the atrioventricular valves have characteristic features that can help diagnosis. The septal leaflet of the tricuspid valve has direct chordal attachments to the ventricular septum, whereas the mitral valve lacks a septal leaflet. The mitral valve adjoins the aortic valve through an area of valvar fibrous continuity, whereas the tricuspid and pulmonary valves are separated by muscle. The paired arrangement of the papillary muscles is a good guide for the mitral valve. The hinge lines (annulus) of the tricuspid and mitral valves are located at different levels. At the septum, there is valvar offset due to the tricuspid valve being hinged at a lower level, closer to the cardiac apex, than the mitral valve. The offset results in a part of the cardiac septum being located in between the right atrium and the left ventricle. Previously described as the "atrioventricular septum," closer anatomic studies have revealed that much of this "septum" is not truly septal but is composed of atrial wall and ventricular wall separated by a fibro-fatty tissue plane that has invaginated from the epicardium. Atrioventricular septal defects, including the so-called primum atrial septal defect, occur in this part of the cardiac septum. There is then a common atrioventricular junction with abnormal formation of the atrioventricular valves (see Chapter 9).

Morphologic distinction of the great arteries is based on origin (or lack) of coronary arteries and the branching patterns upstream from the semilunar valve. Typically, the pulmonary trunk bifurcates into the left and right pulmonary arteries. In contrast, the aorta usually has three branches arising from its arch.

Having determined the morphology of each chamber, segmental analysis considers the connections across the atrioventricular junctions and those across the ventricular–arterial junctions (Figure 3.2). Connection refers to the anatomic linkage between atrial and ventricular chambers and between ventricular chambers and great arteries. "Connection" of adjoining chambers is

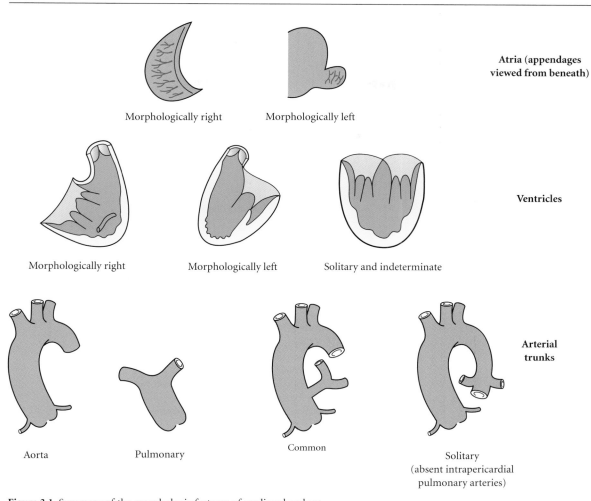

Atria (appendages viewed from beneath)

Morphologically right   Morphologically left

Ventricles

Morphologically right   Morphologically left   Solitary and indeterminate

Arterial trunks

Aorta   Pulmonary   Common   Solitary (absent intrapericardial pulmonary arteries)

Figure 3.1 Summary of the morphologic features of cardiac chambers.

usually, but not always, synonymous with "drainage." In certain rare physiologies, drainage is abnormal even though the connection is normal.

For the convenience of readers new to the morphologic approach, Table 3.1 lists some examples of the common short-hand terms and eponyms to show how the defects are described using sequential segmental analysis.

Steps in sequential segmental analysis

Atrial arrangement

The first step in analysis is the determination of atrial arrangement (also known as "situs"). According to the

morphology of the atrial appendages, there are four variants of arrangement (Figure 3.3); see also Chapter 6:

Atrial arrangements

- **Usual arrangement** ("situs solitus") denotes normality and is by far the most common. These have the atrial appendages in their normal positions
- **Mirror-image arrangement** ("situs inversus") is present when the morphologic right atrial appendage is on the left side while the morphologic left atrial appendage is on the right side
- **Right isomerism**
- **Left isomerism**

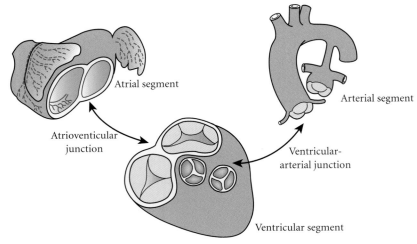

Atrial segment

Atrioventricular
junction

Arterial segment

Ventricular-
arterial junction

Ventricular segment

Figure 3.2 The three segments of the heart are analyzed sequentially.

Table 3.1 Examples of how commonly occurring lesions can be described using the sequential segmental method of nomenclature

Commonly used term	Sequential segmental analysis
Atrial septal defect (ASD)	**Usual atrial arrangement, concordant AV and VA connections** + atrial septal defect (oval fossa defect)
Ventricular septal defect (VSD)	**Usual atrial arrangement, concordant AV and VA connections** + perimembranous inlet ventricular septal defect
Atrioventricular septal defect (AV canal)	**Usual atrial arrangement, concordant AV and VA connections** + atrioventricular septal defect with common valvar orifice
Coarctation	**Usual atrial arrangement, concordant AV and VA connections** + coarctation
Fallot's tetralogy (with anomalous LAD and right aortic arch)	**Usual atrial arrangement, concordant AV and VA connections** + perimembranous outlet ventricular septal defect with subpulmonary stenosis (tetralogy of Fallot), overriding aorta, right ventricular hypertrophy, pulmonary valvar stenosis, anomalous origin of LAD from right coronary artery, right aortic arch
Transposition of the great arteries (d-TGA) with VSD, aortic stenosis and coarctation	**Usual atrial arrangement, concordant AV and discordant VA connections** + perimembranous ventricular septal defect, aortic stenosis, coarctation
Congenitally corrected transposition (l-TGA) with VSD, PS, and Ebstein malformation	**Usual atrial arrangement, discordant AV and discordant VA connections** + perimembranous ventricular septal defect, subpulmonary stenosis, Ebstein malformation
Tricuspid atresia with transposition and coarctation	**Usual atrial arrangement, absent right AV connection and discordant VA connection** + morphologic left atrium to morphologic left ventricle, ventricular septal defect, coarctation
Situs inversus, dextrocardia, double outlet right ventricle (DORV) with valvar PA	**Mirror-image atrial arrangement, concordant AV connection and double outlet VA connection from the right ventricle** + muscular inlet VSD, valvar pulmonary atresia, heart in right chest, apex to right

For each example, segmental analysis of atrial arrangement, atrioventricular (AV) connection, and ventricular–arterial (VA) connection are in bold. Examples of associated lesions are included, illustrating how analysis provides the initial building block on which specific details are added.

ASD, atrial septal defect; LAD, left anterior descending coronary artery; PA, pulmonary atresia; PS, pulmonary stenosis; RV, right ventricle; VSD, ventricular septal defect.

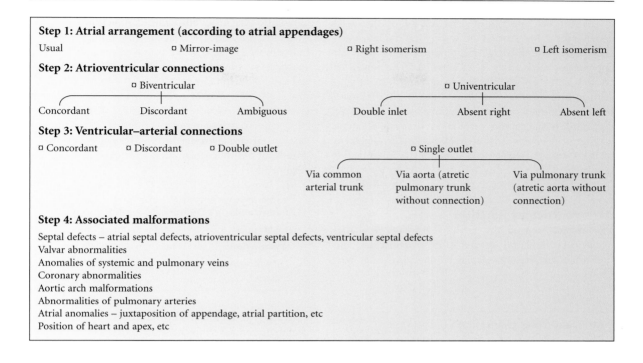

Step 1: Atrial arrangement (according to atrial appendages)

Usual   □ Mirror-image   □ Right isomerism   □ Left isomerism

Step 2: Atrioventricular connections

□ Biventricular   □ Univentricular

Concordant   Discordant   Ambiguous   Double inlet   Absent right   Absent left

Step 3: Ventricular–arterial connections

□ Concordant   □ Discordant   □ Double outlet   □ Single outlet

Via common arterial trunk   Via aorta (atretic pulmonary trunk without connection)   Via pulmonary trunk (atretic aorta without connection)

Step 4: Associated malformations

Septal defects – atrial septal defects, atrioventricular septal defects, ventricular septal defects
Valvar abnormalities
Anomalies of systemic and pulmonary veins
Coronary abnormalities
Aortic arch malformations
Abnormalities of pulmonary arteries
Atrial anomalies – juxtaposition of appendage, atrial partition, etc
Position of heart and apex, etc

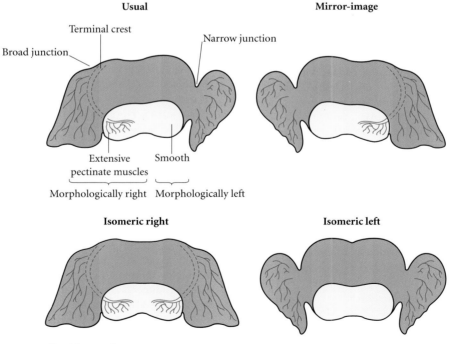

Figure 3.3 Arrangement of atrial appendages.

The last two variants of arrangement of the atrial appendages are present, as the description implies, when the hearts have bilateral morphologic right and left appendages, respectively (see Chapter 17). Arrangement of the atrial appendages frequently corresponds to arrangement of the branching pattern of the main bronchi. Although previously described as syndromes of visceral heterotaxy, the correlation between isomeric arrangement of the atrial appendages and arrangement of the abdominal organs and status of the spleen is not consistent.

Atrioventricular junction

The second step in the analysis examines the atrioventricular junction in terms of biventricular and univentricular atrioventricular connections (see also Chapter 6).

Atrioventricular connections

- **Biventricular atrioventricular connections** describe the arrangement whereby each atrium is connected to its own ventricle, albeit that one of the ventricles may be hypoplastic or the atrioventricular valve is imperforate.
- **Univentricular atrioventricular connections** by contrast describe hearts where only one ventricle is connected to the atrial mass.

Biventricular atrioventricular connections

When the atrial appendages are lateralized (either usual arrangement or mirror-image arrangement), there are two variations of biventricular atrioventricular connection: concordant and discordant (Figure 3.4a). In the setting of isomeric arrangement of the atrial appendages, however, the atrioventricular connections are described as ambiguous (Figure 3.4b) since the atrioventricular junctions are neither entirely concordant nor discordant.

Biventricular atrioventricular connections

- **Concordant** (Figure 3.4a): when the atria are connected to the appropriate ventricles
- **Discordant** (Figure 3.4a): when the atria are connected to inappropriate ventricles (see Chapter 14)
- **Ambiguous** (Figure 3.4b): atrial connections are neither entirely concordant nor discordant

---

Univentricular atrioventricular connections

Univentricular atrioventricular connections describe hearts in which the atria are connected primarily to one ventricle (see Chapters 15 and 16). Most frequently, there is a second but smaller ventricle in the ventricular mass that is also described as a rudimentary ventricle since it lacks the inlet portion. Univentricular atrioventricular connections can exist in combination with any of the four variants of atrial arrangement. There are two major groups of univentricular atrioventricular connections (Figure 3.5).

Univentricular atrioventricular connections

- **Double inlet**
- **Absent atrioventricular connection** subdivided into:
  - Absent right connection
  - Absent left connection

Hearts with **double inlet connections** have both atrial chambers connected to the same ventricle (see Chapter 16). The receiving ventricle is usually large and described as dominant. Most frequently, the dominant ventricle is of left ventricular morphology, recognized by its fine apical trabeculations. Accompanying the dominant ventricle, there is usually a right ventricle in the anterior portion of the ventricular mass. This right ventricle is usually small and rudimentary. Occasionally, the dominant ventricle is of right morphology. In these cases, the rudimentary left ventricle is located on the diaphragmatic aspect of the ventricular mass. It may be very small or even slit-like. Very rarely, the receiving ventricle is of indeterminate morphology with very coarse trabeculations. This is a solitary ventricle, the truly univentricular heart.

In contrast to double inlet connections, **absence of an atrioventricular connection** describes hearts in which only one atrium is connected to the ventricular mass (Figure 3.5) (see Chapters 15 and 16). This situation arises when either the right- or left-sided atrium ends blindly in a muscular floor at the atrioventricular junction. Absence of a right atrioventricular connection usually exists with the left-sided atrium opening to a dominant morphologic left ventricle. Again, in these cases, a rudimentary right ventricle is located in the anterior part of the ventricular mass. On the other hand, absence of the left atrioventricular connection usually occurs with the right-sided atrium connected to a dominant right ventricle, while the rudimentary morphologic

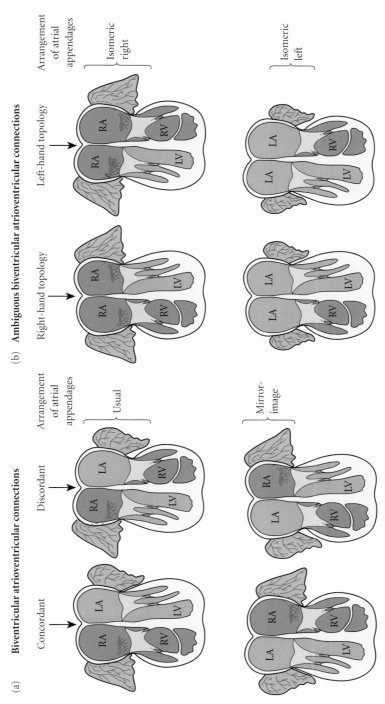

Figure 3.4 Biventricular atrioventricular connections occurring with usual and mirror-image atrial arrangements (a), and with isomeric arrangements of the atrial appendages (b).

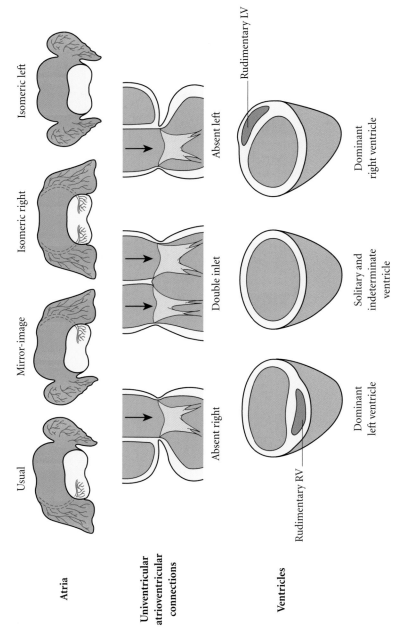

Figure 3.5 Univentricular atrioventricular connections can occur with any of the four variants of atrial arrangement and three variants of ventricular morphology. LV, left ventricle; RV, right ventricle.

left ventricle is sited on the diaphragmatic aspect of the ventricular mass.

While consideration of the atrioventricular connections is a vital step in sequential analysis, the morphology of the atrioventricular valves should not be ignored. For instance, note should be taken of any straddling and overriding, and the presence of an imperforate valve or of any valvar stenosis. A straddling valve is one that has its tension apparatus (chords, papillary muscle or both) inserted in both ventricles on either side of the ventricular septum. Often, a straddling valve also overrides the septum. Override is defined as commitment of the valvar orifice across the septal crest to both ventricles. The proportion of overriding may change the type of atrioventricular connection from a biventricular form to a univentricular form, and *vice versa* (see Chapter 6). An imperforate valve should be distinguished from absence of an atrioventricular connection since there is the potential for connection when a valvar membrane interposes between atrial and ventricular chambers.

Ventricular–arterial junctions

The third step in segmental analysis is to examine the connections across the ventricular–arterial junction.

Ventricular–arterial connections

- **Concordant**

- **Discordant:** as with atrioventricular connections, these can be concordant or discordant when two identifiable great arteries are present and each arises from one ventricular chamber (see Chapter 14)

- **Double outlet ventricle:** when both great arteries arise from the same ventricle, this situation is described as double outlet from the right, the left, or the indeterminate ventricle (see Chapter 15)

- **Single outlet ventricle:** occasionally, the blind origin of one of the great arteries cannot be traced back to a specific ventricle. When this occurs, as in some cases with aortic atresia (see Chapter 16) or pulmonary atresia (see Chapter 15), the term single outlet is used (see above2). Single outlet is also used to describe the connection existing in the settings of common arterial trunk or solitary arterial trunk where there is only one arterial valve (see Figure 3.1)

Again, the morphology of the arterial valves should be noted. The proportion of overriding of an arterial valve needs to be taken into account. The 50% rule is used in adjudicating ventricular–arterial connections. Where there is more than 50% override, the connection is termed double outlet rather than concordant.

Associated malformations

Finally, segmental analysis is not complete until all the associated malformations have been examined and listed. These are:
- Septal defects;
- Valvar abnormalities;
- Coronary abnormalities;
- Anomalies of systemic venous connection;
- Anomalies of pulmonary venous connection;
- Aortic arch anomalies;
- Anomalies of pulmonary arteries;
- Position of the heart and apex, etc.

Further reading

Brandt PWT, Calder AL. Cardiac connections: the segmental approach to radiologic diagnosis in congenital heart disease. *Curr Prob Diagn Radiol* 1977;7:1–35.

Carvalho JS, Ho SY, Shinebourne EA. Sequential segmental analysis in complex fetal cardiac abnormalities: a logical approach to diagnosis. *Ultrasound Obstet Gynecol* 2005; 26:105–111.

de la Cruz MV, Nadal-Ginard B. Rules for the diagnosis of visceral situs, truncoconal morphologies and ventricular inversions. *Am Heart J* 1972;84:19–32.

Ho SY, McCarthy KP, Josen M, Rigby ML. Anatomic-echocardiographic correlates: an introduction to normal and congenitally malformed hearts. *Heart* 2001;86 (Suppl 2): 3–11.

Ho SY, Rigby ML, Anderson RH. *Echocardiography in the Heart Made Simple*. London: Imperial College Press, 2005, pp. 29–47.

Shinebourne EA, Macartney FJ, Anderson RH. Sequential chamber localization-logical approach to diagnosis in congenital heart disease. *Br Heart J* 1976;38:327–340.

Tynan MJ, Becker AE, Macartney FJ, Quero-Jimenez M, Shinebourne EA, Anderson RH. Nomenclature and classification of congenital heart disease. *Br Heart J* 1979;41:544–553.

Van Praagh R. The segmental approach to diagnosis in congenital heart disease. In: *Birth Defects*, original article series 8, no.5. Baltimore: Williams & Wilkins, 1972, p. 4.

4 History and clinical examination

Lee Beerman

University of Pittsburgh School of Medicine and Children's Hospital of Pittsburgh of UPMC, Pittsburgh, PA, USA

History

In pediatric cardiology, the history is an extremely important diagnostic tool. The family and patient should be asked open-ended questions to allow them to provide as much information as possible without undue influence from the clinician. However, the clinician must guide the history and obtain all key elements.

The exact symptoms that a patient with heart disease experiences vary with the patient's age as well as the underlying disease. Some symptoms are common and should always be explored.

Important symptoms to elicit in an infant

- Abnormal breathing
- Difficulty feeding
- Diaphoresis/sweatiness on crying/feeding
- Failure to thrive
- Episodes of cyanosis or pallor (see Chapter 41)
- Chest pain, which may masquerade as colic (see Chapter 38)

It should be noted that chronically cyanotic infants or children may not appear blue to the parents; episodic cyanosis is less frequently overlooked. Infants with heart failure almost always have an increased respiratory rate, often associated with labored breathing or grunting. If an experienced caregiver reports that an infant is breathing more rapidly than expected, cardiac disease should always be considered. Additionally, infants with heart failure frequently have difficulty with feeding. They may become tired and fall asleep quickly with their feeds, only to awaken still hungry. Prolonged feeding may be associated with diaphoresis. Poor weight gain may be one of the first signs of heart failure.

Symptoms to ask older children and their families about

- Abnormal breathing
- Cyanosis
- Exercise tolerance
- Chest pain (see Chapter 38)
- Palpitations (see Chapter 39)
- Tachycardia (see Chapter 24)
- Lightheadedness and syncope (see Chapter 37)

It is extremely important to determine if any of these signs or symptoms are precipitated by exertion, as they often are if cardiac disease is present. The patient and parents may be in denial about the patient's limitations, but asking how well the patient keeps up with other children of his or her age is often the best way to assess exercise tolerance.

If there is a complaint of **chest pain** the patient should always be asked if the pain is "pleuritic" with exacerbation on breathing or movement of the chest (see Chapter 38). With the exception of pericarditis, "pleuritic-type" chest pain is much more likely to be musculoskeletal in origin than cardiac in nature. Similarly, if the pain is not related to exertion, it is extremely unlikely to be cardiac. In fact, cardiac chest pain is extremely rare in children.

Syncope is a particularly common symptom in adolescents. Although serious arrhythmias may cause sudden loss of consciousness, syncope in the pediatric population is more commonly due to vasovagal reactions or postural hypotension than to cardiac disease (see Chapter 37). A careful history is often the key to the diagnosis of this complaint and needs to address the setting in which the syncope occurred, the presence of a prodrome, duration

Pediatric Heart Disease: A Practical Guide, First Edition. Piers E. F. Daubeney, Michael L. Rigby, Koichiro Niwa, and Michael A. Gatzoulis.
© 2012 Blackwell Publishing Ltd. Published 2012 by Blackwell Publishing Ltd.

of the event, and the suddenness of onset and recovery (see Chapters 23, 24, and especially 37). The patient should always be questioned about postural lightheadedness, and salt and fluid intake assessed.

A detailed past medical history, complete review of systems, including any current medications or drugs, social history, and family history should, of course, be performed. A careful family history is particularly important because of the inherited nature of some cardiac diseases (see Chapter 1), such as hypertrophic cardiomyopathy (see Chapter 19), genetic arrhythmia syndromes (e.g. long QT syndrome) (see Chapter 24), and certain congenital heart defects. Emphasis should be placed on the onset of heart disease in family members younger than 40 years of age, sudden collapse or cardiac arrest, or congenital heart disease in close relatives. The frequent response that "someone in the family had a heart murmur" is rarely rewarding unless a specific cardiac diagnosis was made.

Clinical examination

A thorough physical examination is fundamental to the evaluation of patients suspected of having heart disease and will often lead to the correct diagnosis. Equally as important, it may rule out heart disease, sparing patients unnecessary anxiety and diagnostic testing.

An acceptable physical examination requires the proper setting, including a comfortable, quiet, well-lit room, and the patient must be as calm and relaxed as possible. In the pediatric setting this often requires patience and determination on the part of the clinician as well as the family. Infants are often quieter and more comfortable in a parent's lap than on an examining table. All organ systems should be assessed with particular attention paid to findings that may be associated with heart disease, such as tachypnea, labored respirations, hepatomegaly or edema. The remainder of this chapter will focus on the cardiac portion of the exam.

Inspection
This should begin with an assessment of the patient's:
• **Overall condition**, e.g. how unwell or well the child appears.
• Presence of **dysmorphic features**, particularly for relatively common genetic syndromes associated with important heart disease, such as:
  ◦ Down (trisomy 21)
  ◦ Marfan (*FBN 1* gene mutations, 15q21)
  ◦ Turner (XO)

  ◦ Noonan (*PTPN11* gene mutations, 12q24)
  ◦ Williams (7q11 deletion)
  ◦ DiGeorge (22q11 deletion).
• **Central cyanosis** by examining the mucosal surfaces of the oropharynx and lips, keeping in mind that cyanosis that is only perioral is peripheral rather than central and does not indicate arterial hemoglobin oxygen desaturation.
• **Pallor** as pale conjunctiva may indicate anemia.
• Presence of **clubbing** in the upper and lower limb nailbeds.
• **Cyanosis and edema** in the extremities. **Jugular venous pulsation**, which can be **difficult to assess** accurately in pediatric patients. In order to visualize the pulsations best, the patient should be in a recumbent position between 15 and 30 degrees. The jugular venous pulsations consist of three waves:
  ◦ a wave from atrial contraction
  ◦ c wave at the onset of ventricular systole after closure of the tricuspid valve
  ◦ v wave from atrial filling during systole and its peak occurs just prior to the opening of the tricuspid valve.
The degree of elevation of the jugular venous pulsations above the level of the heart can be used as an estimate of right atrial pressure. Abnormally large a waves, cannon waves, can be seen with the simultaneous atrial and ventricular contractions that occur during atrioventricular dissociation, such as with a junctional rhythm or third-degree heart block. Large v waves are present with severe tricuspid regurgitation.
• **Pulsations in the neck** can also represent arterial systolic waves. These waves differ from jugular venous pulsations in that the arterial wave does not vary with changes in position. They also can be differentiated by auscultating the heart and determining their timing in relation to the heart cycle, or by light pressure at the base of the neck to obliterate venous pulsations.
• The **precordial area** should also be inspected. A parasternal lift or prominent apical impulse should be noted. Displacement of the apical impulse from the fourth or fifth intercostal space along the mid-clavicular line usually reflects cardiomegaly.
• Presence of **scars**, e.g. central sternotomy, left or right lateral thoracotomy or drain sites.

Palpation
Precordial motion should be assessed by palpation.
• The point of maximal impulse (PMI) can be a misleading term, as it may be caused by a parasternal or apical impulse. In the normal patient, the PMI, or more

precisely the **apical impulse**, is usually palpable, but may not be evident in very obese or muscular individuals. The apical impulse corresponds to left ventricular systole and is normally a brief outward movement well localized to the fourth or fifth intercostal space in the mid-clavicular line. This impulse should be assessed with the patient supine, but the patient may be rolled to the left lateral decubitus position if it is difficult to feel. The apical impulse may be displaced or more pronounced and prolonged with left ventricular hypertrophy or volume overload. Conversely, it may be diminished with ventricular dysfunction, obesity, or pulmonary disease that leads to hyperinflated lungs.

• A **left parasternal lift or "heave"** is usually due to the right ventricular impulse. In neonates, who have a relatively large right ventricle, a mild left parasternal lift can be a normal finding. However, a marked lift in a neonate may be an important clue to the presence of severe congenital heart disease, such as hypoplastic left heart syndrome. Outside the newborn period, a parasternal lift usually indicates right ventricular volume or pressure overload, but may be normal in very asthenic individuals.

• A **thrill** is a vibratory sensation associated with a loud murmur. Any patient with a loud murmur should be palpated over the areas of auscultation. A thrill is most reliably felt with the portion of the palm over the distal metacarpals.

There are several other abnormal pulsations that may help with diagnosis:

• **Pulmonary artery pulsations** may be palpable in very thin young children as a normal finding, but a localized lift at the left parasternal region associated with a palpable closure of the second heart sound may indicate pulmonary hypertension. These findings may also be present with congenital defects resulting in anterior leftward displacement of the aorta, such as in congenitally corrected transposition of the great arteries.

• **Prominent suprasternal notch pulsations** may be present with severe aortic insufficiency or coarctation of the aorta.

• A **pulsatile mass in the neck** may indicate a cervical aortic arch.

Pulses should be palpated in all four extremities. The most important pulses to assess are:

• Carotids (except in infants with relatively inaccessible necks);
• Brachials;
• Femorals.

It is important to characterize the amplitude of the pulses. Increased pulses, sometimes associated with pal-

pable palmar or digital pulses, indicate a wide pulse pressure from increased cardiac output or diastolic run-off from the aorta due to a patent ductus arteriosus or aortic insufficiency. Weak pulses may indicate severe aortic stenosis or decreased stroke volume due to myocardial dysfunction. The pulses should also be assessed for symmetry. Significantly diminished, delayed, or absent femoral pulses in the setting of normal or strong upper extremity pulses are diagnostic of coarctation of the aorta.

Auscultation

The **first heart sound (S1)** is produced by the closure the mitral and tricuspid valves. It is usually a single sound and loudest at the low left sternal border or apex. Although rarely discussed and infrequently recognized, the first heart sound may be narrowly split in many normal children, with the second component representing tricuspid valve closure.

• A prominently split S1 is usually due to right bundle branch block, but may also occur with Ebstein anomaly.

• The first heart sound may be loud with increased left ventricular contractility, short PR interval, late mitral valve closure in patients with mitral stenosis, or if the tricuspid valve closure is unusually forceful as in patients with an atrial septal defect.

• A soft S1 may be due to a long PR interval, depressed myocardial contractility, or obesity.

The **second heart sound (S2)** represents aortic and pulmonary valve closure and is normally loudest at the base of the heart. The aortic component normally precedes the pulmonary component, and in the normal patient S2 is more widely split on inspiration than on expiration ("deelupp" versus "dlupp"). In young children S2 may be persistently split with expiration when supine, but becomes single during expiration when upright.

• A widely split S2 is usually due to a delay in right ventricular systole, as with right bundle branch block or prolongation of right ventricular ejection time caused by pulmonary stenosis or increased flow across the right ventricular outflow tract.

• Fixed splitting of S2 (loss of respiratory variation) is most common with an atrial septal defect.

• Paradoxical splitting of S2, becoming single with inspiration and separating with expiration, is usually due to delayed aortic closure with left bundle branch block, or to early closure of the pulmonic valve when the right ventricle is "pre-excited" in individuals with Wolff–Parkinson–White syndrome.

• A single S2 is heard when the aortic and pulmonic components occur nearly simultaneously, as is often the

case with pulmonary hypertension, when the pulmonic component is inaudible due to severe pulmonic stenosis or pulmonary atresia, or when the aorta is anterior (as in transposition of the great arteries or tetralogy of Fallot).
• A loud pulmonic component of S2, regardless of the degree of splitting, can be an important finding, indicating pulmonary hypertension.
• A soft S2 is most commonly due to body habitus, but may also be due to severe pulmonic stenosis or poor ventricular contractility. A pericardial effusion may cause both S1 and S2 to be soft.

A **third heart sound (S3)** is a low frequency sound in early diastole and is a common finding in normal children. A loud S3 by itself does not imply cardiac disease in children, but when present in association with other evidence of heart failure it should be considered a gallop.

A **fourth heart sound (S4)** is a late diastolic sound which occurs when atrial systole results in a rapid rise in ventricular pressure due to decreased ventricular compliance. This is an uncommon and always abnormal finding in children. Hypertrophic cardiomyopathy is the most common cause, but an S4 also may be associated with other causes of ventricular hypertrophy or an acutely non-compliant ventricle due to ischemia or myocarditis.

Abnormal heart sounds include ejection sounds, sometimes referred to as clicks, and opening snaps. Ejection sounds occur in early systole and originate from a stenotic or abnormal semilunar valve or a dilated great artery root.
• A pulmonary ejection sound is loudest at the high left sternal border, high pitched, and varies markedly with respirations, being loudest with expiration and softer or absent with inspiration.
• An aortic ejection sound is almost always best heard at the apex. It does not vary with respiration and is not as high pitched as the pulmonary ejection sound, usually sounding like the second component of a split S1.
• The presence of an ejection sound can help differentiate valvar aortic or pulmonic stenosis from obstruction at the subvalvar or supravalvar level.
• Mid-to-late systolic apical clicks may be single or multiple and are usually due to mitral valve prolapse.
• Opening snaps occur in early diastole and are related to mitral stenosis. They are extremely uncommon in children.

Murmurs result from turbulent blood flow. The initial evaluation for murmurs should begin by auscultating over the following areas:
• High right sternal border;
• High, mid and low left sternal edge;
• Apex;
• Neck;
• Back.

Murmurs should be assessed in a systematic manner.

Assessment of murmurs

• **Timing:** Murmurs are systolic, diastolic or continuous:
  ○ Systolic murmurs can be early, mid, late or holosystolic (pan-systolic)
  ○ Diastolic murmurs also may be early, mid, late or pan-diastolic
  ○ Continuous murmurs begin in systole and spill over into diastole, but do not have to last throughout diastole
  ○ Most systolic murmurs can be described as either ejection-type (crescendo–decrescendo, diamond-shaped) or holosystolic (pan-systolic)
  ○ Ejection murmurs, such as with aortic stenosis, normally do not extend throughout systole
  ○ Holosystolic, or regurgitant, murmurs, like mitral insufficiency, last throughout systole.
• **Shape:** Murmurs can be crescendo, decrescendo, crescendo–decrescendo (commonly referred to as "ejection-type"), or plateau.
• **Location:** Defined by where the murmur is loudest. In general, ejection murmurs are loudest above an imaginary line between the nipples; pan-systolic murmurs are loudest below this line.
• **Radiation**, e.g. to the back in pulmonary stenosis or carotids in aortic stenosis.
• **Pitch:** Can provide important clues to its cause. Murmurs can be low, medium, or high pitched (blowing).
• **Loudness:** On a scale of 1–6:
  ○ Grade 1 – barely audible
  ○ Grade 2 – easily heard but not loud
  ○ Grade 3 – loud without a thrill
  Grades 4–6 are reserved for murmurs with a thrill:
  ○ Grade 4 – only heard with the diaphragm of the stethoscope flush with the chest wall
  ○ Grade 5 – audible with the diaphragm held at an angle to the chest wall
  ○ Grade 6 – heard with the diaphragm completely off the chest.
• **Quality:** Innocent murmurs are "vibratory", "musical," or "like a twanging string." Murmurs due to outflow tract obstruction and some ventricular septal defects have a harsh quality. A "machinery" murmur describes a continuous murmur heard in some patients with a patent ductus arteriosus. Aortic insufficiency, although normally producing a high-pitched blowing murmur, sometimes has the quality of a "cooing dove." "Honking" murmurs are characteristic of mitral valve prolapse.

Table 4.1 Differential diagnosis of systolic murmurs

Site	Cause	Clinical findings
High right sternal border	Innocent	Aortic flow murmur: soft, little radiation
	Aortic stenosis	Harsh, radiates to neck, ±ejection sound, carotid thrill
High left sternal border	Innocent	Pulmonary flow murmur: soft, little radiation
	Pulmonic stenosis	Harsh, radiates to axillae and back, ±ejection sound
	Atrial septal defect	Widely split and fixed S2, ±mid diastolic murmur LLSB
	Coarctation	Radiates to left axilla and back, decreased femoral pulses
Mid/low left sternal border	Innocent	Still's murmur: characteristic "vibratory" quality
	Ventricular septal defect	Medium-to-high pitched, often harsh
	Tricuspid regurgitation	High pitched, varies with respirations
	Subaortic or subpulmonic stenosis	Harsh, radiates to upper sternal border
Apex	Mitral regurgitation	High pitched, radiates to axilla, mid-systolic click with mitral valve prolapse
Back	Peripheral pulmonic stenosis	High pitched, common in first 6 months, resolves
	Pulmonic stenosis	Much louder anteriorly
	Coarctation	Audible anteriorly and decreased femoral pulses

LLSB, lower left sternal border.

Murmurs are extremely common in childhood and adolescence. Most are physiologic and not associated with structural heart disease. These common "normal" murmurs are usually referred to as functional or innocent.

It is helpful to have a general differential diagnosis for murmurs based on the characteristics listed above. Table 4.1 lists the common auscultatory sites of systolic murmurs with a simple differential diagnostic scheme to help separate innocent from "organic" murmurs. The only common innocent murmur that is not systolic is a venous hum. This is a physiologic continuous murmur with diastolic accentuation heard over the clavicles. This murmur is due to rapid venous return through the internal and external jugular veins enhanced by gravity, and is **only** heard in the sitting position.

Murmurs can be further differentiated by their timing and auscultatory shape. The various patterns of the most common murmurs are illustrated along with a brief differential diagnosis in Figure 4.1.

It is often helpful to perform dynamic auscultation to identify an innocent murmur. The patient should be auscultated in the squatting position and then again after standing up. This maneuver results in a dramatic decrease in venous return due to venous pooling in the legs and increased systolic emptying of the left ventricle because of the decrease in arterial resistance when the patient is standing. A Valsalva maneuver accomplishes the same physiologic changes, but it is often difficult for a younger child to perform this maneuver effectively. Innocent murmurs are critically dependent on the volume of flow and usually become softer or even disappear when the patient stands; while murmurs due to mitral valve prolapse or hypertrophic subaortic stenosis become louder because of the decreased size of the left ventricle.

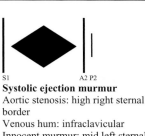

Systolic ejection murmur
Aortic stenosis: high right sternal
border
Venous hum: infraclavicular
Innocent murmur: mid left sternal border

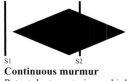

Continuous murmur
Patent ductus arteriosus: high
left sternal border/infraclavicular
Arteriovenous fistula: anywhere

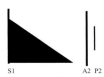

Pansystolic murmur
Ventricular septal defect: mid/low
left sternal border
Mitral regurgitation: apex
Tricuspid regurgitation: low left sternal
border

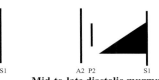

Early diastolic murmur
Aortic regurgitation: left sternal border (high
pitched)
Pulmonic regurgitation: left sternal border
(medium pitched)

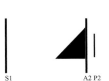

Decrescendo early systolic murmur
Small ventricular septal defect:
mid/low left sternal border

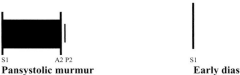

Mid-to-late diastolic murmur
Mitral stenosis: apex
Tricuspid stenosis: low left sternal
border

Late systolic murmur
Mitral valve prolapse: apex

Figure 4.1 Characterization of murmurs by timing and shape.

Further reading

Advani N, Menahem S, Wilkinson JL. The diagnosis of innocent
murmurs in childhood. *Cardiol Young* 2000;10:340–342.
Park SC, Beerman LB. Cardiology. In: Zitelli BJ, Davis HW, eds.
Atlas of Pediatric Physical Diagnosis, 4th edn. Philadelphia:
Mosby, 2002, pp. 127–152.

Pelech AN. Evaluation of the pediatric patient with a cardiac
murmur. *Pediatr Clin North Am* 1999;46:167–188.
Zuberbuhler JR. *Clinical Diagnosis in Pediatric Cardiology*. New
York: Churchill-Livingstone, 1981.

5 Basic non-invasive investigations

Lee Beerman

University of Pittsburgh School of Medicine and Children's Hospital of Pittsburgh of UPMC, Pittsburgh, PA, USA

Chest radiography

Chest X-rays (CXRs) play a critical role in the evaluation of children with heart disease. Findings on CXR can be useful in differentiating pulmonary disease from heart disease, as well as aiding in the diagnosis of specific cardiac lesions or processes such as congestive heart failure or cyanotic heart disease.

The CXR should be examined systematically with particular reference to several key features.

> **Key features of the CXR**
> - Cardiac size and shape
> - Location of the heart and visceral situs
> - Great artery appearance
> - Pulmonary vascularity
> - Skeletal abnormalities
> - Parenchymal lung changes

Assessment of the **cardiac size and shape** is important in the interpretation of a CXR. The size of the heart is evaluated by determining the cardiothoracic ratio; calculated by dividing the width of the heart by the width of the chest at the level of the diaphragm. Assuming that the film is taken at or near a full inspiration, the ratio is normally less than 0.5. In addition to the overall size of the heart, one should assess the heart borders and general shape. Figure 5.1 demonstrates the anatomic chambers that are visible on the normal posteroanterior (PA) view. One should be able to identify the right atrial, right ventricular, pulmonary artery, left ventricular, and aortic borders. Specific chamber enlargement is better defined by echocardiography, but the CXR findings may be suggestive. With some congenital heart diseases the cardiac silhouette may have a classic configuration, such as a boot-shaped heart with tetralogy of Fallot. These classic CXR findings will be further discussed in the lesion-specific chapters.

Pulmonary vascularity should be assessed in all cardiac patients. The pulmonary vascular markings may be normal, increased, or decreased (Figure 5.2). Increased pulmonary vascular markings may be due to increased pulmonary blood flow or pulmonary venous congestion. The former is present with left-to-right shunts or cyanotic lesions with unobstructed pulmonary blood flow, while the latter results from left ventricular failure, pulmonary venous obstruction, cor triatriatum or mitral valve stenosis. Decreased pulmonary markings are caused by lesions associated with diminished pulmonary blood flow due to obstructive lesions in the right heart and right-to-left shunting, such as tricuspid atresia, tetralogy of Fallot, critical pulmonary stenosis, or pulmonary atresia. Normal pulmonary vascularity may be present with a variety of cardiac anomalies that are not associated with intracardiac shunting.

The CXR is an important tool in the assessment of **sidedness of the heart** and visceral situs.

- In most patients the heart is on the left side and abdominal situs is normal with the liver on the right side, and the stomach bubble and spleen are on the left – situs solitus or usual atrial arrangement. The airway has a normal branching pattern of the right and left bronchi. The right bronchus has an early take-off of the upper lobe branch and is eparterial (superior to the right pulmonary artery), while the left bronchus has a

Pediatric Heart Disease: A Practical Guide, First Edition. Piers E. F. Daubeney, Michael L. Rigby, Koichiro Niwa, and Michael A. Gatzoulis.
© 2012 Blackwell Publishing Ltd. Published 2012 by Blackwell Publishing Ltd.

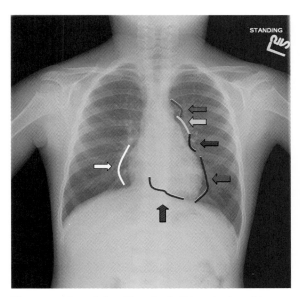

Figure 5.1 Normal chest X-ray in the PA projection with borders marked. White arrow, right atrial border; purple arrow, right ventricular border; red arrow, aortic notch; yellow arrow, pulmonary artery; blue arrow, left atrial border; green arrow, left ventricular border.

long main stem component and is hyparterial (inferior to the left pulmonary artery). However, the heart may be on the right side (dextrocardia) or in the middle (mesocardia).

• With **heterotaxy syndromes** there is isomerism of the airway with both main stem bronchi having either a right or left branching pattern (see Chapter 17). Since the atrial appendage morphology almost always follows the anatomy of the ipsilateral bronchus, bilateral right sidedness is usually referred to as right atrial isomerism. On the other hand, bilateral left bronchi indicate left atrial isomerism. Atrial isomerism is usually associated with complex congenital heart disease, a midline liver, and abnormal splenic anatomy. Asplenia and polysplenia syndromes are highly associated with right and left atrial isomerism respectively. The incidence of heart disease is much higher when there is discordance between the sidedness of the heart and visceral situs, such as dextrocardia with normal situs or a left-sided heart (levocardia) with situs inversus.

• In patients with **complete situs inversus** both the heart and the stomach bubble are on the right and the heart is usually normal.

Assessing the **great artery appearance** on CXR can also be very helpful in cardiac diagnosis. Prominence of

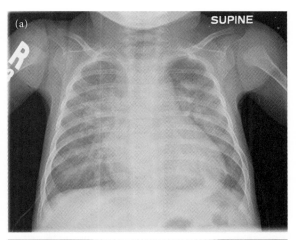

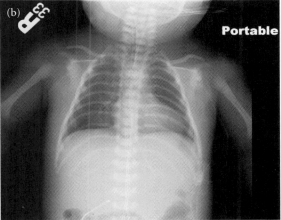

Figure 5.2 (a) Increased pulmonary vascular markings and cardiomegaly in an infant with a ventricular septal defect and congestive heart failure. (b) Decreased pulmonary vascular markings in an infant with a double outlet right ventricle with subvalvar and valvar pulmonary stenosis.

the main pulmonary artery segment at the left upper heart border can be seen with increased pulmonary blood flow, pulmonary hypertension, or post-stenotic dilation due to pulmonic valve stenosis. On the other hand, a diminutive segment suggests a small pulmonary outflow tract such as is seen in tetralogy of Fallot ("absent pulmonary bay" or "boot-shaped heart"). A dilated ascending aorta associated with aortic valve stenosis or primary root enlargement displaces the shadow of the superior vena cava rightward. The side of the aortic arch provides an important clue to the presence of congenital heart disease. For example, a right aortic arch (Figure 5.3) is seen in 25% of patients with tetralogy of Fallot and

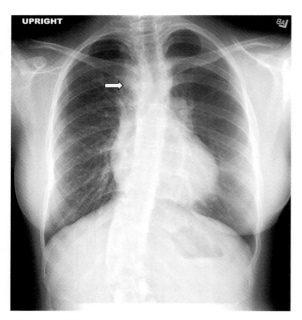

Figure 5.3 CXR of a right aortic arch (arrow) in a patient with truncus arteriosus and scoliosis.

related lesions. Determination of the side of the arch is by ascertaining the bronchus around which the aorta loops (left arch over left bronchus, right arch over right bronchus). This is facilitated by noting deviation of the trachea to the opposite side. The thoracic descending aorta is almost always on the same side as the arch, and this structure can be recognized as it obscures either the right or left side of the vertebral bodies.

The presence of **thoracic skeletal abnormalities** may provide a clue to the presence of certain heart defects. Vertebral anomalies are associated with several syndromes that have a high prevalence of congenital heart defects, e.g. VACTERL association. Pectus excavatum or carinatum, scoliosis, and straight back syndrome are more prevalent in patients with Marfan syndrome and mitral valve prolapse.

Electrocardiography

An electrocardiogram (EKG) is a useful tool in the assessment of congenital and acquired pediatric heart diseases as well as arrhythmias. This test uses a series of electrodes attached to the surface of the body to measure the electrical activity of the heart. The leads are divided into limb leads (I, II, III, aVR, aVL, and aVF) and precordial leads

(V1, V2, V3, V4, V5, V6, and in children an additional right-sided lead V4R). These leads represent vectors which measure the direction and magnitude of electrical activity. A positive deflection represents electrical activity in the same direction as the lead and a negative deflection represents activity in the opposite direction. By convention, the paper on which the EKG is recorded is run at 25 mm/s and the deflection magnitude is calibrated at 10 mm/mV, although these values can be adjusted while obtaining the tracing. The paper is divided into a grid with each small box measuring 1 mm and each larger box measuring 5 mm. Therefore, each small horizontal box on the EKG represents 0.04 s and each large box represents 0.2 s.

Features of an EKG

- P wave reflects atrial depolarization (atrial repolarization is not seen on the standard EKG because it has very low voltage and is obscured by ventricular depolarization)
- QRS complex represents ventricular depolarization
- T wave represents repolarization
- PR interval represents the conduction time from the sinoatrial node to activation of the ventricles
- QRS duration corresponds to the time it takes for the entire ventricular mass to depolarize
- QT interval represents the time from ventricular activation to completion of repolarization

---

In order to interpret the EKG correctly, a systematic approach should be taken. Since normal values vary with age, it is important to refer to age-specific normative data when interpreting a pediatric EKG.

Rate and rhythm

The **heart rate** can easily be calculated from the EKG. If the rhythm is very regular, the RR interval should be measured and divided into 60 s to determine the beats per minute (bpm). For instance, if the RR interval is 1 s (five large boxes), then the heart rate is 60 bpm. Alternatively, the number of large boxes between successive R waves can be divided into 300 for the heart rate in beats per minute. For instance, if the RR interval contains five large boxes, then the heart rate is 300/5 = 60 bpm. If there is not a 1:1 relationship between the P and R waves, separate calculations should be made for both the atrial and ventricular rates. When the rhythm is irregular with varying RR intervals, this calculation is inaccurate and the number of beats in at least a 6-s period should be counted and multiplied by 10. The range of normal resting heart rates is from 60 to 100 bpm in an older child or adult, but there is considerable variation in infants and younger children. Heart rates that are too slow for age indicate bradycardia and rates that exceed the upper limits of normal are considered tachycardia.

In addition to determining the heart rate, the **rhythm** should be assessed. Most patients will be in a normal sinus rhythm, which is defined by a normal P wave axis, a constant PR interval, and a P wave associated with and preceding every QRS. For a detailed discussion of abnormal rhythms refer to Chapters 23 and 24.

Axis

The frontal plane axis of the P wave, the QRS complex, and the T wave should be assessed as described in the paragraph below. Atrial depolarization begins in the superior lateral aspect of the right atrium and travels inferiorly and to the left. Therefore the P wave should be positive in leads I and aVF. The normal P wave axis is between 30 and 90 degrees. If the P wave is negative in I and aVF, atrial depolarization originates from the low left atrium, and if it is positive in I but negative in aVF there is a low right atrial rhythm.

The QRS axis varies with age, reflecting the change in the relative right ventricular size and mass as pulmonary vascular resistance drops after birth; and it is crucial to compare this measurement to age-specific normal data. There are several methods used to assess the frontal plane QRS axis using the limb leads. All of them involve two simple principles:

1. If the sum of the R (positive) and S (negative) deflections in a lead is positive, the axis will be in the positive hemisphere of that lead; conversely if the sum is negative, it will be in the negative hemisphere.

2. If the sum of the R and S deflections in a lead is zero (that is, isoelectric), the axis will be perpendicular to that lead.

The simplest method is to divide the frontal plane into four quadrants and to use the polarity of leads I and aVF to determine in which quadrant the axis lies. See Figure 5.4 for an illustration of the quadrant analysis technique. An alternative method is to determine the sum of the positive and negative deflections in two perpendicular leads, such as I and aVF. These values can then be plotted on graph paper and the exact vector of the QRS axis can be drawn.

Most normal children have a frontal plane axis in the range of 0–90 degrees, or have a mild right axis deviation up to 120 degrees. The presence of a moderate right axis deviation (120–180 degrees) lends support to the diag-

nosis of right ventricular hypertrophy. An axis between 0 and −90 degrees is termed a left axis deviation and suggests certain cardiac defects, such as an atrioventricular septal defect, tricuspid atresia, or varieties of a single ventricle or Noonan syndrome. A north-west axis, one between 180 and 270 degrees, is frequently seen with atrioventricular septal defects or other lesions with severe right ventricular hypertrophy. When the axis is around −90 degrees (+270 degrees), it may be termed a superior axis.

The T wave axis should correspond to the QRS axis. Discordance in the QRS and T wave axis can be due to myocardial injury, strain, or hypertrophy.

Intervals

There are numerous intervals that are measured on the standard EKG (Figure 5.5):

• The **PR interval** is prolonged with first-degree heart block and is shortened with ventricular pre-excitation.

• A slurred onset of the **QRS complex**, representing a delta wave, associated with a short PR interval is diagnostic of Wolff–Parkinson–White syndrome.

• Prolongation of the QRS indicates a conduction disturbance. If the QRS is >0.12 s in an adolescent or >0.10 s in a child, a complete right bundle (rSR' pattern in V1) or left bundle (rR' pattern in V6) branch block is present. A widened QRS can also be seen with severe hypertrophy, electrolyte disturbances, or certain drugs.

• The **QT interval** is the only measurement that does not vary with age, but it does vary markedly with heart rate. Therefore, the measured QT interval should be adjusted for heart rate by dividing it by the square root of the preceding RR interval. The resulting value is referred to as the corrected QT interval, or QTc. Prolongation of the QTc interval can be secondary to electrolyte abnormalities (particularly potassium, magnesium or calcium), certain medications, or to a genetic abnormality causing defects in the function of the cardiac ion channels (long QT syndrome; see Chapter 24).

Morphology

The final step in interpreting an EKG is to analyze the morphology of the different waves. Abnormalities can be indicative of chamber enlargement, hypertrophy, conduction abnormalities, myocardial injury, or arrhythmias.

• The **P wave** should be less than 2.5 mm in height and 0.10 s in duration.

  ◦ Right atrial enlargement results in a peaked P wave ≥3 mm. This is usually most notable in lead II.

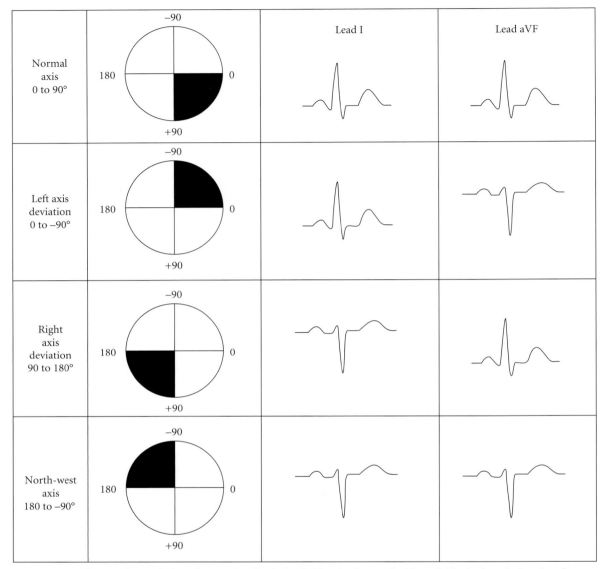

Figure 5.4 Quadrant analysis technique for assessing the QRS axis. The simplest method is to divide the frontal plane into four quadrants and use the polarity of leads I and aVF to determine in which quadrant the axis lies.

○ Left atrial enlargement results in a prolonged P wave that is bifid in lead II or has a broad negative component, >0.04 s, in lead V1.

○ Ectopic atrial beats can be recognized by distortion of the P wave appearance.

• The **QRS morphology** varies greatly with age. In infants there are significantly more right-sided forces than later in life. Therefore, newborn and infant EKGs have more pronounced R waves in the anterior precordial leads than EKGs obtained in older children or adolescents (Figure

5.6). Abnormally large QRS voltages indicate ventricular hypertrophy:

○ Right ventricular hypertrophy: the R wave is larger than normal in V1 and the S wave is larger than normal in V6.

○ Left ventricular hypertrophy: the findings are reversed with a large R in V6 and large S in V1.

One should reference age-adjusted normal data when assessing ventricular hypertrophy. Also, it should be noted that R waves modestly taller than the normal range

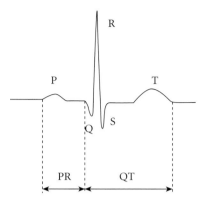

Figure 5.5 Normal EKG intervals: PR and QT intervals.

for age in the left precordial leads are present in some normal children. In the setting of a bundle branch block, the EKG is not reliable in the assessment of ventricular hypertrophy. Diffusely low QRS voltages may be seen with myocarditis, pericardial effusion or obesity.

• The **ST segment** is flat or gently upsloping in most normal subjects. Some adolescents may have mild ST elevation, a normal variant known as early repolarization. The ST segment elevation of early repolarization is characterized by an upward concavity. This must be differentiated from myocardial injury or ischemia, which result in elevated but flat or convex ST segments or ST depressions. With myocardial ischemia due to a coronary lesion the pattern of ST segment abnormalities should be consistent with the distribution of one of the coronary arteries. If there are diffuse ST segment abnormalities, pericarditis or myocarditis is more likely.

• The **T wave** is normally upright in the right precordial leads in the first week of life, but subsequently becomes inverted. By adolescence the T wave again is normally upright in the right precordial leads, although even normal adults may have T wave inversion in V1–3 (particularly African–American women). When T wave inversion is seen in other leads or is associated with ST segment depression, it may reflect myocardial injury, strain, or hypertrophy. T waves also may be diffusely flattened or enlarged, most commonly due to electrolyte abnormalities.

EKG monitors
Holter monitoring
A Holter monitor (24-h tape) is a portable EKG that can be used for documentation of suspected arrhythmias and is most effective if the patient is having daily symptoms. This monitor keeps a continuous two- to three-lead recording of the patient's heart rhythm for 24–48 h. A Holter monitor allows for analysis of the rhythm over the entire monitoring period. The patient should keep a record of any symptoms he or she experiences while wearing the monitor. This device can be instrumental in diagnosing arrhythmias and correlating them with symptoms.

Event monitoring
A cardiac event monitor is the preferred type of monitor for patients with less frequent symptoms. One type of event monitor only records for 30–60 s when activated by the patient. The other type is a continuous loop monitor that records a rolling 4–6 min, without storing the data in memory until the patient activates a record button. Some of the newer units automatically record and store rhythms that are outside programmed upper and lower rates. These types of monitors have the advantage over a Holter monitor of being less bulky and able to monitor for longer periods of time (generally 1 month). The disadvantage is that the patient must be symptomatic during any arrhythmia to trigger the recorder, unless the device has an auto-activation function.

Implantable loop recorder
This type of monitor has proven useful for patients who have troublesome but very infrequent symptoms. This is a very small device that is implanted subcutaneously in the left parasternal area and allows continuous rhythm monitoring for 12–18 months. The device can be triggered by the patient for symptoms, or it will auto-activate for heart rates outside a designated range. The data are subsequently downloaded with a device programmer.

Exercise testing
Exercise testing can provide useful data regarding cardiovascular performance and the significance of an arrhythmia. This is performed using either a treadmill or stationary bicycle. The patient must be old enough to be able to use the equipment safely, follow instructions, and cooperate enough to give a good effort (normally >5–7-years old). Electrode leads are placed and continuous monitoring of the 12-lead EKG and frequent blood pressure measurements are obtained. Patients are encouraged to exercise to maximal capacity. The test can be performed with or without spirometry and respiratory gas exchange analyzers, termed an **MVO$_2$ or VO$_2$ test**; the additional equipment allows assessment of pulmonary function as well as better quantification of cardiovascular and pulmonary reserve. The testing is performed according to specific protocols (e.g. Bruce protocol) with

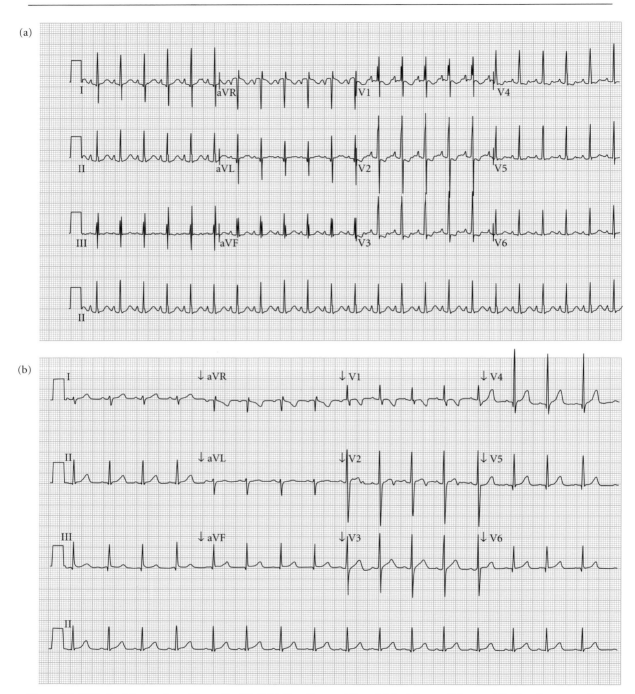

Figure 5.6 EKGs for (a) a newborn (4-month old), (b) infant (3-year old), and (c) adolescent (14-year old). Note the progressive decrease in R wave in V1 from infancy through childhood and adolescence.

(c)

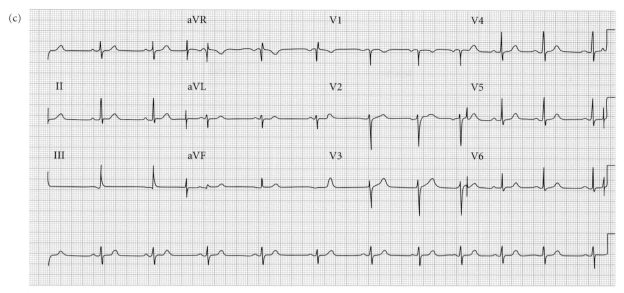

Figure 5.6 (*Continued*)

the level of work required increased at fixed time intervals, adjusting the speed and elevation on the treadmill or resistance on the bicycle. The patient's blood pressure and EKG are monitored for arrhythmias, ST or T wave changes, or an abnormal blood pressure response.

Tilt table testing

A tilt table test is occasionally used in the evaluation of syncope and can be helpful in differentiating vasovagal syncope from other causes (see Chapter 37). The patient is strapped onto a supine table with a footplate and EKG leads are placed to allow for continuous monitoring of the heart rate. The blood pressure is also monitored either by automated cuff measurement, a finger or wrist digital monitor providing a continuous waveform, or rarely, via an arterial line. The patient is placed in a supine position for 10–15 min and then the table is tilted upright to 70 degrees. The patient is left in this position for 20–30 min unless there is a reproduction of symptoms, profound hypotension, or bradycardia. If the test is negative it may be repeated after sublingual nitroglycerine or with an isoproterenol (isoprenaline) infusion. Reproduction of symptoms associated with a dramatic drop in the heart rate and/or blood pressure is indicative of vasovagal syncope. The utility of this test is limited by the significant number of false-positive and false-negative results.

Further reading

Davignon A, Rautaharju P, Boiselle E, Soumis F, Megelas M, Choquette A. Normal ECG standards for infants and children. *Pediatr Cardiol* 1980;1:123–131.

Deal BJ, Johnsrude CL, Buck SH. *Pediatric ECG Interpretation*. Malden, MA: Blackwell Futura Publishing, 2004.

Dubin D. *Rapid Interpretation of EKGs*, 6th edn. Tampa, FL: Cover Publishing, 2000.

Park SC, Beerman LB. Cardiology. In: Zitelli BJ, Davis HW, eds. *Atlas of Pediatric Physical Diagnosis*, 4th edn. Philadelphia: Mosby, 2002, pp. 127–152.

Stephens P Jr, Paridon SM. Exercise testing in pediatrics. *Pediatr Clin North Am* 2004;51:1569–1587.

6 Echocardiography and Doppler

Michael L. Rigby

Royal Brompton Hospital, London, UK

Sound is transmitted as a longitudinal wave of alternating regions of compression and rarefaction within the medium through which it travels. Ultrasound as used in medical imaging applications is generally defined as frequencies above 20 000 Hz – higher than is audible by the human ear. Sound velocity will vary depending on the medium through which it is traveling and is represented by the formula:

$$\text{Velocity (meters / second)} =$$
$$\text{Frequency (Hertz)} \times \text{Wavelength (meters)}$$

In body tissues, the velocity of sound is relatively constant at 1540 m/s and the frequency range used for medical applications is 2–12 MHz. Corresponding wavelengths, therefore, are in the range of 0.8–1.6 mm. This relatively narrow range of wavelengths establishes a fundamental limit to spatial resolution with a given transducer frequency because any point must be separated by more than one wavelength in order to be resolved. When sound travels through a homogeneous medium, some of the energy is absorbed but the remainder is reflected. The overall intensity of reflection is determined by the angle of incidence of the ultrasonic beam, greatest when perpendicular to the interface. The higher the frequency of ultrasound, the less will be the penetration in the tissues. Hence, in the clinical setting, transducers with higher frequencies are used for smaller patients, while those with lower frequencies can be employed with increasingly large patients.

Production of images

The transducer used to obtain ultrasonic images contains crystals capable of producing short pulses of ultrasound at their own natural frequency. Knowing the velocity of ultrasound, the distance from the crystal to any interface is readily determined according to the time required for the reflected sound to return to the crystal. Therefore, each ultrasonic pulse, encountering numerous interfaces, gives rise to a series of reflected echoes returning at time intervals corresponding to their depths. In this way, each pulse from the crystal demonstrates a line of information that corresponds to the structures encountered by the sound beam.

• For a typical **M-mode** trace, the frequency of repetition of the pulse is approximately 1000/s. The M-mode display plots the line of information on the vertical axis, with time on the horizontal axis producing the typical graphic display. Thus, M-mode echocardiography provides excellent temporal resolution of moving structures because the frequency of repetition of the pulse is several times greater than the heart rate.

• **Conventional cross-sectional or two-dimensional echocardiography** is the construction of images using multiple individual lines of information produced in the same way as described for the M-mode trace. The entire image is produced one line at a time, and typically 64 or 128 lines of information are required to produce one

Pediatric Heart Disease: A Practical Guide, First Edition. Piers E. F. Daubeney, Michael L. Rigby, Koichiro Niwa, and Michael A. Gatzoulis.
© 2012 Blackwell Publishing Ltd. Published 2012 by Blackwell Publishing Ltd.

image or frame. Multiple frames are constructed in real-time each second, the limiting factor being the time necessary for the echoes from each pulse to return to the transducer. At depths of 5–15 cm, it is possible to achieve frame rates of 28–50/s. In most instances, this rate will be slower than the underlying heart rate, impairing to some degree the temporal resolution.

Imaging the heart and arterial and venous connections

Cross-sectional echocardiography is an essential part of the investigation of patients with congenital and acquired heart disease. In many instances, no other imaging techniques or methods of investigations such as cardiac catheterization are required to complete the diagnosis. Particularly in infants and young children, cardiac surgery can be undertaken on the basis of ultrasonic imaging. The only limiting factors to precise diagnosis are the resolution of the equipment used, the cooperation of the patient, and the experience of the operator. It is important that investigations are undertaken in a warm and comfortable environment with suitable distractions such as videos, lights, and music. A simultaneous recording of EKG is always used to permit the timing of events during the cardiac cycle. More detailed physiologic measurements will be assisted by phonocardiography to record the precise closure time of the semilunar and atrioventricular valves.

The heart can be examined in certain basic planes by applying the transducer to four major sites:
- Subcostal region;
- Cardiac apex;
- Left parasternal edge between the second and fourth intercostal spaces;
- Suprasternal notch.

In this chapter, the steps necessary to obtain the diagnosis by echocardiography are discussed.

Subcostal sections

These are obtained by combining clockwise and counterclockwise rotation of the transducer directed more posteriorly to show the atria, the venous connections, and the atrioventricular junction, and more anteriorly to image the ventricular–arterial connections and great arteries (Figure 6.1).

Apical and parasternal sections

From the apical and parasternal positions, four-chamber, long axis, and short axis sections of the ventricles and great

arteries are obtained with the patient rotated to the left by about 30 degrees from the supine position (Figure 6.2).

Suprasternal sections

From the suprasternal notch and with hyperextension of the neck, it is possible to image the aortic arch in its entirety, the proximal right and left pulmonary arteries, the pulmonary venous connections to the left atrium, and the brachiocephalic and superior caval veins (Figure 6.3).

Determination of atrial arrangement

By recording horizontal abdominal sections at the level of the 10th to 12th thoracic vertebrae, the relationship of the abdominal great vessels can be used to infer thoracic, and therefore, atrial arrangement (Figure 6.4). The aorta can be recognized by its pulsations synchronous with the arterial pulse or cardiac apex. The inferior caval vein expands with inspiration. When these horizontal sections show symmetrical positions of the aorta and inferior caval vein anterior to the spine, lateralized atrial arrangement can be assumed.

Relationships of the abdominal great vessels

- **Usual atrial arrangement (situs solitus)** (see Chapter 3; Figure 6.4a): the inferior caval vein is on the right and the aorta on the left.

- **Mirror-image arrangement (situs inversus)** (Figure 6.4b): the aorta is on the right with the inferior caval vein to the left. Thus the morphologic right atrium is on the side of the inferior caval vein.

- **Right and left isomerism** (Figure 6.4c and d). Neither the abdominothoracic organs nor atrial chambers are lateralized. Instead, the whole body shows evidence of symmetry and both atria have similar characteristics giving two other alternatives for atrial arrangement, known as left and right isomerism (see Chapters 3 and 17):

  ○ **Right isomerism**, the aorta and inferior caval vein are both on the same side of the spine with the vein in a slightly anterior position (Figure 6.4c)

  ○ **Left isomerism**, the inferior caval vein is absent in the majority of cases and instead the systemic venous return from the abdomen to the heart is via an azygos vein. In this situation, horizontal sections just below the diaphragm will reveal a centrally placed aorta closely aligned to a venous structure slightly posterior (Figure 6.4d).

In some hearts with lateralized atrial arrangement, there can also be absence of the inferior caval vein and therefore attention should also be given to the connection of the hepatic veins. When there is lateralized

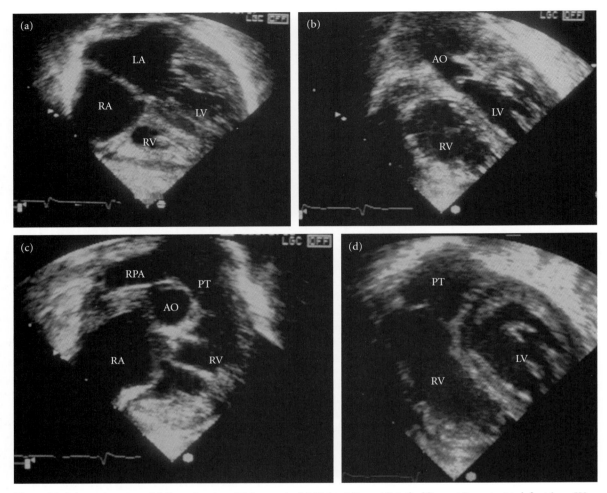

Figure 6.1 Subcostal sections. (a) Four chamber. (b) Long axis. (c) Right oblique. (d) Left oblique. AO, aorta; LA, left atrium; LV, left ventricle; PT, pulmonary trunk; RA, right atrium; RPA, right pulmonary artery; RV, right ventricle.

arrangement (solitus or inversus) or right isomerism, some or all of the hepatic veins drain to the inferior caval vein. In the presence of left atrial isomerism, the hepatic veins almost always drain directly to the atria (see Chapter 17). This pattern also permits the detection of left isomerism in those cases when the inferior caval vein is present. The course of the hepatic veins can be traced with subcostal paracoronal imaging planes.

Types of atrioventricular connection

The type of atrioventricular connection is determined from parasternal, apical, and subcostal four-chamber sections.

Types of atrioventricular connection

Biventricular

- Concordant
- Discordant
- Ambiguous (with right or left atrial isomerism)

Univentricular

- Absent right
- Absent left
- Double inlet:
  - With separate left and right atrioventricular valves
  - With common atrioventricular valve

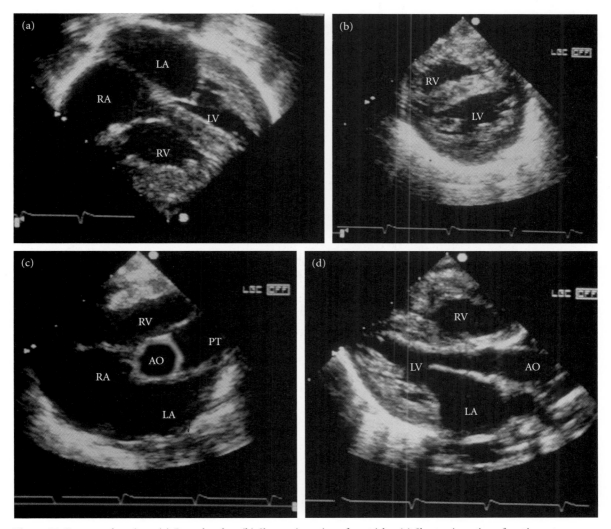

Figure 6.2 Parasternal sections. (a) Four chamber. (b) Short axis section of ventricles. (c) Short axis section of aortic root. (d) Long axis section of left ventricle. AO, aorta; LA, left atrium; LV, left ventricle; PT, pulmonary trunk; RA, right atrium; RV, right ventricle.

Biventricular atrioventricular connection

For hearts with a biventricular atrioventricular connection (each atrium connecting to a separate ventricle):
• The tricuspid valve, an integral part of the morphologically right ventricle, has chordal attachments to the right ventricular aspect of the ventricular septum.
• The mitral valve chords, by contrast, usually attach only to two discrete left ventricular papillary muscles and do not insert into the septum.

Thus, in most hearts with a biventricular atrioventricular connection, the demonstration of the presence or absence of chordal attachments to the septum allows the morphology of the atrioventricular valves and the ventricles to be determined. It may also be possible to determine the morphology of an atrioventricular valve by examining the hinge point of the attachment of its septal leaflet. The septal leaflet of the tricuspid valve is attached slightly nearer to the apex of the heart than the

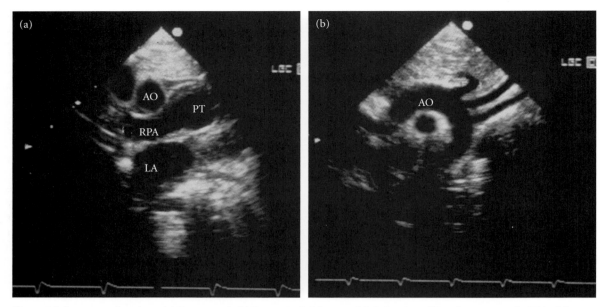

Figure 6.3 Suprasternal sections. (a) Paracoronal. (b) Parasagittal. AO, aorta; LA, left atrium; PT, pulmonary trunk; RPA, right pulmonary artery.

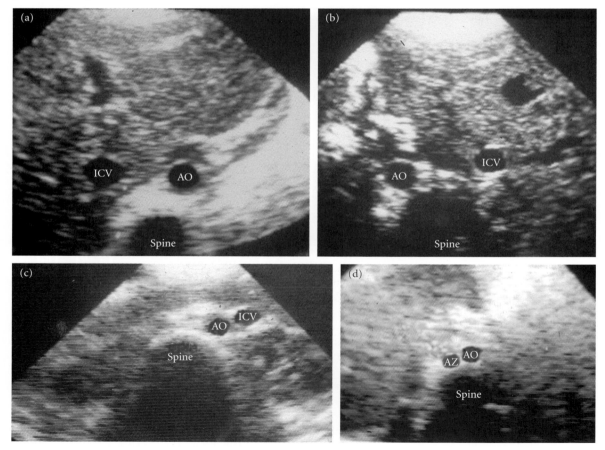

Figure 6.4 Horizontal abdominal sections beneath the diaphragm. (a) Situs solitus. (b) Situs inversus. (c) Right isomerism. (d) Left isomerism. AO, aorta; AZ, azygos vein; ICV; inferior caval vein.

corresponding leaflet of the mitral valve. This offsetting of the atrioventricular valves enables the mitral and tricuspid valves to be distinguished and consequently, ventricular morphology to be determined. Offsetting will no longer be evident when there is a perimembranous ventricular septal defect (VSD), but there are other methods of identifying ventricular morphology. For example, short axis sections may identify the three-leaflet arrangement of the normal tricuspid valve, which contrasts with the two leaflets of the mitral valve. Also, a smooth trabecular pattern and two discrete papillary muscles typify the left ventricle, while the right ventricle is coarsely trabeculated with unequal papillary muscles and with a moderator band at the apex. Once the morphology of the ventricles and the atrial arrangement have been determined, the type of atrioventricular connection (**concordant, discordant or ambiguous**) can be described. The diagnosis, however, is better described as "left (or right) atrial isomerism with a biventricular atrioventricular connection" than "ambiguous atrioventricular connection."

Univentricular atrioventricular connection

The atrioventricular connection is described as univentricular in a significant minority of hearts in which the atria connect predominantly or exclusively to only one ventricle. The possible connections are **double inlet ventricle, absence of the right-sided atrioventricular connection**, and **absence of the left-sided connection** (see Chapters 3, 15, and 16). Four-chamber sections demonstrate a univentricular connection.

• For hearts with an **absent right atrioventricular connection** (usually classical tricuspid atresia), there is no potential connection between the floor of the right atrium and the ventricular mass; atrioventricular sulcus tissue interposes between them.

• Similarly, when there is **absence of the left atrioventricular connection**, the atrioventricular sulcus can be demonstrated between the floor of the left-side atrium and the ventricular mass.

• When both atria are shown to connect directly to one ventricle, either through separate right and left atrioventricular valves or (less frequently) through a common valve, the atrioventricular connection is described as **double inlet**.

Most hearts in which the atrioventricular connection is univentricular also possess a second smaller ventricle, which is often described as "rudimentary"; usually rudimentary ventricles will be demonstrated to the right or left of the dominant ventricle in apical, parasternal, and subcostal four-chamber sections. A rudimentary right ventricle found in a heart with a univentricular connection to a left ventricle will be either left or right sided, but always anterosuperior in parasternal long and short axis sections and in some of the subcostal views. When there is a univentricular atrioventricular connection to a right ventricle, similar sections will demonstrate a posteroinferior rudimentary left ventricle. The identification of the anterior or posterior position of the rudimentary ventricle is the most reliable echocardiographic guide to the morphology of the dominant ventricle. Occasionally there is no second rudimentary ventricle identified; it may then be assumed that the atria are connected to a solitary and indeterminate ventricle, although rarely the rudimentary ventricle may be present but too small in size to be visualized by echocardiography.

Mode of atrioventricular connection

The term "mode" of atrioventricular connection is used to describe the morphology of the valves guarding the atrioventricular junction (see Chapter 3). Cross-sectional echocardiography is particularly suited to the demonstration of abnormalities of the atrioventricular valves, usually by means of four-chamber sections. An imperforate valve allows potential anatomic communication but no flow between an atrium and a ventricle. Characteristically, the valve is seen to balloon into the ventricle during atrial systole. It is not unusual for hypoplastic tensor apparatus to be seen attached to the ventricular aspect of the valve membrane. When there is an **overriding** and/or **straddling valve** (see Chapter 3), there is almost always malalignment between the atrial and ventricular septal structures and a VSD will be present. In order to describe the valve as straddling, tensor apparatus must be seen to arise from both ventricles. The degree of override of the straddling atrioventricular valves can vary, and this determines the precise atrioventricular connection present. A continuous spectrum of anomalies occurs between an overriding valve orifice being almost entirely committed to a ventricle already connected to the other atrium and it being almost exclusively committed to a ventricle not having any other atrioventricular connection. Cross-sectional echocardiography readily allows the distinction between biventricular and univentricular connections in hearts with an overriding valve, and it is the 50% rule that is invoked to make this distinction. In the presence of a common valve, more than 75% of the valve annulus must be connected to one ventricle in order to describe the connection as univentricular.

> **Ventricular–arterial connections**
> - Concordant
> - Discordant
> - Double outlet:
>   - Right ventricle
>   - Left ventricle
>   - Solitary indeterminate ventricle
> - Single outlet:
>   - Common arterial trunk
>   - Pulmonary atresia
>   - Aortic atresia

Types of ventricular–arterial connection

In order to determine the ventricular–arterial connection it is necessary first to identify the morphology of the ventricles using the methods described in Chapter 3. Then the nature of the arterial trunks must be determined. The aorta is identified from its arch and the head and neck vessels. The pulmonary trunk is recognized by its bifurcation into left and right branches. Probably the most common type of single outlet is that associated with pulmonary atresia and VSD (see Chapter 15); the only outlet from the ventricular mass is then through the aorta with the pulmonary arteries being supplied either via an arterial duct or by systemic-to-pulmonary collaterals. A common arterial trunk is a single great artery which gives rise directly in its ascending part to coronary and pulmonary arteries and the ascending aorta (see Chapter 16). A solitary arterial trunk can occur with pulmonary atresia and total absence of intrapericardial pulmonary arteries, and it will not then be possible to distinguish between a solitary aorta and a common arterial trunk with pulmonary atresia.

In practice, it is relatively easy in infants to demonstrate the origin of the pulmonary trunk and its bifurcation by recording subcostal outlet sections. Similarly, it is usually possible to demonstrate the aorta and aortic arch from the same position. Thus, in complete transposition (see Chapter 14), for example, the diagnosis can most often be established using this approach. In older children, the great arteries are not so readily demonstrated in this fashion, but nonetheless the ventricular–arterial connection can usually be established by combining subcostal, parasternal, and apical long axis sections of the ventricles and great arteries together with suprasternal or high parasternal long axis sections of the aorta and the

pulmonary arteries. The diagnosis of abnormalities of ventricular–arterial connection associated with a VSD are most reliably established by parasternal long axis sections which show both ventricles, the ventricular septum, and the origin of both great arteries. The demonstration of an overriding arterial trunk in which more than 50% is connected to the same ventricle as the other great artery permits the diagnosis of a double outlet ventricle.

Comparison of Doppler techniques

The Doppler principle as applied to sound is simply that the frequency of sonic waves changes as they are reflected from a moving target, increasing as the target approaches the receiver and diminishing as it moves away. This change in frequency is called the Doppler shift and has important cardiologic applications. It can be applied to an ultrasonic pulse striking a moving pool of red cells, the back-scattered pulses exhibiting a shift in frequency compared with the emitted pulse from the transducer. The shift depends upon the velocity and direction of blood flow, the angle between the beam and blood flow, and the velocity of sound in the body tissues.

The three basic types of Doppler are complementary to each other and measure blood flow velocities in different ways.
- For the evaluation of high-flow velocities, the method of choice is **continuous wave Doppler**, since it does not give rise to aliasing. Although it does not permit gating for precise localization of the target, modern equipment with a steerable cursor line and a focused beam allows precise alignment, assuring appropriate velocity measurements. Continuous wave Doppler is better than pulse wave Doppler for measuring high velocities.
- **Pulse wave Doppler**, in contrast, enables measurements of flow at a known depth, allowing more precise calculations, but it is limited by the maximal measurable velocity.
- **Color flow Doppler** is qualitative, providing spatial information not obtained with other methods. By permitting visualization of the disturbed blood, it facilitates the alignment of the continuous wave Doppler beam. The visual effect of color flow provides a method of rapidly screening for abnormal velocities within the heart and allows the demonstration of abnormalities such as atrioventricular valve regurgitation, stenosed or regurgitant semilunar valves, and atrial or ventricular septal defects.

Quantitative Doppler measurements

When a fluid flows through a rigid tube, the volume of flow can be derived from the velocity and the cross-sectional area of the tube. When a constant volume of fluid passes through a narrow area in the tube, a high of velocity must be generated distal to the restriction.

Examples of typical Doppler-derived measurements are:
- Systolic gradient in aortic and pulmonary stenosis;
- Diastolic gradient in mitral stenosis;
- Pressure drop across a VSD and patent ductus arteriosus;
- Systolic pressure drop from the right ventricle to the right atrium;
- Diastolic pressure drop from the pulmonary artery to the right ventricle;
- Diastolic pressure drop from the aorta to the left ventricle;
- Right ventricular and pulmonary arterial systolic pressure;
- Pulmonary-to-systemic flow ratio in left-to-right shunts.

The Bernoulli equation

According to the simplified Bernoulli equation, the most important principle of quantitative Doppler echocardiography, the pressure drop across a discrete obstruction can be expressed by the equation:

$$P_1 - P_2 = 4V^2$$

where P_1 is the pressure proximal to and P_2 the pressure distal to the obstruction in mmHg; V is the velocity of flow distal to the obstruction in m/s.

In spite of the fact that arteries are not rigid tubes, that an obstructive lesion is not necessarily a discrete narrowing, and that the flow of a given volume of blood is not constant, this equation can be used in clinical practice to measure the pressure drop across stenotic or regurgitation valves, and across a VSD, arterial duct, or other communication.

It is important to emphasize that the Doppler-derived pressure gradient is the peak instantaneous pressure drop and not the peak-to-peak gradient obtained at cardiac catheterization. The pressure drop derived from Doppler velocities will be greater than the peak-to-peak gradient in every case, although the difference is most marked when there is mild obstruction and less apparent when there is severe obstruction.

The expanded Bernoulli equation

The Bernoulli equation assumes the velocity of blood flow proximal to an obstruction is small when compared with that found distally. When the proximal velocity is greater than 1 m/s (e.g. with multiple levels of obstruction), the expanded Bernoulli equation is used:

$$P_1 - P_2 = 4\left(V_2^2 - V_1^2\right)$$

Mean pressure gradients

The mean pressure gradient, the average of all the instantaneous pressure gradients throughout the period of flow, is calculated by tracing the outer border of the Doppler velocity profile with a digitizing system built into the ultrasonic equipment. Mean pressure gradients may give a better estimate of the severity of obstructive lesions such as aortic or mitral stenosis.

Applications of quantitative Doppler

Almost all of the applications described below involve the use of the Bernoulli equation.

Assessment of pulmonary or aortic stenosis

In isolated pulmonary or aortic valve stenosis (see Chapters 10 and 11), the simplified Bernoulli equation is usually sufficient for measurement of the systolic gradient (Figure 6.5a). When there is more than one site of obstruction, e.g. infundibular and valvar pulmonary stenosis, the expanded Bernoulli equation should be used.

Right ventricular systolic pressure from tricuspid regurgitation

Tricuspid regurgitation is commonly identified by color flow Doppler. Using four-chamber sections, the right ventricular systolic pressure can be derived from the peak instantaneous systolic gradient between the right ventricle and right atrium, calculated from the peak velocity of tricuspid regurgitation; the profile is similar to that of mitral regurgitation (Figure 6.5b). The right atrial systolic pressure is assumed to be 5 mmHg. In the absence of pulmonary stenosis, it can be assumed that the right ventricular and pulmonary arterial systolic pressures are equal.

Right ventricular systolic pressure from flow across a ventricular septal defect

The peak instantaneous systolic pressure drop across a VSD (see Chapter 9) permits the estimation of right ventricular systolic pressure when left ventricular systolic pressure is assumed to be equal to the systemic blood

(a)

(b)

(c)

(d)

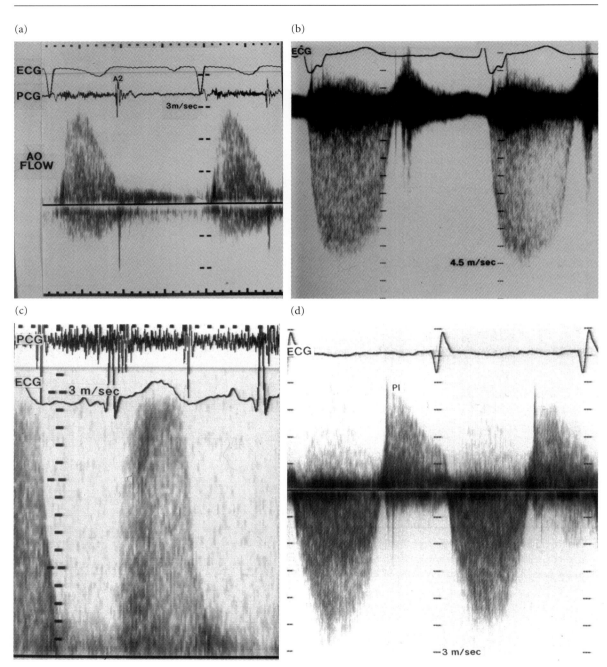

Figure 6.5 (a) Continuous wave Doppler of mild aortic stenosis. (b) Continuous wave Doppler recording of mitral regurgitation with a flow velocity of 4.5 m/s. With the similar velocity of tricuspid regurgitation there would be a high right ventricular systolic pressure indicating either pulmonary stenosis or pulmonary hypertension, or perhaps a large and non-restrictive ventricular septal defect (VSD). (c) Continuous wave Doppler recording from a moderately large VSD in which the flow velocity from the left to right ventricle is 3 m/s. (d) Continuous wave Doppler recording in mild pulmonary stenosis with pulmonary regurgitation in which the end-diastolic gradient between the pulmonary artery and the right ventricle is low. The systolic flow is below the baseline while the diastolic velocity is above it.

pressure (Figure 6.5c). Again it can be assumed that the right ventricular and pulmonary arterial systolic pressures are equal in the absence of any pulmonary stenosis. For patients with an isolated VSD, a calculated pressure drop of 60 mmHg or more is almost always indicative of a relatively small and restrictive VSD. For patients with equal systolic pressures in the right and left ventricle, the gradient derived from Doppler flow measurements is often as high as 20–25 mmHg.

Pulmonary artery systolic pressure from flow through an arterial duct

Using the simplified Bernoulli equation, the pressure drop between the aorta and pulmonary artery across a patent ductus (see Chapter 9) allows the estimation of the pulmonary artery pressure in systole and at end-diastole.

Diastolic pulmonary arterial pressure from pulmonary regurgitation

Trivial pulmonary regurgitation is often detected by color flow Doppler. This will permit the measurement of the end-diastolic gradient between the pulmonary artery and the right ventricle (Figure 6.5d). The right ventricular end-diastolic pressure will be similar to the venous pressure (usually approximately 5 mmHg). In some circumstances, particularly in cases of tetralogy of Fallot

following surgery, pulmonary atresia with an intact ventricular septum, and critical pulmonary stenosis (see Chapter 15), the end-diastolic pressure might be elevated significantly.

Mitral regurgitation

Mitral regurgitation (see Chapter 11) will always be evident from color flow Doppler. The characteristic Doppler trace of mitral regurgitation is similar to that observed in tricuspid regurgitation. The estimation of the degree of regurgitation is usually qualitative but can broadly be assessed as mild, moderate, or severe.

Mitral stenosis

Measuring the severity of mitral stenosis (see Chapter 11) depends on the diastolic pressure drop from the left atrium to the ventricle with the Bernoulli equation applied to the maximal velocity of flow. The Doppler profile can assist in the estimation of severity by observing the rate of decline of the peak velocity (Figure 6.6).

Aortic coarctation

The instantaneous peak systolic gradient correlates well with the severity of coarctation of the aorta (see Chapter 12). More importantly, however, is the velocity profile during systole and diastole. This reaches a peak during

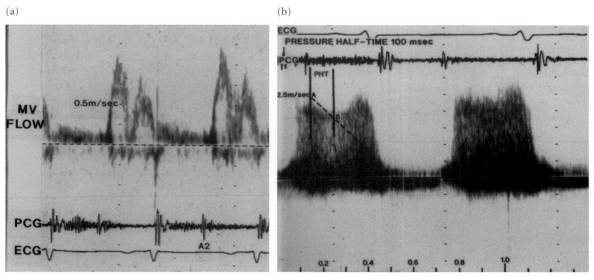

(a)   (b)

Figure 6.6 (a) Pulsed wave Doppler recording from a normal mitral valve in which the E wave precedes the A wave.
(b) Continuous wave Doppler recording in mitral stenosis illustrating the use of the pressure half-time to estimate the severity.

(a)

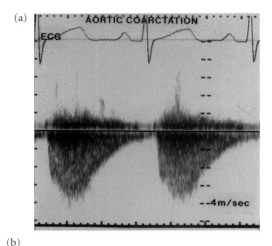

(b)

Figure 6.7 (a) Typical continuous wave Doppler recording in the proximal descending aorta in coarctation. (b) M-mode recording of the left ventricle illustrating the measurements of end-systolic and end-diastolic dimensions as well as posterior left ventricular wall thickness and right ventricular end-diastolic dimension. LVDD, left ventricular diastolic dimension; LVPW, left ventricular posterior wall; LVSD, left ventricular systolic dimension; RVDD, right ventricular diastolic dimension.

systole and then gradually declines during diastole until the onset of the next systole (Figure 6.7a). When coarctation is associated with aortic stenosis, the expanded Bernoulli equation should be used.

Measurement of systemic and pulmonary blood flow

Aortic and pulmonary flow can be calculated from the mean blood flow velocity, the cross-sectional area of the vessel, and the R–R interval on the EKG.

Transesophageal echocardiography

Transesophageal echocardiography is complimentary to conventional transthoracic imaging in the diagnosis and monitoring of congenital heart disease in infants and children. It can be used to monitor intraoperative cardiac function. It has a fundamental role in the documentation of the adequacy of surgical repair on the operating table and in the early postoperative period it provides a better window on the heart than conventional transthoracic imaging (see Chapter 34). It is indispensable in the monitoring of interventional cardiac catheterization procedures, such as closure of atrial or ventricular septal defects. Transesophageal studies are carried out either under general anesthesia or with sedation.

Three-dimensional echocardiography

Three-dimensional echocardiograms are derived from a series of two-dimensional images and display the heart in a completely different format. They can be used to display the borders of atrial or ventricular septal defects *en face*, the anatomic details of ventricular inflow or outflow tract obstruction, and the measurement of ventricular volumes and derived indices of ventricular function. Good quality three-dimensional imaging can only be derived from clear two-dimensional studies.

Measurement of ventricular function

Various indices of systolic and diastolic ventricular function, particularly of the left ventricle, can be derived from an M-mode (Figure 6.7b) or cross-sectional echocardiogram by measuring cavity size at end-systole and end-diastole, and by assessing the Doppler flow profile across the mitral valve. One of the most useful measurements of left ventricular systolic function is the shortening fraction (SF; normal range 28–38%). This is defined as:

$$SF = [(LVEDD - LVESD) / LVEDD] \times 100$$

where LVEDD is the left ventricular end-diastolic dimension and LVESD is the end-systolic dimension.

When there are regional wall motion abnormalities, ejection fraction (EF) will provide a better estimate of overall systolic function of the left ventricle:

$$EF = [(LVEDV - LVESV) / LVEDV] \times 100$$

where LVEDV is the left ventricular end-diastolic volume and LVESV is the end-systolic volume. The volumes are most commonly calculated from cross-sectional images of the left ventricle that involve assumptions about the shape of the ventricle.

It should be noted that both the shortening fraction and the ejection fraction, though commonly used as measures of left ventricular function in everyday practice, are not independent of preload and afterload. Thus, they do not necessarily reflect intrinsic contractility of the myocardium. Numerous load-independent measures of ventricular performance have been described using echocardiography, but are outside the scope of this text.

Further reading

Lai WW, Mertens L, Cohen M, Geva T. *Echocardiography in Pediatric and Congenital Heart Disease: From Fetus to Adult.* New York: Wiley-Blackwell, 2009.

7 Diagnostic cardiac catheterization and angiography

Michael L. Rigby

Royal Brompton Hospital, London, UK

For almost every patient undergoing cardiac catheterization, the diagnosis will already have been established by echocardiography; additional information might have been gained from magnetic resonance imaging (MRI) or computed tomography (CT). The rationale for further investigation will be to obtain specific information such as intracardiac pressures, pulmonary artery pressure, pulmonary vascular resistance, and the quantification of intracardiac shunts. It is usual to perform angiography, particularly for the imaging of peripheral pulmonary arteries, the aorta, aortopulmonary collaterals, pulmonary and systemic veins, and the coronary arteries. The frequency of cardiac catheterization relative to the number of patients undergoing cardiac surgery varies considerably from center to center. Currently, however, the most frequent indication is for interventional cardiac catheterization (see Chapter 33). Improved echocardiography and MRI (see Chapters 6 and 8) have significantly reduced the need for diagnostic cardiac catheterization and inevitably an increasing minority of pediatric cardiologists now undertakes the highly specialized techniques of diagnostic and therapeutic catheterization.

Indications

Diagnostic cardiac catheterization and angiography are most frequently indicated in those children who have undergone previous palliative cardiac surgery (and in whom further surgery is planned) such as:
• Banding of the pulmonary trunk;
• Blalock–Taussig shunt;
• Norwood operation for hypoplastic left heart syndrome;
• Damus–Kaye–Stansell operation;
• Glenn operation;
• Unifocalization operations for systemic-to-pulmonary collaterals in pulmonary atresia.

Cardiac catheterization is often performed when a revision operation is needed following:
• Repair of tetralogy of Fallot with pulmonary stenosis or pulmonary atresia;
• Common arterial trunk;
• Complete transposition of the great arteries;
• Total anomalous pulmonary venous connection.

Another indication is to perform myocardial biopsy in some cases of cardiomyopathy or following heart transplantation (see Chapter 35). It is unusual to perform cardiac catheterization prior to corrective surgery for many conditions, including total anomalous pulmonary venous connection, atrioventricular septal defects, atrial septal defects, ventricular septal defects, tetralogy of Fallot, complete transposition of the great arteries, and double outlet right ventricle.

Angiography is used in many situations, such as the demonstration of systemic-to-pulmonary collaterals, imaging of the coronary arteries in hearts with pulmonary atresia and an intact ventricular septum, and the delineation of pulmonary and systemic venous connections in hearts with atrial isomerism. Cardiac catheterization is also required if there is a clinical indication to measure pulmonary vascular resistance and to assess the effect of pulmonary vasodilators such as oxygen, nitric oxide, adenosine, or sildenafil.

Pediatric Heart Disease: A Practical Guide, First Edition. Piers E. F. Daubeney, Michael L. Rigby, Koichiro Niwa, and Michael A. Gatzoulis.
© 2012 Blackwell Publishing Ltd. Published 2012 by Blackwell Publishing Ltd.

This is, of course, not an exhaustive list of the indications for diagnostic cardiac catheterization. Cases will always be assessed individually, and there are so many variations of the more common congenital heart malformations and so many individually rare conditions that it is inappropriate to make too many generalizations.

Techniques and equipment

Cardiac catheterization involves the insertion of small catheters into the various cardiac chambers, arteries, and veins. In most cases a percutaneous (Seldinger) technique is used, and the most common sites of entry are the femoral vein and artery together with the internal jugular or subclavian vein. Rarely, percutaneous entry of the brachial or subclavian artery may be necessary. Occasionally catheterization is performed following cut-down on the axillary artery and vein or even the carotid artery, and in the newborn infant the umbilical artery or vein can be used. In patients with absence or thrombotic occlusion of the inferior caval vein, direct puncture of a hepatic vein can be performed through the abdominal wall, allowing the introduction of catheters into the intrahepatic inferior caval vein near to the junction with the right atrium.

When percutaneous puncture of an artery or vein is performed, a short valved sheath inserted into the vessel allows the passage of catheters to the heart. The back-stop valve will prevent blood loss from arterial sites and air embolism through venous sheaths. When vascular cut down has been performed the catheter is usually inserted directly into the blood vessel, which is then repaired at the end of the procedure. For arterial catheterization or when large catheters or sheaths are introduced into veins, anticoagulation with heparin reduces the risk of vascular thrombosis. A pediatric cardiologist who performs cardiac catheterization will be familiar with all the techniques described above.

There is considerable variation in the type and shape of catheters available. The decision on the French size of the intravenous or intra-arterial sheath and catheters and the shape and configuration of the catheters themselves will depend on what particular information is required by the operator. A detailed description is beyond the scope of this book. In many cases arterial catheterization is not essential because the left side of the heart can be accessed with a venous catheter passed through an atrial or ventricular septal defect or with the left atrium entered via a transeptal puncture. In general, the smallest French size catheter that will accomplish the goals of catheteriza-

tion is chosen and the range will be from 4 to 7 Fr. Catheter manipulation is dependent on hand–eye coordination, knowledge of the anatomy of the underlying congenital heart malformation, and an awareness of the various types of catheters and guidewires available.

Hemodynamics

Cardiac catheterization may be performed:
• To obtain pressure measurements in the cardiac chambers, arteries, and veins;
• To measure blood oxygen levels and blood gases at various sites;
• To determine cardiac output;
• To quantify left-to-right or right-to-left shunts;
• To measure pulmonary vascular resistance.

The pressure at the catheter tip is transmitted via the catheter and tubing to a transducer, converted to an electrical signal and then passed to a multichannel recorder and by an optical beam to photographic paper. Physiologic recorders have multiple channels for recording not only pressures but also EKG and other signals. An oscilloscope allows continuous inspection of the tracing as it is being generated. Pressures are compared to atmospheric pressure in the middle of the heart, which is defined as 0 mmHg. By convention it is assumed that the middle of the heart is the midway point between the back of the thorax and the top of the sternum whilst the patient is lying in a supine position.

Normal pressures in mmHg (approximate average values)	
Right atrium	3 (mean)
Right ventricle	24/0/5 systolic/beginning diastole/end-diastolic
Pulmonary artery	24/10/13 (systolic/diastolic/ mean)
Pulmonary artery wedge	8 (mean)
Left atrium	8 (mean)
Left ventricle	95/0/6 (systolic/beginning diastole/end-diastolic)
Aorta	95/55/68 (systolic/diastolic/ mean)

A detailed description of the pressure waves at various sites is beyond the scope of this chapter. It is worth noting however that the normal right ventricular and pulmonary arterial systolic pressures are 20–25% of those in the left ventricle and aorta, and the left atrial pressure is higher than the right. A pulmonary artery wedge pressure is a good estimate of pulmonary venous pressure (usually the same as the left atrial pressure) and the pulmonary venous wedge pressure can be used in the estimation of pulmonary artery pressure when it is impossible to make a direct measurement. The normal atrial pressure trace is composed of A and V waves. The A wave represents atrial systole and follows immediately after the P wave on the surface EKG. The V wave occurs at the end of systole and probably represents continued atrial filling against a closed tricuspid or mitral valve. Normally, the right atrial pressure has a dominant A wave which is slightly higher than the V wave, whereas the left atrium has a higher V wave. The A wave has the same value as the corresponding ventricular end-diastolic pressure.

The **right atrial pressure** is elevated in:
- Pericardial tamponade;
- Tricuspid atresia;
- Pulmonary atresia with intact ventricular septum;
- Abnormal connection of the right atrium to a systemic ventricle;
- Large left-to-right atrial shunts;
- Decreased right ventricular compliance found in right ventricular hypertrophy and diastolic dysfunction;
- Tricuspid stenosis;
- Tricuspid insufficiency.

The **left atrial pressure** is elevated in:
- Left-to-right shunts in ventricular septal defect and patent arterial duct;
- Mitral stenosis;
- Mitral regurgitation;
- Absent left atrioventricular connection with restrictive interatrial communication;
- Decreased left ventricular compliance.

Mitral stenosis produces a large A wave whereas mitral regurgitation gives rise to a large V wave.

The **right ventricular systolic pressure** is elevated in:
- Volume overloading caused by, for example, a significant ventricular septal defect or atrial septal defect;
- Pulmonary hypertension;
- Pulmonary stenosis;
- Tetralogy of Fallot: due to the large non-restrictive ventricular septal defect, the right ventricular systolic pressure will be identical to that in the left ventricle and aorta;
- Conditions where the right ventricle is connected to the aorta, such as complete transposition, congenitally corrected transposition, and double outlet right ventricle: right ventricular systolic pressure is likely to be identical to aortic pressure.

The **left ventricular systolic pressure** is elevated in:
- Aortic stenosis;
- Coarctation of the aorta;
- Systemic hypertension.

Oxygen levels

In the cardiac catheterization laboratory, spectrophotometric methods are used to determine the percentage of hemoglobin saturated with oxygen. Spectrophotometers measure the amount of light or optical density transmitted through an opaque tube or cuvette at a given wavelength by oxygenated and deoxygenated hemoglobin. The amount of light absorbed is proportional to the concentration of oxyhemoglobin and deoxyhemoglobin. This method ignores the small amount of oxygen dissolved in plasma.

Normal intracardiac oxygen saturation data	
Superior caval vein	67–87%
Right atrium	69–87%
Coronary sinus	42–55%
Inferior caval vein	62–88%*
Right ventricle	67–86%
Pulmonary artery	67–86%
Pulmonary vein	97–99%
Left atrium	95–99%
Aorta	95–99%

*Measurements from the inferior caval vein can be unreliable because of streaming of blood from the hepatic veins (low saturation) or renal veins (high saturation), and should be interpreted with caution.

Calculations used in diagnostic cardiac catheterization

Various indices can be derived from the basic pressure and saturation data measured during catheterization and, while much useful information can be obtained, it should be recognized that the results of many of the calculations are at best approximations because of the inherent errors in much of the methodology, particularly in the measurement of oxygen consumption. Even if special techniques are used to refine the methods, it should be recognized that the resulting derived data only reflect the physiologic situation at the time the measurements were made. The effects of sedation, anesthesia, and so on influence them. They certainly do not reflect what the physiologic state may be during normal exercise. Nonetheless, it is conventional and useful to derive certain measurements from data obtained routinely during cardiac catheterization.

- Systemic flow index (Qs) (L/min/m²)
- Pulmonary flow index (Qp) (L/min/m²)
- Pulmonary/systemic flow ratio (Qp/Qs)
- Left-to-right shunt (%)
- Right-to-left shunt (%)
- Effective pulmonary blood flow L/min/m²
- Pulmonary resistance (Rp)
- Systemic resistance (Rs)

Although there are several methods of measuring blood flow, including indicator and thermal dilution methods, we are concerned here with the measurement of blood flow using oxygen saturation measurements. This makes use of the Fick principle, which states that the blood flow through an organ is given by the oxygen consumption of that organ (in unit time) divided by the difference in the oxygen content of blood flowing into and out of that organ. For example, pulmonary blood flow is given by:

$$\frac{\text{Oxygen consumption}}{\text{Pulmonary vein oxygen content} - \text{Pulmonary artery oxygen content}}$$

By assuming that over a period of time the oxygen taken up in the lungs is equal to the oxygen consumed by the body in metabolic processes, the systemic flow is given by:

$$\frac{\text{Oxygen consumption}}{\text{Systemic arterial oxygen content} - \text{Systemic (mixed) venous oxygen content}}$$

Oxygen consumption

This is the amount of oxygen taken up by blood passing through the lungs in unit time. It is assumed to equal the amount of oxygen used in metabolic processes during the same time. It can be obtained by direct measurement in the catheterization laboratory or from the tables of normal values.

Oxygen capacity

This is the amount of oxygen that can combine (as oxyhemoglobin) with $100\,\text{mL}$ ($=1\,\text{dL}$) of the patient's blood when fully saturated (mL/100 mL, mL/dL or vol%). This does not include the amount of oxygen in physical solution in the plasma. It is obtained by multiplying the hemoglobin in g/dL by the factor 1.34, which represents the maximum amount of oxygen that can be combined with 1 g of hemoglobin.

$$\text{Capacity}(\text{mL/dL}) = \text{Hb}(\text{g/dL}) \times 1.34$$

Oxygen saturation (%)

This is the amount of oxygen bound to hemoglobin in relation to its capacity.

Oxygen content

This is the actual amount of oxygen present in a given sample of blood. It represents both oxygen present as oxyhemoglobin and oxygen in physical solution, the latter being insignificant when breathing room air and becoming more significant the greater the concentration of inspired oxygen. Plasma content can be ignored for up to 33% inspired oxygen.

When breathing 33–100% oxygen:

$$\text{Oxygen content}(\text{mL/dL}) = \text{Hb}(\text{g/dL}) \times 1.34 \times \text{O}_2 \text{ saturation}(\%) + \text{pO}_2(\text{kPa}) \times 7.5 \times 0.003$$

Calculation of flows using the Fick principle
Pulmonary flow (L/min)

$$Qp = \frac{\text{O}_2 \text{ consumption}(\text{mL/min})}{[\text{O}_2 \text{ content pulmonary veins}(\text{mL/dL}) - \text{O}_2 \text{ content pulmonary artery}(\text{mL/dL})] \times 10}$$

Systemic flow (L/min)

$$Qs = \frac{\text{O}_2 \text{ consumption}(\text{mL/min})}{[\text{O}_2 \text{ content aorta}(\text{mL/dL}) - \text{mixed venous O}_2 \text{ content}(\text{mL/dL})] \times 10}$$

Effective pulmonary flow

$$\frac{\text{O}_2 \text{ consumption}(\text{mL/min})}{[\text{O}_2 \text{ content pulmonary veins}(\text{mL/dL}) - \text{mixed venous O}_2 \text{ content}(\text{mL/dL})] \times 10}$$

This is the amount of blood to which oxygen can be added during passage through the lungs, thus excluding blood that is already fully saturated; the most common example of a condition with a high pulmonary artery saturation is complete transposition of the great arteries.

Calculation of shunts

Left-to-right shunt (%) =

$$\frac{\text{Pulmonary artery saturation} - \text{Mixed venous saturation}}{\text{Pulmonary vein saturation} - \text{Mixed venous saturation}}$$

Right-to-left shunt (%) =

$$\frac{\text{Pulmonary vein saturation} - \text{Systemic arterial saturation}}{\text{Pulmonary vein saturation} - \text{Mixed venous saturation}}$$

Pulmonary-to-systemic blood flow ratio

This is probably the most useful shunt calculation. As most of the variables cancel each other out:

$$Qp/Qs = \frac{\text{Aortic saturation} - \text{Mixed venous saturation}^*}{\text{Pulmonary venous saturation} - \text{Pulmonary artery saturation}}$$

Pulmonary vascular resistance (PVR; Wood units)

$$\frac{\text{Pulmonary artery mean pressure} - \text{Left atrial mean pressure}}{Qp}$$

Hypoxia, hypercapnia, and acidosis can cause an increase in pulmonary vascular resistance and should be avoided during the collection of data which should be obtained under stable conditions.

Systemic and pulmonary flow index

It is conventional to correct flows for body surface area. When oxygen consumption is indexed for body

surface area, further indexing is not required. In such cases the unit of PVR is Wood units $\cdot$ m^2 (i.e. not divided by m^2).

Angiography

Modern catheter laboratories have either one X-ray tube mounted on a single C-arm or two C-arms in a biplane design. Angiograms are rarely exposed using merely anteroposterior and lateral projections. The acquisitions are usually made with axial angiography for which the C-arms are ideally suited. Examples of angiograms are shown in Figures 7.1–7.4. The movie images obtained during the injection of contrast medium can be stored on ciné film or digitally. Digital information can be stored on a central server within a hospital and retrieved by pediatric cardiologists and cardiac surgeons through their office PC.

Radiation exposure

The radiation exposure to both patient and personnel from diagnostic and therapeutic cardiac catheterization is considerable. It is therefore extremely important that personnel involved, and especially the cardiologists performing the catheterization, understand the risks of radiation and aim to limit the radiation exposure to as low as reasonably possible. Radiation exposure should be audited for every patient and when acceptable levels are exceeded internal hospital review undertaken. In practice, complications of radiation are rare but they include tissue injury and cataracts, genetic effects, and carcinogenesis, both to the patient and laboratory staff. Transient skin erythema is the most common complication encountered but more permanent skin damage can occur. It is important to remember that the effects of radiation are cumulative; this has implications for patients having a number of cardiac catheter procedures over the years and for cardiologists performing frequent investigations. Fetal exposure should be avoided and patients at risk of being pregnant should have a pregnancy test prior to catheterization. The following principles are used to reduce radiation risk for both patient and laboratory personnel:

• Fluoroscopic and cinéangiographic times are kept as short as possible;
• Smallest possible radiation dose is used during acquisition of images;
• Forward planning to minimize number of ciné runs;

---

*The best estimates of mixed venous saturation when calculating shunts are either $[(\text{SVCsat} \times 3) + \text{IVCsat}]/4$ or merely SVC saturation or the average of SVC, low IVC, and high IVC saturations, where IVC is inferior caval vein and SVC is superior caval vein.

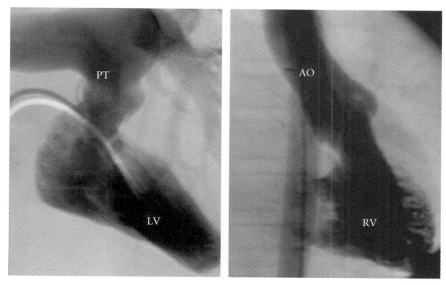

Figure 7.1 Left and right ventricular angiograms from a patient with usual atrial arrangement, discordant atrioventricular connection, and discordant ventricular–arterial connection. The pulmonary arteries are dilated. The aorta is left sided. AO, aorta; LV, left ventricle; PT, pulmonary trunk; RV, right ventricle.

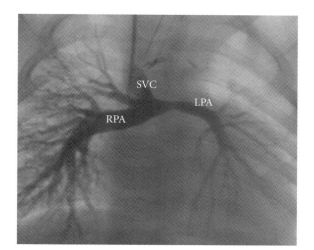

Figure 7.2 Pulmonary arteriogram via a bidirectional cavo-pulmonary anastomosis revealing hypoplasia of the left pulmonary artery. LPA, left pulmonary artery; RPA, right pulmonary artery; SVC, superior caval vein.

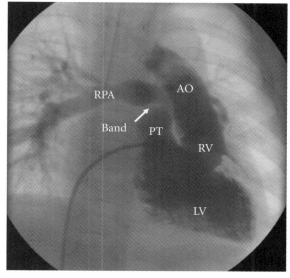

Figure 7.3 Left ventricular angiography in a patient with a double inlet left ventricle and left-sided rudimentary right ventricle with a discordant ventricular–arterial connection and previous pulmonary artery banding. AO, aorta; LV, left ventricle; PT, pulmonary trunk; RPA, right pulmonary artery; RV, right ventricle.

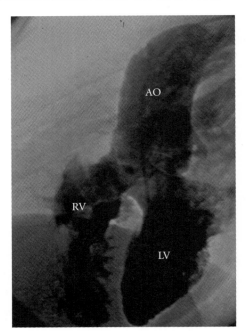

Figure 7.4 Left ventriculogram in a patient with a perimembranous outlet ventricular septal defect and pulmonary atresia. The aorta overrides the ventricular septum. AO, aorta; LV, left ventricle; RV, right ventricle.

• Laboratory personnel should wear lead aprons, thyroid shields, and eye glasses;
• X-ray shield of leaded glass should be placed between the operators and image intensifier;
• All laboratory staff should wear film badges beneath and outside the lead apron at all times to determinetheir monthly cumulative radiation dose;
• Regular audit of procedures and radiation doses are the responsibility of a dedicated radiation protection officer.

Contrast agents

The contrast agents used during angiography are iodine based with the basic chemical structure of a benzene ring with three iodine atoms. Low osmolality contrast media or isotonic contrast media are always used in infants and children. Complications and reactions to contrast media are now unusual. The most common effects are vasodilatation resulting in flushing, hypotension, and a transient rise in temperature. Cardiac arrhythmias, bradycardia, cardiac ischemia, negative inotropic effects, pulmonary hypertension, acute renal dysfunction, and nausea and vomiting are all encountered. Anaphylactoid or allergic-like reactions are rare but can lead to death from circulatory collapse or severe bronchospasm.

Adverse events

Adverse events are particularly prone to occur during cardiac catheterization. In addition to those associated with radiation exposure and the injection of contrast media already described, the major other complications include:
• Tachy- and brady-arrhythmias (e.g. SVT, VT, VF, complete heart block);
• Heart perforation and cardiac tamponade or hemorrhagic pleural effusion;
• Arterial or venous thrombosis;
• Excessive internal or external bleeding, including abdominal hemorrhage;
• Dissection of major arteries and veins;
• Intramyocardial injection of contrast medium;
• Hypotension;
• Renal failure;
• Cardiac arrest;
• Failure to obtain the required information.

For neonates and infants, potential problems, which should be avoided, include hypothermia, hypoglycemia, excessive hypoxia, acidosis, and electrolyte disturbance.

There are also specific complications of interventional cardiac catheterization, including rupture of the aorta, pulmonary arteries or major veins, as well as embolization of closure devices and stents (see Chapter 33). Cardiologists and anesthetists involved in diagnostic and therapeutic catheterization and other catheter laboratory personnel will be prepared to deal promptly with any of these adverse events. The catheter laboratories should be near to the operating rooms and intensive care unit, and cardiac surgeons should be close at hand.

It is important to be aware that accidents in medicine are rarely due to a single error and are usually system failures. The general attributes of safe organizations are:
• Culture of constructive doubt and skepticism;
• Climate of openness and equality of respect;
• Freedom to challenge, question or advise;
• Procedural counterchecks and revisions;
• Performance monitoring;
• Constant search for improvement;
• Vigorous adverse event reporting;
• No blame culture;

• Accept human error is inevitable;
• Value experience.

Incorporating these attributes into a hospital environment is the best way of minimizing errors, complications, and adverse events in general, and maintaining the highest standards.

Further reading

Lock JE, Keane JF, Perry SB. *Diagnostic and Interventional Catheterisation in Congenital Heart Disease,* Second Edition. Boston: Kluwer Academic Publishers, 2000.

8 Advanced cardiac imaging

Michael Cheung

Murdoch Childrens Research Institute and The Royal Children's Hospital, Melbourne, VIC, Australia

Echocardiography is likely to remain the mainstay of cardiac imaging and assessment in children with congenital heart disease for the foreseeable future. In contrast to adults undergoing echocardiography, the problem of adequate imaging windows is less of an issue in the majority of pediatric patients. The portability of ultrasound machines, access to an echocardiography service, and relative technical ease of performing studies in children further increase its applicability. There are, however, complementary assessment techniques which may provide additional information from both a clinical and a research perspective. Since there is increasing overlap of imaging modalities with comparable information being provided, in particular by magnetic resonance imaging (MRI) and computed tomography (CT), the relative merits of these two techniques will be briefly discussed initially. This chapter will go on to describe the increasing role of cardiovascular MRI and briefly present the roles of CT and nuclear imaging in children with congenital heart disease.

MRI compared to CT

These two competing technologies have developed rapidly over the past decade. This is largely related to significant advances in computing power and developments in MRI and CT hardware. Both now provide excellent 3D anatomic imaging of the cardiovascular system (Figures 8.1 and 8.2) and can also provide information about ventricular function. MRI is more versatile than CT. It can differentiate between tissues and give a broad range of structural and functional information without ionizing radiation and, in many instances, without the need for contrast agent, but CT offers more rapid acquisition of images with higher spatial resolution. A complete 3D dataset with coverage of the entire thorax can be obtained within a few seconds. This is an advantage over MRI where data acquisition is more time-consuming and requires more patient cooperation. Because of this limitation, MRI studies in younger children are more likely to need general anesthesia or sedation. Other thoracic structures outside the cardiovascular system, e.g. lungs, airways, and bones, are well-imaged by CT, whereas these are currently relatively poorly visualized by MRI. Furthermore the spatial resolution obtained with CT is potentially greater than that with MRI.

An obvious disadvantage with CT is the use of ionizing radiation, which is a major concern in developing children and those needing repeated assessment. There are, however, occasions when CT may be a more appropriate imaging modality than MRI, e.g. in sick patients where rapid acquisition of anatomic information is required and functional assessment is less important. Patients with implanted pacemakers may undergo CT scans, whilst this remains a contraindication to MRI, although there are early reports of patients with pacemakers safely undergoing MRI scans. A major strength of cardiac MRI in the assessment of patients with congenital heart disease is the ability to quantify blood flow, which is not possible using CT.

Cardiovascular MRI

Improvements in hardware, including magnet technology and computer processing power, and software have significantly increased the applications of cardiovascular MRI in congenital heart disease. Previously, assessment was largely limited to 2D anatomic imaging, and lengthy assessments of blood flow; however, rapid imaging sequences have now made it possible to obtain functional data in patients with fast heart rates with relatively high

Pediatric Heart Disease: A Practical Guide, First Edition. Piers E. F. Daubeney, Michael L. Rigby, Koichiro Niwa, and Michael A. Gatzoulis.
© 2012 Blackwell Publishing Ltd. Published 2012 by Blackwell Publishing Ltd.

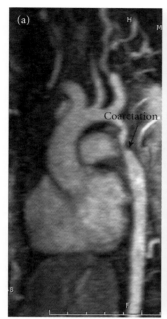
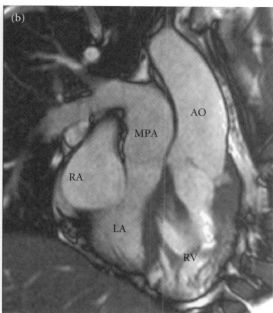

Figure 8.1 Magnetic resonance imaging. (a) Coarctation of the aorta. The aortic arch tapers, becoming hypoplastic and tortuous. There is a coarctation distal to the take-off of the left subclavian artery. (b) Congenitally corrected transposition of the great arteries. There are discordant atrioventricular connections, with the right atrium (RA) being connected to the left ventricle (LV) and the left atrium to the right ventricle (not shown). There are discordant ventricular arterial connections, with the left ventricle being connected to the main pulmonary artery (MPA) and right ventricle (RV) being connected to the aorta (AO). Note that the two great arteries ascend in parallel rather than in a normal spiraling fashion. (Courtesy of Dr Philip Kilner.)

Comparison of cardiac MRI and CT	
MRI	CT
3D Imaging of cardiovascular anatomy	3D Imaging of cardiovascular anatomy
Ventricular function (routine)	Ventricular function (possible)
Assessment of blood flow	Flow assessment not possible
Relatively lower spatial resolution	High spatial resolution
Poor visualization of other thoracic structures	Good imaging of other thoracic structures
Low incidence of contrast reaction	Higher incidence of contrast reaction
More likely to need general anesthesia/sedation	Fewer studies under general anesthesia/ sedation
Pacemakers currently remain a contraindication.	Pacemakers not an issue
No ionizing radiation	Ionizing radiation

temporal resolution in a single breath-hold. Ciné imaging and flow quantification are the main techniques employed in children. There are additional sequences, beyond the scope of this chapter, which provide information such as assessment of myocardial viability, myocardial perfusion, and tissue characterization.

Basic principles

Briefly, images are obtained by transmitting a radio signal of a certain frequency into the body of a patient while lying in a strong magnetic field (typically 1.5–3 Tesla). During and immediately following this brief radio pulse, a sequence of relatively weak magnetic field gradients and gradient changes is applied in three orthogonal directions. Spectral analysis of the frequencies, amplitudes, and phases of the radio signal re-emitted from the body, relative to the radio pulse(s) and gradient applications used, enables the reconstruction of magnetic resonance images and velocity maps. In simple terms, what has happened is that the spins (or rather the precession of spins) of the protons that make up the hydrogen nuclei in the body, mainly in water and fat, have been aligned, tuned, and

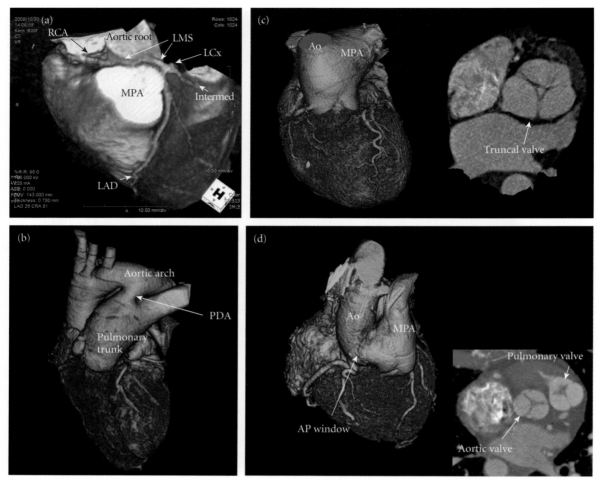

Figure 8.2 CT Angiography. (a) Anomalous course of the left coronary artery. The left mainstem (LMS) coronary artery arises from the right facing sinus with the right coronary artery (RCA). It then travels between the aortic root and the main pulmonary artery where it is being compressed. It then divides into the left circumflex (LCx) and left anterior descending (LAD) coronary arteries. (b) Large arterial duct. PDA, patent ductus arteriosus. (c) Common arterial trunk type I with the main pulmonary artery (MPA) arising from the ascending aorta (Ao). The single truncal valve is clearly seen in the cross-sectional view. (d) Aorto-pulmonary (AP) window. Two separate semilunar valves are clearly seen in the cross-sectional view. (Courtesy of Dr Mike Rubens.)

retuned by the magnetic fields. Only those nuclei in a slice tuned, initially, to a particular frequency will resonate with the radio pulse of the same frequency. The spins of these energized nuclei are then re-tuned in x and then y directions with respect to the slice, and the re-emitted signal is analyzed. As x and y magnetic gradients cannot be applied simultaneously, the process is not simple, and other texts should be referred to for further information. The appli-cation of magnetic gradients tends to generate noise, and ear protection is usually needed during an MRI scan.

Phase velocity mapping

Although there are a number of different methods, assessment of blood flow is mainly performed by a tech-nique known as phase-contrast velocity encoding. In this technique, magnetic gradient changes are used not only to locate the sources of re-emitted radio signal in space, but also to encode the velocities of the displacements of nuclei in one or more directions. For speed of acquisition, only one direction is usually encoded, and the most useful and accurate direction is generally through the plane of the slice.

Ciné imaging

A major advantage of MRI over echocardiography is the ability to image structures in any desired plane. With careful planning of imaging slices, planes exactly aligned to reference anatomic landmarks can be prescribed. Protocols have been developed in collaboration with radiologists and echocardiographers in order to standardize imaging planes. Furthermore, slices of a chosen thickness can be used to cover the entire ventricular cavity, enabling accurate measurement of ventricular volume using Simpson's rule of discs. Tracing of the epicardial and endocardial contours of the ventricle also permits a measurement of the myocardial volume and hence myocardial mass. Indeed, MRI has become the gold standard non-invasive method of assessment of ventricular volumes for both the left and right ventricles. Although MRI has become widely accepted as the best technique currently available for assessment of right ventricular volume, it must be said that analysis of data with manual tracing of the endocardial border may be technically difficult, particularly in heavily trabeculated ventricles. The much finer trabeculations of the left ventricle make this much less of an issue in assessment of left ventricular function. The ciné images obtained by MRI will otherwise be familiar to those experienced in echo imaging.

One technical advantage of echocardiography over MRI currently is that of real-time acquisition with high temporal resolution and good spatial resolution of certain structures and boundaries. While tissue contrast can be good, spatial resolution is generally poorer with MRI, and this becomes even more of an issue in patients with small hearts. MRI data are typically collected over several heart beats and the data analyzed to reconstruct the frames of a ciné acquisition. This is not the same as real-time acquisition, and the images tend to be degraded by arrhythmias. Although real-time MRI is commercially available on most systems, the temporal resolution is poor.

Flow quantification

Currently, the ability to quantify flow is the major strength of MRI over other techniques in the assessment of patients with congenital heart disease. An imaging slice perpendicular to the direction of blood flow is generally used and velocities of flow through this plane are measured using the phase-contrast technique. The same imaging sequence allows a measurement of the luminal area, thus permitting a calculation of the volume of blood flow. Since the phase-contrast technique also gives information about the direction of blood flow through the plane of interest, the relative amounts of regurgitant and forward flow can be determined. This method has been of great value in the assessment of valvar regurgitation, e.g. in patients with tetralogy of Fallot with chronic pulmonary regurgitation. It is also possible to measure the velocities of jets, as long as adequate signal can be recovered from voxels located within a coherent jet core. Application of the simplified Bernoulli equation allows pressure differences across stenoses to be estimated:

$$\text{Pressure drop} = 4 \times (\text{velocity})^2$$

Myocardial viability and tissue characterization

Adjustment of sequence parameters allows the visualization and differentiation of certain tissues within the body. For example, areas of fat can be specifically highlighted or suppressed. Similarly, areas of edema and inflammation or fibrosis can be focused upon. These techniques are of importance in the assessment of cardiomyopathy and myocarditis, and also the delineation of cardiac tumors.

Of major interest to adult cardiologists is the assessment of myocardial viability in patients with ischemic heart disease. Important prognostic information can be derived from stress MRI with the infusion of dobutamine or adenosine, for example, during ciné imaging similar to stress echocardiography. Additional information regarding viability is provided by delayed enhancement following gadolinium infusion. This technique visualizes myocardial scar tissue with high spatial resolution, allowing the extent of infarcted tissue to be determined. The role of this technique in patients with congenital heart disease is being explored.

Computed tomography

Helical rotation of the X-ray tube within the CT gantry around the patient allows detection of the X-ray beams transmitted through the patient. The patient is passed through the gantry to cover the area of interest. Iodinated contrast agents are injected intravenously and data acquisition is timed to coincide with peak enhancement of the structures of interest. This technique is useful for rapid anatomic imaging of vascular structures within the thorax and also visualization of the airways.

Multidetector row CT

The introduction of multidetector row CT systems in 1998 significantly reduced the scan time required to cover a particular volume of tissue. Simultaneous acquisition of n sections results in an n-fold increase in speed if all other parameters are unchanged. There is also the additional advantage of an increase in the longitudinal spatial resolution of the scan. Further reduction in scan time will be possible with the development of dual-source CT systems which use two X-ray sources and detectors at the same time.

EKG-gated CT

A further advantage of the increased scanning speed is the ability to image the heart without motion artifact. With EKG-gating, only scan data acquired during a particular phase of the cardiac cycle are used to reconstruct an image to provide ciné imaging and information about ventricular volume. X-ray dosage is significantly increased using this technique however, and it is also not suitable for use in patients with fast or irregular heart rates. This technique is therefore currently largely restricted to use in adult patients.

Nuclear cardiology

Radionuclide-labeled compounds have been used for over three decades for the study of cardiac function. Different techniques allow assessment of myocardial perfusion, viability, metabolism, and also ventricular function. The basic principle is that the radionuclides are either extracted by the myocardium or remain within the blood pool. The emitted gamma rays are detected by a scintillation camera which generates photons. The photons are converted to an electrical pulse which is proportional in size to the number of gamma rays emitted. These techniques, except for radionuclide angiography, are rarely used in the management of patients with congenital heart disease.

Radionuclide angiography

This technique employs technetium (^{99m}Tc)-labeled red blood cells to assess ventricular function. Broadly, there are two approaches to radionuclide angiography. First-pass angiography examines the initial transit of a radio-

nuclide bolus through the central circulation. More widely used, however, is the technique of equilibrium radionuclide angiography, whereby, with prior calibration using a labeled blood sample, ventricular volume can be measured since radioactivity is proportional to the volume of labeled red cells. Patient cooperation is important using this method since the acquisition of nuclear data is coupled to EKG-gating and sampling is over several hundred heart beats. Data are obtained in multiple views in order to detect regional wall motion abnormalities and accurately assess ventricular volume. Emission tomographic imaging of the intracardiac blood pools is also possible and may have advantages over planar imaging in patients with congenital heart disease.

Myocardial perfusion

This area of assessment is of much greater importance in the study of patients with ischemic heart disease. There are also patients with congenital heart disease, e.g. unrepaired congenitally corrected transposition of the great arteries or anomalous origins of coronary arteries, who have been shown to have myocardial perfusion defects (Figure 8.3). Single photon-emitting radioisotopes, such as thallium-201 (^{201}Tl) or ^{99m}Tc-labeled compounds, that accumulate within the myocardium in proportion to regional perfusion and viability are used to examine regional myocardial blood flow.

The images are most commonly acquired using **single photon emission computed tomography (SPECT)** for which the gamma camera rotates around an arc to acquire a series of planar images from which three-dimensional data sets can be reconstructed. EKG-gating allows myocardial function as well as perfusion and visibility to be assessed.

Myocardial metabolism

Currently the gold standard for assessment of myocardial metabolism remains **positron emission tomography (PET)**. Positron-emitting radionuclide isotopes of carbon (^{11}C), fluorine (^{18}F), nitrogen (^{13}N), and oxygen (^{15}O) can be incorporated into a wide variety of substrates (e.g. glucose, lactate, acetate, palmitate) utilized in diverse metabolic pathways. Using this technique it is possible to quantify myocardial blood flow, myocardial oxygen consumption, and myocardial utilization of fatty acids and glucose.

Since the radionuclides have a short half-life, a major limitation of this method is the need for an on-site cyclotron to generate the isotopes. Access to PET is therefore limited.

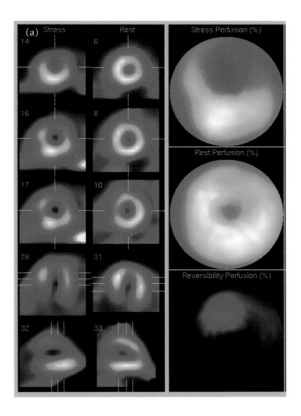

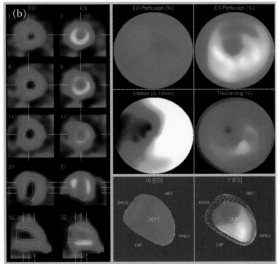

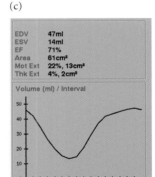

EDV	47ml
ESV	14ml
EF	71%
Area	61cm²
Mot Ext	22%, 13cm²
Thk Ext	4%, 2cm²

Figure 8.3 Nuclear cardiology imaging. Taken from a 4-year-old boy with anomalous origin of the left coronary artery from the right facing sinus and anomalous course between the aortic root and pulmonary trunk. He had exercise-induced angina. (a) Stress (left) and rest (center) myocardial perfusion tomograms in selected planes with corresponding polar plots (right). There is a profound inducible perfusion abnormality of the anterior wall, extending anterolaterally and compatible with left anterior descending territory. The resting images show mild reduction of counts anteroapically, compatible with partial thickness scarring. (b, c) The EKG-gated resting tomograms show normal global left ventricular function with a left ventricular ejection fraction of 71%. The end-diastolic (green) and end-systolic (red) contours show septal akinesis, confirmed in the polar plot of motion (center) but with preserved thickening shown in the thickening polar plot (center right). This pattern is typical of the findings after sternotomy. However, the anterior wall has hypokinesis and reduced thickening compatible with the partial thickness scarring. (Courtesy of Professor Richard Underwood.)

Summary

There is considerable overlap in the information that can be provided by these techniques. Broadly speaking, the main techniques used at a clinical level are MRI and CT. The relative merits of these two approaches have been discussed. The major concern regarding exposure to ionizing radiation means that MRI is used more frequently in the follow-up of patients with congenital heart disease, even when taking into account the need for sedation or anesthesia in younger patients. Echocardiographic assessment of cardiac anatomy and function will remain the main diagnostic investigation of choice; however, complementary and additional information can be provided by these alternative imaging modalities.

Further reading

Brenner DJ. Estimating cancer risks from pediatric CT: going from the qualitative to the quantitative. *Pediatr Radiol* 2002; 32:228–223; discussion 242–244.

Grotenhuis HB, *et al.* Magnetic resonance imaging of function and flow in postoperative congenital heart disease. In: Higgins CB, de Roos A, eds. *MRI and CT of the Cardiovascular System*, 2nd edn. Philadelphia: Lippincott Williams & Wilkins, 2005.

Helbing WA, Niezen RA, Le Cessie S, van der Geest RJ, Ottenkamp J, de Roos A. Right ventricular diastolic function in children with pulmonary regurgitation after repair of tetralogy of Fallot: volumetric evaluation by magnetic resonance velocity mapping. *J Am Coll Cardiol* 1996;28:1827–1835.

Kim RJ, Wu E, Rafael A, Chen EL, Parker MA, Simonetti O, Klocke FJ, Bonow RO, Judd RM. The use of contrast-enhanced magnetic resonance imaging to identify reversible myocardial dysfunction. *N Engl J Med.* 2000;343:1445–1453.

Manning WJ, Pennell DJ. *Cardiovascular Magnetic Resonance.* Edinburgh: Churchill Livingstone, 2002.

Reddy A, *et al.* Congenital heart disease: magnetic resonance evaluation of morphology and function. In: Higgins CB, de Roos A, eds. *MRI and CT of the Cardiovascular System*, 2nd edn. Philadelphia: Lippincott Williams & Wilkins, 2005.

Roest AA, Helbing WA, Kunz P, *et al.* Exercise MR imaging in the assessment of pulmonary regurgitation and biventricular function in patients after tetralogy of Fallot repair. *Radiology* 2002;223:204–211.

Russell RR, 3rd, Zaret BL. Nuclear cardiology: present and future. *Curr Probl Cardiol* 2006;31:557–629.

9 Left-to-right shunts

Phil Roberts

Children's Hospital at Westmead, Sydney, NSW, Australia

In the normal cardiac cycle pulmonary blood flow (Qp) is equal to the systemic blood flow (Qs). When some of the blood destined for systemic circulation enters the pulmonary arteries before the peripheral capillary bed, a left-to-right shunt is present and consequently Qp > Qs.

Left-to-right shunts can occur at atrial, ventricular, pulmonary venous, great artery, and arteriovenous levels. The resultant pathophysiology depends on the response of the pulmonary vascular bed to the size of the shunt and the effects of any elevated pressure that the pulmonary vasculature is exposed to (Figure 9.1). The most important long-term pathology that may develop from a large left-to-right shunt is an irreversible increase in the pulmonary vascular resistance secondary to muscular hypertrophy of the pulmonary arterial system. When the pulmonary vascular resistance exceeds the systemic resistance, the shunt reverses, becoming predominantly right to left with resultant systemic arterial desaturation. This situation is called the **Eisenmenger syndrome** (see Chapter 22) and carries with it a guarded long-term prognosis and reduced life expectancy. The justification for surgical or catheter intervention in this group of malformations is not only the treatment of symptoms but also to prevent late complications, including the Eisenmenger syndrome.

Causes of left-to-right shunts

- Partial anomalous pulmonary venous connection (PAPVC)
- Interatrial communication or atrial septal defect (ASD)
- Atrioventricular septal defect (AVSD)
- Ventricular septal defect (VSD)
- Aortopulmonary (AP) window
- Patent arterial duct or patent ductus arteriosus (PDA)
- Systemic arteriovenous fistula

From the site of the shunt it is possible to predict clinical features and what special investigations will show:

- **Shunts at an atrial or venous level** are low pressure and will involve the passage of excess blood through the whole of the right heart, thus causing volume overload of both the right atrium and ventricle. This will be reflected on the EKG, CXR, echocardiogram, and MRI. Significant pulmonary hypertension is uncommon but prolonged right atrial loading predisposes to atrial arrhythmias while right ventricular failure may also be part of the natural history.
- **Shunts at a ventricular or great artery level**, e.g. complete AVSD, VSD, and PDA), by causing an increase in pulmonary blood flow, give rise to left ventricular volume loading. For large defects the pulmonary vasculature is exposed to high pressures, the main contributing factor to the cascade of events leading to pulmonary vascular disease and the Eisenmenger syndrome (see Chapter 22).

Clinical features common to all left-to-right shunts

The approach should always be history, examination, and special investigations, of which the most easily obtainable and useful comprise EKG, CXR, and echocardiogram. In general, infants and children with an ASD or partial anomalous pulmonary venous drainage are relatively symptom-free. Moderate-to-large interventricular or interarterial communications, by giving rise to a large left-to-right shunt, usually cause congestive heart failure during the second month of life as the pulmonary vascular resistance falls from the elevated level found at birth.

It is unusual for an ASD or PAPVC to cause respiratory distress and failure to thrive during infancy. Many older children and adolescents claim to be symptom-free

---

Pediatric Heart Disease: A Practical Guide, First Edition. Piers E. F. Daubeney, Michael L. Rigby, Koichiro Niwa, and Michael A. Gatzoulis.
© 2012 Blackwell Publishing Ltd. Published 2012 by Blackwell Publishing Ltd.

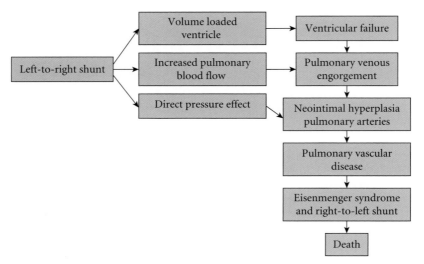

Figure 9.1 Sequence of events leading to pulmonary vascular disease.

but formal testing often identifies impaired exercise performance.

A large VSD, complete AVSD, large PDA, or aortopulmonary (AP) window will usually cause:
- **Tachycardia**;
- **Respiratory distress** with varying degrees of:
  - Tachypnea
  - Nasal flare
  - Use of accessory respiratory muscles
  - "Head bobbing"
  - Tracheal, intercostal, and subcostal recession during early infancy.

These result in feeding difficulties and failure to thrive; the latter is due to a combination of poor caloric intake and increased caloric demand associated with an increased respiratory effort. An important feature of heart failure is hepatomegaly but peripheral edema and fine basal lung crepitations of pulmonary venous congestion and edema are less common than in adults. Older children surviving infancy without treatment will manifest poor exercise tolerance caused by high pulmonary blood or progressive pulmonary vascular disease.

There may be a third heart sound (gallop rhythm). A loud pulmonary component of the second heart sound is indicative of pulmonary hypertension, but it is important to understand this is not the same as an irreversibly raised pulmonary vascular resistance. With longstanding large left-to-right shunts, an improvement in symptoms may be related to either a reduction in the size of the shunt (e.g. VSD becoming smaller) or more ominously,

an increasing pulmonary vascular resistance limiting the left-to-right shunt.

Eisenmenger syndrome (see also Chapter 22)

Now uncommon in the developed world, Eisenmenger syndrome is best defined as irreversible pulmonary hypertension resulting from excessive pulmonary blood flow and exposure of the pulmonary arterioles to excessive high pressures. It is characterized by:
- Loud and even palpable P2;
- Central cyanosis and finger clubbing;
- Right ventricular heave;
- Right-sided S4;
- Pulmonary ejection click;
- High pitched early diastolic murmur (high velocity pulmonary regurgitation).

Specific lesions

Atrial septal defects

An ASD is a direct communication between the two atria and can be associated with PAPVC. In the fetus right-to-left shunting across a defect in the oval fossa is a normal finding. It allows blood from the inferior caval vein, with a higher oxygen content than that from the superior caval vein, to enter the left side of the heart and perfuse predominantly the myocardium and brain. After birth the flap valve of the oval fossa closes as the left atrial pressure rises. The true atrial septum is represented only by the oval fossa with the remainder being made up of an infolding of the atrial wall. It can be argued therefore that the only true "ASD" is one within the oval fossa (secundum defect). The term "**interatrial communication**," which is the direct translation in most languages, allows the avoidance of unnecessary argument about what is and is not an ASD.

Types of interatrial communication (Figure 9.2)

- Secundum (oval fossa)
- Superior sinus venosus
- Inferior sinus venosus
- Coronary sinus
- Primum

Incidence and etiology

Approximately 30% of the population has a patent foramen ovale (PFO), which may only be probe patent and as such it should not be considered an abnormality. The shunt from a PFO is never of any direct consequence; however, interventional closure can be justified in the setting of paradoxical emboli and stroke. The role of PFO in migraine is unclear, but it is an increased risk factor for paradoxical emboli and "the bends" in deep sea divers.

Located in the oval fossa, secundum defects are the commonest type and have the potential for spontaneous

closure during infancy in a few. Two separate defects may be encountered, but multiple small defects (fenestrations) are more common and often associated with an aneurysm of the oval fossa. Sinus venosus defects are characterized by a bi-atrial connection of one of the caval veins due to a deficiency in the infolding of the atrial wall. In a superior sinus venosus ASD the right superior caval vein (SVC) and right upper pulmonary vein override the defect; the right upper pulmonary vein has an anomalous connection to the superior caval vein at its junction with the atria. Inferior sinus venosus defects are rare. The bi-atrial connection of the superior or inferior caval vein may result in central cyanosis because of the streaming of blood into the left atrium.

A primum defect (also known as a partial AVSD) is invariably associated with a trileaflet left atrioventricular (AV) valve (see AVSD section below and also Figure 9.4). This does not resemble the normal mitral valve; the zone of apposition of the superior and inferior bridging leaflets is sometimes described as a "cleft" and often leads to valve insufficiency. The degree of regurgitation will affect the timing of presentation and severity of symptoms.

Coronary sinus defects are uncommon; they result from partial unroofing of the coronary sinus at its junction with the atrial septum.

Clinical features

Symptoms seldom occur during childhood and if they do, additional pathology should be sought. The pulse is

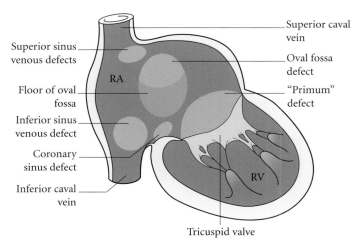

Figure 9.2 Various types of atrial septal defect as seen from the right side of the heart. RA, right atrium; RV, right ventricle. (Adapted from Gatzoulis MA, Swan L, Therrien J, Pantely GA, eds. *Adult Congenital Heart Disease, A Practical Guide*, 2005, with permission from Blackwell Publishing Ltd.)

regular with loss of respiratory variation. There is a normal first heart sound with a fixed split of the second heart sound. An ejection systolic murmur is audible at the upper left sternal edge (increased pulmonary flow) and a mid-diastolic murmur may be audible at the lower left sternal edge from the increased flow across the tricuspid valve. With primum defects there may be a pansystolic murmur radiating from the apex to axilla secondary to the left AV valve regurgitation.

Investigations
• **EKG:** May show loss of sinus arrhythmia with an rSR pattern in V1 and a rightward mean frontal QRS axis.
• **CXR:** May show increased pulmonary vascular markings, prominent central pulmonary arteries, and mild cardiomegaly.
• **Echocardiography:** Diagnostic.

Treatment
For isolated ASDs the risk of infective endocarditis is extremely small and medical therapy with diuretics is extremely unusual. Definitive intervention is usually justified on the basis of improving long-term health in adult life. Closure is delayed until 3–4 years of age unless associated defects dictate otherwise. Surgical closure has been performed for more than five decades and carries a high success and low complication rate. For secundum defects only, transcatheter device closure can now be performed in the majority and often as a day-case procedure.

Late complications and long-term outcome (see also Chapter 31)
Following ASD closure during the first two decades, life expectancy approaches normal in the majority, although a few will develop atrial arrhythmias. Untreated patients and some undergoing late closure are at significant risk of atrial arrhythmias, right heart failure, pulmonary vascular disease, and premature death in the fifth or sixth decades.

Ventricular septal defects
VSDs, although usually occurring in isolation, are also an integral part of many congenital heart malformations including, for example, tetralogy of Fallot, common arterial trunk, and double outlet right ventricle. Defects are described as opening to the inlet, apical trabecular, or outlet of the right ventricle, or as being confluent when they are large and open to more than one component.

Types of ventricular septal defect (Figure 9.3)

• **Muscular defects** have a completely muscular border and can be multiple

• **Perimembranous defects** are partly bordered by the membranous septum and have tricuspid–aortic valve fibrous continuity

• **Doubly-committed defects** have, as part of their border, fibrous continuity between the leaflets of the semilunar (arterial) valves or else are overridden by a common arterial valve (common arterial trunk)

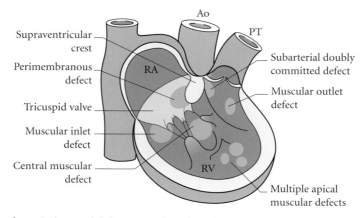

Figure 9.3 Various types of ventricular septal defect as seen from the right side of the heart. Ao, aorta; PT, pulmonary trunk; RA, right atrium; RV, right ventricle. (Adapted from Gatzoulis MA, Swan L, Therrien J, Pantely GA, eds. *Adult Congenital Heart Disease, A Practical Guide*, 2005, with permission from Blackwell Publishing Ltd.)

Up to 80% of isolated defects will close spontaneously during the first three decades. Typically these are perimembranous inlet or small muscular defects.

Incidence and etiology

VSDs are one of the most common congenital cardiac malformations, accounting for at least 20% of all defects.

Clinical features

• Small "restrictive" defects produce a significant pressure gradient between the ventricles and are accompanied by a small shunt (Qp:Qs ≤ 1.5:1).
• Moderately restrictive VSDs are associated with a moderate shunt (Qp:Qs 1.5–2.5:1) and pose a moderate hemodynamic load on the left ventricle.
• Large VSDs result in a large shunt (Qp:Qs ≥ 2.5:1) if the pulmonary vascular resistance is low and produce a significant hemodynamic burden on the left ventricle.

Symptoms directly attributable to a VSD are seldom present before 1 month of age as the neonatal pulmonary vascular resistance is high at birth, falling gradually during the first 4–6 weeks of life. Symptoms before 1 month of age suggest additional anomalies; left heart obstructive lesions should be excluded. The first heart sound is normal and the pulmonary component of the second heart sound is accentuated in the presence of pulmonary hypertension. Typically, small VSDs produce the loudest murmur, which is classically a pan-systolic murmur heard best along the left sternal edge and may be associated with a thrill. If the shunt is large, the cardiac apex may be displaced and there may be an apical diastolic murmur and third heart sound from the increased flow across the mitral valve. It is important to note that if the defect is large with no pressure difference between the left and right ventricles, then the murmur will be unremarkable and even absent. Tiny defects close to complete closure cause a short early systolic murmur at the lower left sternal edge at any age. Perimembranous or doubly committed defects may cause aortic valve prolapse leading to insufficiency. Occasionally discrete subaortic stenosis will develop when there is a perimembranous VSD.

Investigations

• **EKG:**
  ○ Small defects are associated with a normal EKG
  ○ Moderate sized defects cause left ventricular hypertrophy with or without left atrial enlargement
  ○ Larger defects are characterized by biventricular hypertrophy

○ When there is pulmonary vascular disease, isolated right ventricular hypertrophy is present.
• **CXR:**
  ○ Cardiomegaly of varying degrees due to left atrial and left ventricular dilatation reflects the amount of left-to-right shunting
  ○ Pulmonary plethora is absent in smaller defects and becomes more pronounced the bigger the defect and greater the left-to-right shunt
  ○ Dilated central ("hilar") pulmonary arteries with small peripheral vessels ("pruning") are characteristic of a raised pulmonary vascular resistance.
• **Echocardiography:**
  ○ Diagnostic in most cases
  ○ Need to document:
   Morphology of the defect
   Presence of additional defects
   Size of the left atrium and ventricle
   Pressure drop between left and right ventricles
   Pressure drop across tricuspid valve in systole
   Pressure drop across pulmonary valve in diastole
   Aortic valve prolapse
   Discrete subaortic stenosis
   Right ventricular outflow obstruction.
• **Cardiac catheterization:**
  ○ Performed as part of transcatheter device closure of a perimembranous or muscular defect
  ○ Occasionally performed to measure pulmonary vascular resistance when it might be too high to permit closure of a defect.

Treatment

• Diuretics with or without additional ACE inhibitors are prescribed for heart failure in early infancy.
• Surgical repair of moderate-to-large defects causing heart failure and failure to thrive is usually performed from 2 to 6 months of age. Later operation may be required in a few patients initially considered not to be candidates for closure who manifest increasing cardiomegaly, left ventricular enlargement, and pulmonary plethora, or who develop aortic valvar prolapse or subaortic stenosis. Mortality and morbidity from surgical closure of a VSD should approach zero.
• Pulmonary artery banding is reserved for infants with multiple defects or for a huge confluent defect considered too large for biventricular repair.
• Transcatheter device closure of some perimembranous inlet or muscular defects in patients beyond early infancy is now performed frequently, but there remains concern

(a)

(b)

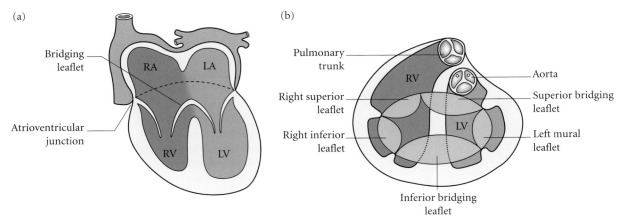

Figure 9.4 Anatomy of atrioventricular septal defect (AVSD). (a) Note the common atrioventricular junction (universal feature of all AVSDs) and bridging leaflet. Balanced complete AVSD with well-developed right and left ventricles, and both atrial and ventricular communications. (b) Heart base as seen from above. Note the five leaflets of a common atrioventricular valve (left mural, superior bridging, right superior, right inferior, and inferior bridging leaflet) guarded by a common atrioventricular junction in a patient with a complete AVSD. Patients with partial or incomplete AVSD (also called primum ASD) have fusion of the atrioventricular valve between the superior and inferior bridging leaflets (yellow central area), producing two separate atrioventricular valves. Note that the left atrioventrioventricular valve has three leaflets as a result. Patients with partial AVSDs have usually only an atrial communication, and occasionally a small but never a large ventricular communication (hence at low risk of developing pulmonary hypertension compared with patients with complete AVSDs). Double dotted line in the center indicates position of the underlying ventricular septum. LA, left atrium; LV, left ventricle; RA, right atrium; RV, right ventricle. (Adapted from Gatzoulis MA, Swan L, Therrien J, Pantely GA, eds. *Adult Congenital Heart Disease, A Practical Guide*, 2005, with permission from Blackwell Publishing Ltd.)

about the risk of early and late complete heart block in muscular inlet and perimembranous defects.

Late complications and long-term outcome (see also Chapter 31)
• Small muscular defects usually close spontaneously and hardly ever give rise to complications.
• Small perimembranous defects often close spontaneously but require annual follow-up because of the risk of aortic valve prolapse, subaortic stenosis, left ventricular-to-right atrial shunting and late left ventricular enlargement.
• Untreated moderate-to-large defects may result in early death in infancy, progressive symptoms of heart failure, increasing cardiomegaly and pulmonary plethora, late atrial or ventricular arrhythmias or pulmonary vascular disease.
• There is always the risk of endocarditis, a risk that is greater in perimembranous defects but remains even following successful closure.

Atrioventricular septal defects
The term "AVSD" refers to a group of anomalies unified by the following morphologic features:
• Deficiency of the AV septum;
• Common AV junction;
• Common AV valve;
• A trileaflet arrangement of the valve leaflets within the left ventricle (Figure 9.4).

AVSDs can all be broadly classified into those with a common valve orifice and those with two valve orifices:
• **AVSD with two valve orifices ("partial AVSD")**: By far the most common variant is an isolated primum interatrial defect ("primum ASD") with a left-to-right obligatory shunt. Other variants include an isolated interventricular communication, primum defect with small ventricular communication, and, rarely, intact atrial and ventricular septal structures. Common to each of these is a trileaflet left AV valve orifice which bears no resemblance to a normal mitral valve.

• **AVSD with common valve orifice ("complete AVSD"):** Usually a more severe form in terms of clinical symptoms, and sometimes called "AV canal defect," there is a primum defect and moderate-to-large ventricular component ("VSD"), both permitting a left-to-right shunt and consequently a high pulmonary blood flow.

Associated anomalies

The most important associated anomalies can occur with a separate or common valve orifice and include:
• Atrial isomerism (visceral heterotaxy syndromes) (see Chapters 3 and 17);
• AV valve insufficiency;
• Ventricular imbalance (relative hypoplasia of the right or left ventricle);
• Left or right ventricular outflow obstruction (see Chapters 10 and 11);
• Tetralogy of Fallot (see Chapter 15);
• Double outlet right ventricle (see Chapter 15).

Incidence and etiology

Accounting for 2% of congenital heart disease, complete AVSD is most commonly (>75%), but not exclusively, encountered in the setting of Down syndrome. Most patients with partial AVSDs (>90%) have normal chromosomes. There is also a strong association of AVSD with atrial isomerism.

Clinical features and investigations
Primum ASD (see also above)

Accounting for 1–2% of all congenital heart disease, the clinical features are identical to those of a secundum ASD, providing there is no major left AV valve regurgitation. Many patients are symptom-free unless there is moderate or severe regurgitation which can alter the clinical profile significantly. There is:
• Fixed splitting of the second heart sound;
• Soft ejection systolic murmur at the upper left sternal edge;
• Sometimes a soft mid-diastolic murmur at the lower left sternal border;
• Apical pan-systolic murmur. If associated with symptoms of tachypnea and heart failure in infancy or early childhood, early surgical repair may be needed;
• Pan-systolic murmur at the lower left sternal edge when there is a small ventricular communication.

Complete AVSD

An infant with a complete AVSD is usually symptom-free at birth, developing increasing symptoms of heart failure after the age of 1 month. Features found are:

• Varying degrees of tachypnea and failure to thrive;
• Hyperactive precordium;
• Loud first heart sound;
• Increased intensity of the pulmonary component of the second heart sound;
• Murmurs:
  ○ None or
  ○ Short ejection systolic murmur or
  ○ Apical pan-systolic murmur.

The severity of symptoms will depend on the size of the ventricular component of the AVSD, the severity of AV regurgitation, and the pulmonary vascular resistance restricting pulmonary blood flow. Patients with a small ventricular component and insignificant AV regurgitation follow a similar course to those with a large ASD or primum ASD. Where the ventricular component of the defect is large or there is significant left AV regurgitation, then the presentation is that of congestive heart failure.

Investigations
• **EKG:**
  ○ Typically there is a superior axis to the mean frontal QRS axis and frequently a prolonged PR interval
  ○ With a primum defect partial, right bundle branch block is common
  ○ Right or biventricular hypertrophy is found with a complete defect.
• **CXR:** During early life the CXR may be normal, but cardiomegaly with a prominent right atrium and pulmonary plethora are the typical findings and are more marked in a complete AVSD.
• **Echocardiography:**
  ○ Precise diagnosis can always be made using echocardiography
  ○ The hallmarks are the common AV junction and absent offsetting of AV valve leaflets
  ○ It is important to identify the sites of left-to-right shunting and to demonstrate any AV valve regurgitation
  ○ Visualization of the common AV valve *en face* is important, particularly to ensure there is an adequate mural leaflet and no accessory orifices.
• **Cardiac catheterization:** Only performed to measure pulmonary vascular resistance prior to surgical repair in a few patients presenting late with a complete AVSD and minimal symptoms.

Management
Primum ASD

Surgical repair is usually performed after 3 years of age in patients who are symptom-free, but much earlier in those with significant left-sided AV valve regurgitation and symptoms.

Complete AVSD
Initial treatment with diuretics and ACE inhibitors in early infancy and surgical repair from 2 to 4 months of age is the norm. Occasionally the initial surgical treatment is banding of the pulmonary trunk, e.g. in patients with additional muscular VSDs or ventricular imbalance. The rapid development of pulmonary vascular disease in the first year is well documented in untreated infants with Down syndrome.

Late complications and long-term outcome (see also Chapter 31)
Late complications following surgical repair include:
• Left AV valve regurgitation requiring revision surgery, sometimes with valve replacement;
• Left AV valve stenosis;
• Subaortic stenosis;
• Complete heart block;
• Atrial arrhythmias;
• Endocarditis.

Patent arterial duct
The arterial duct arises from the left pulmonary artery close to the bifurcation of the pulmonary trunk and connects to the anterolateral aspect of the descending aorta at its junction with the aortic arch. Its major role is in fetal life, allowing the majority of blood flowing into the pulmonary trunk to bypass the lungs and enter the descending aorta. The PDA occurs most commonly in isolation but may complicate any congenital heart malformation. While a left-sided duct is by far the most common, it may be right-sided or even bilateral (Figure 9.5). A right aortic arch is sometimes associated with a left duct which arises from the left innominate artery.

Incidence and etiology
The normal duct usually closes within a few hours or days after birth, but delayed closure is particularly common in premature infants and prematurity is an important etiologic factor for continuing patency into later life. In preterm infants a large duct is associated with early mortality, necrotizing enterocolitis, intracerebral hemorrhage, and the development of chronic lung disease (bronchopulmonary dysplasia). Data from the pre-antibiotic era suggest an increased risk of endocarditis.

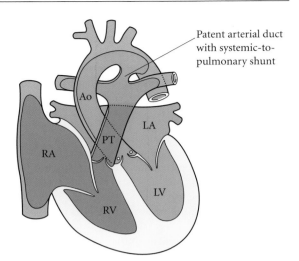

Figure 9.5 Patent arterial duct with left-to-right shunting. Ao, aorta; LA, left atrium; LV, left ventricle; PT, pulmonary trunk; RA, right atrium; RV, right ventricle. (Adapted from Gatzoulis MA, Swan L, Therrien J, Pantely GA, eds. *Adult Congenital Heart Disease, A Practical Guide*, 2005, with permission from Blackwell Publishing Ltd.)

Accounting for approximately 10% of all congenital heart disease, PDA has a female–to-male ratio of 3:1.

Clinical features
These depend on the size of the duct, the degree of left-to-right shunting, and the pulmonary vascular resistance. Patients with a small duct are symptom-free and may have a systolic murmur only or soft continuous murmur at the upper left sternal edge. With increasing ductal diameter in infancy, tachypnea, poor weight gain, recurrent chest infections, and overt congestive heart failure become more pronounced. Typical findings are:
• Bounding peripheral pulses with a wide pulse pressure;
• Hyperactive precordium;
• Systolic thrill;
• Continuous murmur at the upper left sternal border which may be loud and described as a "machinery murmur";
• No murmur in patients with a large duct or raised pulmonary vascular resistance, or in some premature infants;
• Rarely encountered are older patients with Eisenmenger syndrome manifesting a loud P2 and cyanosis of the feet with clubbing of the toes due to a right-to-left shunt ("differential cyanosis").

Investigations

- **EKG:**
  - If the arterial duct is small, the EKG may be normal
  - Larger defects will result in EKG features of left ventricular hypertrophy often with T wave inversion in the left-side precordial leads (V5 and V6). Right ventricular hypertrophy is indicative of a raised pulmonary artery pressure.
- **CXR:** Varies from normal to exhibiting cardiomegaly and pulmonary plethora or pulmonary edema if the duct is large.
- **Echocardiography:**
  - Diagnostic; a large left-to-right shunt causes enlargement of the left atrium and ventricle
  - Doppler allows measurement of the systolic and diastolic pressure drop between the aorta and pulmonary artery, and estimation of pulmonary artery pressure.

Management

There is a good chance of spontaneous closure in the preterm infant. In the preterm infant in the first month of life, the use of prostaglandin synthetase inhibitors is indicated. If this fails and the infant remains symptomatic, then surgical ligation or transcatheter closure are options.

In the term infant spontaneous closure after the age of 3 months is unlikely. For a small duct with no associated murmur ("silent duct") no intervention is required and there is not considered to be a risk of endocarditis. For symptoms and signs of pulmonary venous congestion, diuretics are the mainstay. For the older infant and child, there are now several coil or plug devices available for transcatheter closure (see Figure 33.2).

Late complications and long-term outcome (see also Chapter 31)

- Life expectancy following closure of the duct is normal in most cases and long-term follow-up is only required for those in whom the pulmonary vascular resistance is raised.
- A small residual duct is uncommon after surgical or transcatheter treatment.
- An untreated large duct may cause pulmonary vascular disease, sometimes by the age of 2 years.
- Calcification of an untreated duct may develop in adult life.
- Scoliosis is an uncommon but well-recognized consequence of a left lateral thoracotomy used for surgical ligation.

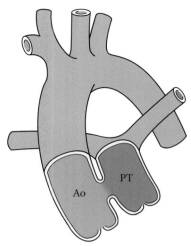

Figure 9.6 Aortopulmonary window. Note the two exits from the heart with a normal aortic and pulmonary valve and a large non-restrictive communication between the two arterial trunks (window) at relatively close proximity to the semilunar valves. Patients require early repair to avoid irreversible pulmonary vascular disease. Ao, aorta; PT, pulmonary trunk. (Adapted from Gatzoulis MA, Swan L, Therrien J, Pantely GA, eds. *Adult Congenital Heart Disease, A Practical Guide*, 2005, with permission from Blackwell Publishing Ltd.)

- Endarteritis is uncommon in the current era and virtually unheard of after complete closure.

Aortopulmonary window

This uncommon anomaly, not associated with 22q deletion, is characterized by a communication between the ascending aorta above the coronary sinuses and the pulmonary trunk (Figure 9.6). In the majority, the defect is large and extends to the right pulmonary artery, which frequently has an anomalous origin from the ascending aorta. Smaller defects are more proximal. Associated anomalies found in half the cases include aortic interruption, aortic coarctation, anomalous origin of one or both coronary arteries from the pulmonary trunk, tetralogy of Fallot with pulmonary atresia, VSD, and aortic atresia.

Clinical features

- Cases with duct-dependent systemic blood flow (aortic interruption and coarctation) present in the early neonatal period with features of low cardiac output.
- Presentation in most patients with a large defect:
  - Severe tachypnea
  - Subcostal recession
  - Poor feeding

◦ Mild cyanosis (common mixing) in the first month of life.
• Examination reveals:
  ◦ Hyperactive precordium
  ◦ Bounding pulses
  ◦ Loud single second heart sound
  ◦ Hepatomegaly
  ◦ Frequently no murmur.
• In the 10% with smaller defects the clinical presentation and signs are similar to a small-to-moderate sized PDA. The most striking finding is a loud continuous murmur, while a supraclavicular thrill is sometimes present.

Investigations

• **EKG:** Biventricular hypertrophy is the most common finding.
• **CXR:** Cardiomegaly, extreme pulmonary plethora, and pulmonary edema are found with large defects.
• **Echocardiography:** Diagnostic in the majority and the only imaging required for diagnosis and surgery.
• **Cardiac catheterization:** Only required if the additional anatomy is unusual, if an assessment of pulmonary vascular is required, or if transcatheter closure is contemplated.

Management

• Surgical repair during the first few weeks of life is required in the majority.
• Smaller defects remote from the right pulmonary artery and coronary arteries may be suitable for transcatheter device closure.

Complications and outcome

Premature death during early infancy in untreated cases is common. Rarely, patients have survived to adult life with pulmonary vascular disease. Following surgical repair of an isolated window, life expectancy approaches normal.

Systemic arteriovenous fistulae

These rare lesions can be hepatic, coronary, or cerebral in origin. There may be single or multiple lesions and in the case of a coronary artery fistula, may be associated with other cardiac anomalies, in particular pulmonary atresia.

Clinical features

The clinical features can be divided into local effects, such as hydrocephalus, and the cardiac signs and symptoms arising from the left-to-right shunt.

• **Symptoms:**
  ◦ Breathlessness with feeding
  ◦ Poor growth.
• **Signs:**
  ◦ Collapsing or bounding pulse
  ◦ Heart sounds are usually normal but a third heart sound may be present
  ◦ Bruit may be heard over the site of the arteriovenous fistula
  ◦ Coronary artery fistula usually causes a continuous murmur.

Investigations

The EKG may show biventricular hypertrophy and the CXR cardiomegaly. Two-dimensional ultrasound with color Doppler over the fistula will demonstrate the lesion. The right heart is usually volume loaded with any significant shunt.

Management

Medical therapy with diuretics is employed whilst definitive treatment is planned. Transcatheter device occlusion with coils or plugs is most commonly used as definitive treatment.

Late complications and long-term outcome

These depend on the size and site of the lesion. Fistulae with large shunts result in high output cardiac failure. Small lesions may be hemodynamically insignificant but still cause local effects. Cerebral lesions can cause hydrocephalus and seizures. Coronary artery fistulae may cause ischemia. They may regress spontaneously.

Further reading

Birk E, Silverman NH Intracardiac shunt malformations. In: Yagel S, Silverman NH, Gembruch U (eds) *Fetal Cardiology*. London: Martin Dunitz, 2003, pp. 201–210.

Freedom RM, Yoo S-J, Mikailian H, Williams WG (eds) *The Natural and Modified History of Congenital Heart Disease*. Oxford: Blackwell Futura, 2004, Chapters 3, 4, 5, 9, 20.

Gatzoulis MA, Webb GD, Daubeney PEF (eds) *Diagnosis and Management of Adult Congenital Heart Disease*, 2nd edition. London: Elsevier, 2010, Chapters 25, 26, 27.

Thanopoulos BD, Brili SD, Toutouzas PK. Patent ductus arteriosus and aortopulmonary window. In: Gatzoulis MA, Webb GD, Daubeney PEF (eds) *Diagnosis and Management of Adult Congenital Heart Disease*, 2nd edition. London: Elsevier, 2010, pp. 256–260.

10 Right-sided malformations

Victoria Jowett

Royal Brompton Hospital, London, UK

Pulmonary stenosis

These are a relatively common group of malformations affecting 7–10% of children with congenital heart disease. Figure 10.1 shows the differing sites of obstruction.

Pulmonary stenosis (PS) may be valvar (90%), supravalvar, or subvalvar. In addition, it may exclusively involve the left and/or right branch pulmonary arteries. Obstruction to the right ventricular outflow results in an increase in right ventricular pressure, which causes the right ventricular muscle to hypertrophy. Secondary infundibular stenosis is frequently found when there is severe pulmonary valve stenosis.

Types of pulmonary stenosis

- Pulmonary valve
- Subpulmonary:
  - Infundibular
  - Double (two)-chambered right ventricle
- Supravalvar
- Stenosis of main left and/or right pulmonary artery (branch stenosis)
- Peripheral left and/or right pulmonary arterial stenoses

Mild branch PS is not an uncommon finding in the neonatal period, reflecting the reduced blood flow to the lungs in the fetal circulation (see Chapter 30). Generally this improves with growth in the first few weeks of life. Branch and/or peripheral stenosis is frequently found in Williams, Alagille, and Noonan syndromes, although for the latter supravalvar stenosis is particularly frequent. Branch PS may be congenital in pulmonary atresia with ventricular septal defect (VSD) (see Chapter 15) and is occasionally found in tetralogy of Fallot (see Chapter 15) or common arterial trunk (see Chapter 16). Pulmonary arterial stenosis may be acquired as a consequence of the Blalock–Taussig (BT) and other systemic-to-pulmonary artery shunts, conduit operations, and the arterial switch procedure (see Chapter 14).

Clinical features

- Mild or moderate – usually asymptomatic.
- Severe – in the neonatal period severe or critical PS may present with cyanosis. This is due to the high right heart pressures causing shunting of blood from right to left across the patent foramen ovale (PFO). The pulmonary blood supply may be dependent on a patent arterial duct in this situation. The right ventricular cavity and tricuspid valve may be hypoplastic.
- Older children with severe PS may have exertional dyspnea and occasionally chest pain, syncope or signs of right heart failure. In the presence of a PFO, they may also have mild cyanosis at rest which becomes more severe on exertion.

Examination

- Ejection click, heard best at the upper left sternal edge, is characteristic of valvar PS.
- Systolic thrill often occurs in moderate-to-severe infundibular, valvar, and supravalve stenosis.
- Physiologic splitting of the second heart sound with inspiration.
- Second heart sound is widely split.
- Reduced intensity of P2; if inaudible the second heart sound will be single.
- Ejection systolic murmur at the upper left sternal edge is louder and longer with increasing severity of PS.
- This murmur may be louder over the back in peripheral pulmonary stenosis (occasionally continuous).

Pediatric Heart Disease: A Practical Guide, First Edition. Piers E. F. Daubeney, Michael L. Rigby, Koichiro Niwa, and Michael A. Gatzoulis.
© 2012 Blackwell Publishing Ltd. Published 2012 by Blackwell Publishing Ltd.

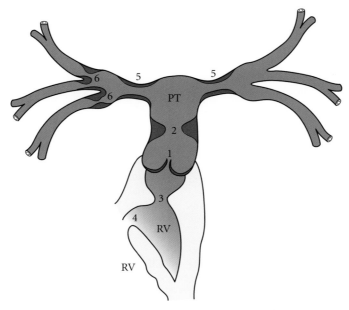

Figure 10.1 Composite diagram showing multiple sites of right heart obstruction. 1, Valvar stenosis; 2, supravalvar stenosis; 3, infundibular stenosis; 4, double (two) chamber right ventricle; 5, branch pulmonary artery stenosis; 6, peripheral pulmonary artery stenosis. PT, pulmonary trunk; RV, right ventricle.

Investigations

- **EKG:**
  - Mild PS – normal
  - Moderate PS – right axis deviation (RAD) and right ventricular hypertrophy (RVH)
  - Severe PS – signs of strain in addition to RVH and RAD.
- **CXR:**
  - Normal heart size
  - Prominent main pulmonary artery in the presence of post-stenotic dilatation
  - Decreased pulmonary vascular markings only in severe PS.
- **Echocardiography:**
  - Pulmonary valve and right ventricular outflow tract are well seen in the subcostal right oblique view and parasternal short axis
  - Valve may appear doming with thickened dysplastic leaflets
  - May be right ventricular hypertrophy and post-stenotic dilatation of the pulmonary artery
  - Color flow Doppler is useful to determine the level of obstruction as in sub- or supra-valvar PS the aliasing may be identified to start below or above the pulmonary valve respectively

  - Continuous wave Doppler across the pulmonary valve measures the peak systolic pressure drop, which is a good estimate of the degree of stenosis. The tricuspid regurgitation jet velocity can be used to estimate the right ventricular systolic pressure.

Management

- **Mild PS:** May remain unchanged or improve with time. Patients are asymptomatic and no intervention is needed.
- **Moderate-to-severe valvar PS:** Defined as a peak systolic gradient across the valve of >50–60 mmHg depending on age. Procedure of choice would be a percutaneous balloon pulmonary valvuloplasty. Branch pulmonary stenosis can also be treated by balloon angioplasty with or without the insertion of stents. The latter are rarely employed under the age of 8 years. Peripheral pulmonary arterial stenoses treated by balloon angioplasty, with or without cutting balloons, may improve segmental pulmonary blood flow but this rarely results in a significant fall in right ventricular pressure.
- **Severely dysplastic valve:** Surgical valvotomy may be more successful. In supra- or sub-valvar PS, surgical enlargement of the pulmonary trunk or resection of infundibular stenosis respectively is required.

- **Critical PS:** In the neonatal period these patients initially require intravenous prostaglandin E2 infusion to maintain patency of the arterial duct. To establish adequate pulmonary blood flow the options are:
  - Balloon pulmonary valvotomy
  - BT shunt with later balloon valvuloplasty or surgical repair.

Late complications and long-term outcome

- Moderate-to-severe branch stenosis and hypoplasia of the pulmonary arteries diagnosed in infancy not infrequently undergoes spontaneous improvement with increasing age.
- Following surgery for PS the majority of patients remain symptom-free without further intervention. Re-intervention is particularly prominent in those patients who have had transannular patch repair due to the development of pulmonary regurgitation.
- Following balloon pulmonary valvuloplasty, the majority of patients can be expected to have a reduction in the pressure gradient across the valve. Freedom from intervention rates in a study from Toronto of 150 children who had the procedure were 90%, 83%, and 77% at 5, 10, and 15 years respectively. In the best hands the outcome in severe or critical PS in early infancy is excellent and the technique can readily be applied in premature infants weighing 1500 g or less.
- Pulmonary regurgitation is usually well tolerated for a number of years but if severe, leads to progressive dilatation of the right ventricle necessitating replacement of the pulmonary valve.
- The risk of atrial or ventricular arrhythmias becomes progressively greater with increasing age, particularly for patients who had severe pulmonary PS or required infundibular resection.

Double chamber right ventricle

This condition, a variant of subpulmonary stenosis deserving its own section, is characterized by muscular subvalvar or mid-cavity right ventricular obstruction (see Figure 10.1). Anomalous muscle bundles divide the right ventricle into a high pressure proximal chamber and a low pressure distal chamber. The embryonic origin of these bundles is not known. They appear to be distinct from the moderator band and may represent accessory septoparietal trabeculations. The bands run either diago-

nally or horizontally across the right ventricular outflow tract but typically from the right atrioventricular junction to the septomarginal trabeculation and moderator band.

Incidence and etiology

This is an uncommon anomaly found in approximately 1% of congenital heart disease. In most patients this condition occurs in combination with other congenital heart defects:

- VSD in particular;
- Tetralogy of Fallot;
- Valvar pulmonary stenosis;
- Double outlet right ventricle.

Double chamber right ventricle (DCRV) may present before or after the primary defect has been repaired. It has been suggested by one study that a superior displacement of the moderator band is associated with an increased incidence.

Clinical features

These vary with the degree of obstruction:

- Right ventricular heave in moderate-to-severe cases;
- Second heart sound normally split;
- P2 may be inaudible;
- Loud ejection systolic murmur over the left sternal border with or without a thrill;
- Cyanosis in very severe cases due to the raised right heart pressures causing right-to-left shunting across the PFO.

Investigations

- **EKG:**
  - Right ventricular hypertrophy
  - Right axis deviation.
- **Echocardiography:**
  - **Subcostal right oblique section** – hypertrophied muscle bundles, typically from the superior part of the right atrioventricular junction to the apex of the right ventricle
  - **Parasternal long axis and short axis sections of right ventricle** – demonstrate muscle bundles and allow Doppler measurements of pressure drop
  - Usually diagnostic in infants and young children, although with increasing age additional types of imaging are required.
- **Other imaging:** Cardiac MRI, CT angiography, and even cardiac catheterization and angiography may be required for precise diagnosis.

Management

Although measures such as balloon dilatation of the right ventricular outflow tract have been attempted, generally patients with this condition require surgical resection of the muscle bundles. DCRV tends to be progressive and if untreated, the obstruction causes further hypertrophy of the anomalous muscle bands, thus increasing the degree of obstruction. Co-existent defects can be repaired at the same time.

Late complications and long-term outcome

Generally the obstruction does not recur after surgery, but there is a late risk of ventricular arrhythmias.

Idiopathic dilatation of the pulmonary artery

This is an uncommon and usually benign condition in which the pulmonary trunk and sometimes the proximal right and left pulmonary arteries are dilated in the presence of normal peripheral lung vasculature. Mild dysplasia of the pulmonary valve is frequently found. The major conditions that need to be excluded are:
• Presence of an abnormal intracardiac or extracardiac shunt;
• Pulmonary hypertension;
• Pulmonary stenosis.

Dilatation of the proximal pulmonary artery with histologic evidence of an arteriopathy is occasionally encountered in congenital heart malformations such as congenitally corrected transposition and tetralogy of Fallot.

Clinical features

Cardiovascular examination may be entirely normal. There may be a soft pulmonary ejection systolic murmur or secondary pulmonary regurgitation giving rise to a soft early diastolic murmur at the left sternal border.

Investigations

The diagnosis of this condition is based on the exclusion of other causes of dilatation of the main pulmonary artery. Investigation should therefore be focused at excluding potential causes.
• **CXR:** Dilatation of the main pulmonary artery with a normal sized heart and normal peripheral vessels.
• **Echocardiography:** Dilatation of the main and branch pulmonary arteries can be demonstrated on transthoracic and transesophageal echocardiography.

• **Additional imaging:** Cardiac MRI or CT angiography is the investigation of choice.

Management

In the absence of other pathology, conservative management is adopted in this condition.

Late complications and long-term outcome

This is generally thought to be a benign abnormality. There is a case report of sudden death in association with idiopathic dilatation of the pulmonary artery which at postmortem was found to be due to pulmonary artery dissection. However, it is possible that this patient had an underlying connective tissue disorder.

Ebstein malformation of the tricuspid valve

Ebstein malformation or anomaly is characterized by apical displacement of the septal and mural (inferior) leaflets of the tricuspid valve (Figures 10.2 and 10.3). The hinge line of the valve leaflet is therefore in the right ventricular cavity rather than at the atrioventricular junction. The result of this is that a portion of the right ventricular cavity becomes "atrialized" (Figure 10.3).

The valve leaflets may appear dysplastic or have other abnormalities.

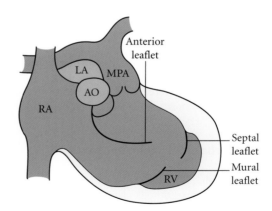

Figure 10.2 Right ventricle (RV) viewed from right oblique section showing Ebstein malformation. There is apical displacement of the mural and septal leaflets of the tricuspid valve with a sail-like anteroseptal leaflet. This produces a large "atrialized" portion of the RV and greatly reduces the actual RV cavity. AO, aorta; LA, left atrium; MPA, main pulmonary artery; RA, right atrium.

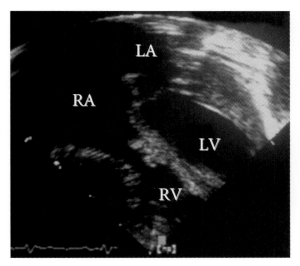

Figure 10.3 Echocardiogram in four-chamber projection showing the right ventricle in Ebstein malformation. There is apical displacement of the mural and septal leaflets of the tricuspid valve producing a large atrialized portion of the right ventricle (RV) and tiny actual right ventricular cavity. LA, left atrium; LV, left ventricle; RA, right atrium.

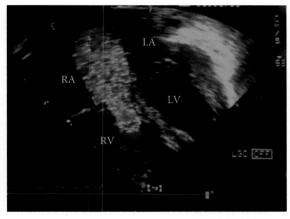

Figure 10.4 Echocardiogram in a four-chamber projection of a child with Ebstein malformation of the tricuspid valve. Tricuspid regurgitation on color flow Doppler. This is of moderate severity and has broad origin at the valvar level. LA, left atrium; LV, left ventricle; RA, right atrium; RV, right ventricle.

Types of valve leaflet and other abnormalities

- Septal leaflet:
  - Occasionally completely absent
  - Almost always displaced into the ventricular cavity
  - Often very short
  - May have a "tubular" attachment to the ventricular septum
  - May be represented by "cauliflower-like" excrescences
- Mural (inferior) leaflet:
  - Hinge point displaced into right ventricle
  - May be very short or virtually absent
  - Sometimes fuses with anterosuperior leaflet
  - Movement may be impaired due to short chords that attach it to the right ventricular wall
- Anterosuperior leaflet:
  - Hinge point always partly at aortic root
  - Significant displacement unusual
  - Often malformed and unusually large with a sail-like movement
  - May be abnormally attached to right ventricular free wall
  - Tricuspid regurgitation of variable severity is a frequent finding (Figure 10.4)

The atrialized portion of the right ventricle becomes extremely thin-walled. Tricuspid regurgitation can lead to dilatation of the atrium which in its most extreme form can result in the wall–to-wall heart sometimes seen in the newborn and often associated with lung hypoplasia.

In addition, the following features may be present to a varying degree:
- PFO/atrial septal defect present in virtually all patients;
- Abnormal location of the right bundle branch resulting in a right bundle branch block appearance on EKG;
- Arrhythmias due to often multiple accessory atrioventricular pathways. This is thought to be secondary to apical displacement of the septal leaflet causing discontinuity of the central fibrous body. Ectopic atrial tachycardia, atrial flutter, and ventricular tachycardia can also occur;
- Fibrosis of right and left ventricular free walls;
- Hypoplasia of the lungs, a poor prognostic feature, is associated with severe cardiomegaly.

Associated defects

Approximately 20% of patients presenting in infancy will have one or more co-existent defects including:
- Pulmonary stenosis;
- Pulmonary atresia;

- Muscular VSD;
- Congenitally corrected transposition of the great arteries (see Chapter 14).

Ebstein malformation with an imperforate valve may occur in pulmonary atresia with an intact ventricular septum (see Chapter 15).

Prevalence and etiology

Ebstein anomaly accounts for 0.5% of congenital heart defects. The etiology is unknown but an increased incidence has been observed in children born to mothers treated with lithium in pregnancy.

Clinical features

In fetal life severe Ebstein malformation may cause fetal hydrops or death. Postnatal presentation is highly variable, depending on the degree of displacement of the tricuspid valve leaflets, degree of regurgitation, and co-existent abnormalities. In the most severe cases, presentation is in infancy with cyanosis due to right-to-left shunting at atrial level; congestive cardiac failure may occur and carries a particularly poor prognosis. There is an interesting group of patients in whom the cyanosis present at birth becomes progressively less severe as the pulmonary vascular resistance falls, ending in a normal arterial oxygen concentration after a few weeks.

Many children are remarkably well and symptom-free, particularly if the tricuspid insufficiency is mild. Older children may present with dyspnea, exercise intolerance, or palpitations. Others may be diagnosed because of an incidental murmur in childhood; in older children and young adults the presenting symptom may be supraventricular tachycardia, while beyond infancy cyanosis is an unusual presentation but it begins to become significant in older patients.

Clinical examination may reveal:
- Cyanosis;
- Raised venous pressure with hepatomegaly in the infant and raised jugular venous pressure in the older child;
- Wide splitting of the first heart sound with a loud tricuspid component ("sail sound");
- Second heart sound may be soft and delayed (right bundle branch block);
- Third heart sound due to the opening of the anterosuperior leaflet;
- Systolic murmur at the left sternal edge of tricuspid regurgitation. The length and intensity of the murmur increases with the degree of regurgitation;
- Diastolic murmur may be present.

Investigations
- **EKG:**
  - Right atrial hypertrophy
  - Right bundle branch block
  - Superior axis may be present
  - First-degree heart block present in 40%
  - Wolff–Parkinson–White in 20%
  - QRS frequently widened due to interventricular conduction delay.
- **CXR:**
  - "Wall-to-wall" appearance of heart with extreme cardiomegaly (due to enlarged right atrium) in severe cases.
  - Near-normal heart size and pulmonary vascular markings in mild cases.
- **Echocardiography:**
  - Detailed imaging of each leaflet of tricuspid valve
  - Relationship of leaflets to atrioventricular junction and their distal attachments
  - Detailed search for co-existent defects

The following views are particularly useful in Ebstein malformation:
  - Subcostal four-chamber view – images mural leaflet and its attachment to diaphragmatic wall of right ventricle
  - Subcostal right oblique – anterosuperior leaflet (attachment to crest of septum and distal attachments within right ventricle seen)
  - Apical four-chamber view – septal leaflet attachments to septum and anterosuperior leaflet attached to aortic root.

Management
Medical management

Initial therapy in a neonate with severe Ebstein malformation is ventilation with high FiO_2 and nitric oxide to dilate the pulmonary vasculature. Prostaglandin E2 (PGE2) is used to maintain patency of the arterial duct. The newborn infant with hypoplastic lungs will be ventilator dependent and has little prospect of survival.

With the physiologic fall in pulmonary vascular resistance over the first few days and weeks of life there may be an improvement in forward flow across the pulmonary valve in some patients, allowing the PGE2 to be stopped. Heart failure is treated with diuretics. If the condition is complicated by arrhythmias, amiodarone or flecainide are commonly used. Paroxysmal arrhythmias may also necessitate the use of anticoagulation.

Patients may deteriorate due to lung hypoplasia or progressive tricuspid regurgitation and right heart failure.

Surgical management

Surgery is performed for symptomatic patients failing medical management. There are a number of options:

• **Palliative systemic-to-pulmonary artery shunt** – can be performed in neonates with Ebstein malformation associated with pulmonary stenosis or atresia.

• **Repair of the tricuspid valve and annuloplasty** – only possible if the ventricle distal to the valve is large enough to support the pulmonary circulation and the valve leaflets are not too dysplastic or adherent.

• **Repair involving vertical plication of the atrialized ventricle and valve leaflet reimplantation after clockwise rotation.**

• **Prosthetic valve implantation** (up to 65% in published series of large numbers of patients).

• **Starnes procedure** – over-sewing of the tricuspid valve to create a tricuspid atresia with a systemic-to-pulmonary arterial shunt. Subsequent management will be that of a heart unsuitable for biventricular repair with eventual total caval pulmonary connection.

Late complications and long-term outcome

The long-term outcome is highly variable. Clearly neonatal presentation with severe Ebstein malformation is associated with a worse prognosis. Beyond infancy, symptoms relate to the severity of tricuspid insufficiency, the presence of arrhythmias, and the degree of cyanosis, which might result from a right-to-left atrial shunt.

As patients become older there is an increasing risk of cyanosis, development of arrhythmias requiring radiofrequency ablation or ablative surgery, and sudden death. Following tricuspid valve repair and annuloplasty, one center has reported a freedom from re-intervention rate of 91% at 5 years, falling to 61% at 15 years, with 89% of patients in NYHA class I or II.

Tricuspid valve stenosis and regurgitation

The normal tricuspid valve is composed of three leaflets: the septal, mural (inferior), and anterosuperior. Each has a hinge point at the atrioventricular junction, tensor apparatus (chordae), and three papillary muscles. Dysplasia (abnormal development) of the valve leads to abnormalities in one or more of the components of the valve and may have the functional consequence of tricuspid stenosis or tricuspid regurgitation. The term dysplasia is also used more generally to refer to abnormal thickening of leaflets of the tricuspid valve. Sometimes

there is dispute clinically about whether there is an Ebstein malformation or simply a dysplastic valve. The differentiation of these conditions should be based on careful inspection of the proximal attachments of the valve that are uniquely displaced towards the apex in Ebstein malformation.

Tricuspid valve stenosis

The tricuspid valve orifice is small (miniaturized) or narrowed, causing obstruction to blood flow from the right atrium to the right ventricle.

Incidence and etiology

This is a condition rarely encountered in pediatric practice. Congenital malformations leading to tricuspid stenosis comprise:

• Shortened chordae;
• Hypoplastic leaflets;
• Parachute deformity with the chordae arising from a single papillary muscle;
• Supravalvular ring;
• Fused commissures;
• Underdeveloped annulus.

Typically stenosis is found in pulmonary atresia with intact ventricular septum (see Chapter 15) and in some cases of critical pulmonary stenosis; occasionally it results from the Rastelli operation or VSD closure and the right atrioventricular valve can become stenotic following repair of a complete AVSD (see Chapter 9).

Clinical features

Increased pressure in the systemic veins results in hepatomegaly and distended neck veins with giant a waves in the jugular venous pulse. A soft mid-diastolic murmur at the lower left sternal edge may be audible.

Investigations

• **EKG:** Right atrial hypertrophy.
• **CXR:** Dilatation of the right atrium.
• **Echocardiography:**
  ◦ The tricuspid valve is best seen in the apical four-chamber view, subcostal oblique, and parasternal long axis angling posteriorly
  ◦ Abnormal valve apparatus may be demonstrated on 2D echo
  ◦ Color flow Doppler will show aliasing across the valve
  ◦ Doppler assessment of the peak gradient and pressure half-time across the valve allows calculation of the gradient and valve area.

Tricuspid regurgitation
Incidence and etiology
Abnormalities in the tricuspid valve that may result in regurgitation include an isolated cleft of the anterosuperior leaflet, hypoplasia of the papillary muscles, tethering of the leaflets due to shortened tendinous chordae, and abnormal or underdeveloped leaflets that do not close adequately in systole. It is common in pulmonary atresia with intact septum (see Chapter 15), Ebstein malformation (see above), and hearts with a discordant atrioventricular connection (see Chapter 14). Functional tricuspid insufficiency in cases of pulmonary hypertension (see Chapters 21 and 22) or right ventricular volume overload (see Chapter 15) is frequently observed. Physiologic trivial regurgitation occurs frequently in the normal heart and transient insufficiency is a well-recognized cause of a neonatal heart murmur. In the fetus, the most severe form causes hydrops and intrauterine death.

Clinical features
• A systolic regurgitant murmur and diastolic rumble at the lower left sternal edge are characteristic findings.
• Loud S3.
• With severe regurgitation there may be pulsatile liver and neck veins due to the phasic increase in right atrial pressure during systole caused by the regurgitation.

Investigations
• **EKG:**
  ◦ Right atrial hypertrophy
  ◦ Right ventricular hypertrophy
  ◦ Right bundle branch block.
• **CXR:** Right atrial enlargement if severe.
• **Echocardiography:** Four chamber and subcostal right oblique (paracoronal) sections almost always demonstrate the severity and allow the measurement of the systolic pressure drop between the right ventricle and atrium.

Management
Abnormalities resulting in stenosis of the valve present in infancy and childhood, and require early intervention. In contrast, tricuspid regurgitation may be well tolerated for many years.

If the regurgitation is severe and the patient symptomatic, there are a number of surgical options available to repair the valve. These include a Kay plication, Vega annuloplasty, and Carpentier ring annuloplasty. Prosthetic valve implantation may also be considered.

Late complications and long-term outcome
Mild-to-moderate tricuspid regurgitation is very well tolerated for many years. Progressive dilatation of the right atrium results in an increased risk of atrial arrhythmias, particularly atrial flutter and ectopic atrial tachycardia.

It is not uncommon for re-intervention to be required following tricuspid valve surgery. Reoperation rates have been reported as 90%, 66%, and 52% after 5, 10, and 15 years respectively.

Further reading

Redington AN, Brawn WJ, Deanfield JE, Anderson RH. *The Right Heart in Congenital Heart Disease*. London: Greenwich Medical Media, 1998.

Double chambered right ventricle
Pongliglione G, Freedom RM, Cook D, Rowe RD. Mechanisms of acquired right ventricular outflow tract obstruction in patients with ventricular septal defect: an angiocardiographic study. *Am J Cardiol* 1982;50:776–780.
Wong PC, Saunders SP, Jonas RA, *et al*. Pulmonary valve-moderator band distance and association with development of double chambered right ventricle. *Am J Cardiol* 1991:68:1681–1686.

Idiopathic dilatation of the pulmonary artery
Andrews R, Colloby P, Hubner PJ. Pulmonary artery dissection in a patient with idiopathic dilation of the pulmonary artery: a rare cause of sudden cardiac death. *Br Heart J* 1993;69:268–269.

Pulmonary stenosis
Garty Y, Veldtman G, Lee K, Benson L. Late outcomes after pulmonary valve balloon dilation in neonates , infants and children. *J Invasive Cardiol* 2005;17:318–322.
Roos-Hesselink JW, Meijboom FJ, Spitaels SE, *et al*. Long-term outcome after surgery for pulmonary stenosis (a longitudinal study of 22–33 years). *Eur Heart J* 2006;27:482–488.

Ebstein malformation
Boston US, Dearani JA, O'Leary PW, *et al*. Tricuspid valve repair for Ebstein's anomaly in young children: A 30 year experience. *Ann Thorac Surg* 2006;81:690–696.
Chen JM, Mosca RS, Altmann K. Early and medium-term results for repair of Ebsteins anomaly. *J Thorac Cardiovasc Surg* 2004;127:990–999.

11 Abnormalities of left ventricular inflow and outflow

Anna Seale

Royal Brompton Hospital, London, UK

Types of left heart anomaly

For simplification, left heart anomalies are categorized into two main groups.

Left heart anomalies

Lesions of left heart outflow

- Obstructive lesions:
  - Supravalvar aortic stenosis
  - Valvar aortic stenosis
  - Subvalvar aortic stenosis
- Other lesions:
  - Aortic valve regurgitation
  - Bicuspid aortic valve
  - Double outlet left ventricle (see Chapter15)

Lesions of left heart inflow

- Obstructive lesions:
  - Mitral valve stenosis
  - Supravalvar mitral membrane
  - Cortriatriatum
  - Pulmonary vein stenosis
- Other lesions:
  - Mitral valve regurgitation
  - Mitral valve prolapse

It is not unusual for malformations of inflow and outflow to occur in the same patient; in addition more than one site of left ventricular inflow or outflow obstruction may be encountered in the same patient. When inflow and outflow obstruction occur together with aortic coarctation, the term "Shone syndrome or complex" is sometimes used, although an exact description of the morphology should always be applied.

Hypoplastic left heart syndrome is described separately in Chapter 16.

Incidence

Bicuspid aortic valve is a common congenital cardiac anomaly occurring in 1–2% of the population with a male predominance (4:1). Mitral valve prolapse is also common (2% of the population).

Valvar aortic stenosis occurs in approximately 5% of all congenital cardiac lesions in liveborn children in the United Kingdom. Hypoplastic left heart syndrome similarly accounts for 3.2%. All other left heart lesions are relatively rare.

Abnormalities of left ventricular outflow

Bicuspid aortic valve

Congenital bicuspid aortic valve is one of the most common congenital heart malformations. It can be associated with other forms of congenital heart disease and in particular coarctation of the aorta. In the normal aortic valve, there are three valve cusps separated along their whole length and hence allowing free movement. In a bicuspid aortic valve there is fusion of two of the three cusps resulting in two functioning leaflets (Figure 11.1).

Although common, this anomaly is often undetected in early life as it does not cause any hemodynamic

---

Pediatric Heart Disease: A Practical Guide, First Edition. Piers E. F. Daubeney, Michael L. Rigby, Koichiro Niwa, and Michael A. Gatzoulis.
© 2012 Blackwell Publishing Ltd. Published 2012 by Blackwell Publishing Ltd.

disturbance. However, bicuspid valves can become stenotic over time and subsequently have clinical significance in adult life. The valves can also be prone to endocarditis and prolapse. A bicuspid aortic valve may be associated with a progressive ascending aortopathy.

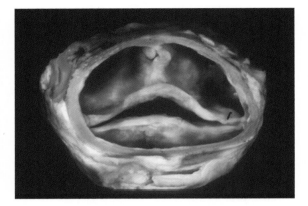

Figure 11.1 Morphologic specimen of a bicuspid aortic valve. Fusion of two cusps (top part) producing an eccentric functional orifice with the third cusp (bottom part); true bicuspid, i.e. two leaflet aortic valve is uncommon. Note limited opening of the valve with thickening of the cusp edges and failure of complete leaflet co-aption, leading to both aortic stenosis and regurgitation. (Reproduced from Gatzoulis MA, Swan L, Therrien J, Pantely GA, eds. *Adult Congenital Heart Disease, A Practical Guide*, 2005, with permission from Blackwell Publishing Ltd.)

If a bicuspid valve is detected in childhood in the absence of obstruction or any other associated congenital heart disease, bacterial endocarditis prophylaxis has traditionally been advised at times of potential bacteremia. This advice has now been modified (see Appendix D). There is however, a very small risk of endocarditis resulting from tooth extraction and other operations. For the patient, such a development can be disastrous in terms of future prognosis and for this reason, some cardiologists continue to advise prophylaxis at times of risk. Assessment of a bicuspid valve (without hemodynamic complication) should occur every 3–5 years by a medical practitioner, looking for signs of stenosis or regurgitation.

Late complications and long-term outcome
See Chapter 31.

Left ventricular outflow tract obstruction (LVOTO)

Obstruction can occur at three levels:

• **Subvalvar LVOTO:** Discrete fibromuscular subaortic stenosis takes the form of a crescent or even complete ring, immediately below the aortic valve (Figures 11.2 and 11.3a). Only rarely present at birth, it is considered by many to be, at least partly, an acquired anomaly and the association with a perimembranous ventricular septal defect (VSD) is well described. Less commonly, there is a tunnel-like obstruction, usually associated with an inherently narrow outflow tract, hypertrophy of the septal myocardium, and fibrous or muscular prolongation of

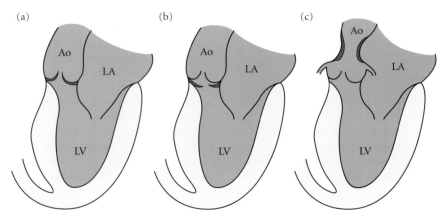

Figure 11.2 Schematic diagram showing the three subtypes of aortic stenosis. (a) Valvar aortic stenosis. (b) Discrete subaortic stenosis. (c) Supravalvar aortic stenosis. Ao, aorta; LA, left atrium; LV, left ventricle.

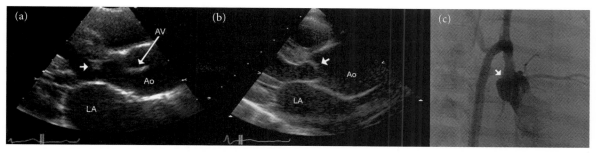

Figure 11.3 The three types of left ventricular outflow tract obstruction (LVOTO). (a) Echocardiogram illustrating discrete subvalvular LVOTO (short arrow). The long arrow indicates the position of the aortic valve. (b) Echocardiogram showing a doming aortic valve in valvar LVOTO (arrow). Note the aortic root dilatation. (c) Angiogram showing supravalvar aortic stenosis (arrow). Ao, aorta; AV, aortic valve; LA, left atrium.

the distance between the aortic valve and the anterior mitral leaflet. Thus, subaortic stenosis can be extremely complex often with additional features such as subaortic malalignment of the infundibular septum and abnormal atrioventricular valve attachments or tissue tags. There is a male predominance of 2:1.

• **Valvar LVOTO:** Although complete fusion of two leaflets produces a bicuspid aortic valve, the normal three-valve cusps can become partially fused along their commissures, beginning from the edge of the leaflet and extending towards the center of the valve, leading to valvar stenosis with a trileaflet or bicuspid valve. In addition, the valve leaflets may be thickened, reducing their mobility (Figure 11.2 and 11.3b). This is the most common form of LVOTO, again with a male predominance of 4:1. Although a bicuspid aortic valve is the most common, the distinction between this and a tricuspid or unicuspid valve may be difficult with echocardiography in some patients.

• **Supravalvar obstruction:** Discrete narrowing at the level of the sinotubular junction is the most common form, but diffuse tubular hypoplasia of the ascending aorta is also encountered, occasionally extending to the arch and descending aorta (Figures 11.2 and 11.3c). This is the least common type of LVOTO and can occur either sporadically, in families (with autosomal dominant inheritance), or in association with Williams syndrome. In the latter, the underlying cause of supravalvar aortic stenosis is a mutation of the *elastin* gene on chromosome 7q11.23. This results in an obstructive arteriopathy of varying severity, most prominent at the aortic sinotubular junction but involving all of the aorta and its branches. Often associated with varying degrees of branch pulmo-

nary arterial stenoses, coarctation of the aorta and renal artery stenosis are also encountered.

Presentation and clinical course in childhood

In all cases presentation depends upon the severity of the lesion and the degree of obstruction caused. Some patients are asymptomatic, particularly when the obstruction is mild. Such patients may present with an incidental heart murmur. At the other end of the spectrum, the patient may present with dyspnea, chest pain, sudden death, and syncope when the obstruction is severe.

In neonates, very severe valvar LVOTO (**critical aortic stenosis**) may lead to collapse following closure of the arterial duct. This is because in critical aortic stenosis there is a "duct-dependent systemic circulation" in which the right ventricle maintains cardiac output and blood flow to the descending aorta. These infants require immediate resuscitation, a prostaglandin E infusion, and transfer to a cardiac center for definitive care. Prenatal diagnosis of critical aortic valve stenosis is an indication for the prophylactic administration of prostaglandin E from birth.

Clinical findings of LVOTO are:
• Ejection systolic murmur heard in the upper right precordium above the nipple line radiating to the carotids;
• Carotid thrill;
• Ejection click, heard best at the apex, in aortic valve stenosis;
• Peripheral pulses may be weak with a narrow pulse pressure in severe obstruction.

Subvalvar and supravalvar obstruction are usually progressive. With increasing obstruction, patients develop aortic valve regurgitation and left ventricular hypertrophy.

In supravalvar aortic stenosis there is often a diffuse arteriopathy involving the systemic, coronary, and branch pulmonary arteries. Coarctation of the aorta, renal artery stenosis, and even coronary artery aneurysms may be found. Branch ("peripheral") pulmonary arterial stenoses, unlike supravalvar aortic stenosis, may resolve with time in many patients. Aortic valve stenosis usually becomes progressively more severe as the patient grows, but the rate of increase is variable and unpredictable.

Investigations
- **EKG:**
  ○ Left ventricular hypertrophy
  ○ ST segment depression depending on severity
  ○ T wave inversion in the left precordial leads when obstruction is severe
  ○ Normal or near-normal EKG does not exclude significant LVOTO.
- **Echocardiography:**
  ○ Mainstay of diagnosis; alone usually sufficient for diagnosis of valvar and subvalvar LVOTO
  ○ Level of left heart obstruction identified by 2D and 3D imaging
  ○ Valve morphology by 2D/3D imaging
  ○ Mechanism of stenosis – tricuspid, bicuspid or unicuspid aortic valve
  ○ Stenosis/regurgitation demonstrated by color flow Doppler
  ○ Severity of stenosis/regurgitation quantified by pulsed and continuous wave Doppler
  ○ Secondary effects of left heart obstruction, e.g. left ventricular hypertrophy
  ○ Systolic and diastolic dysfunction require evaluation by M-mode, tissue Doppler, and mitral valve Doppler inflow pattern
  ○ Associated forms of congenital heart disease, including mitral stenosis (any type), left heart hypoplasia, coarctation of the aorta and **Shone complex** – an association of multiple levels of left ventricular inflow and outflow obstruction.
- **Additional imaging:**
  ○ Cardiac catheterization, CT angiography, and cardiac MRI
  ○ Often needed in supravalvar stenosis to confirm/exclude tubular hypoplasia of the aorta, origin of stenosis of the head and neck arteries, coronary artery stenosis, and peripheral pulmonary artery stenoses. Care should be taken as these patients are notoriously unstable under general anesthesia, which should be avoided if possible.

Management
The management of supravalvar and subvalvar obstruction is surgical. Timing of surgery is important because both lesions may progress. Factors that are taken into consideration include the severity of the obstruction, symptoms, associated aortic regurgitation, ventricular hypertrophy, and function.

Indications for considering intervention in left ventricular outflow obstruction
- Symptoms caused by LVOTO
- Asymptomatic LVOTO with peak-to-peak **catheter** gradient >50 mmHg
- Asymptomatic LVOTO with left ventricular systolic dysfunction
- Aortic regurgitation in supravalvar and subvalvar LVOTO
- Left ventricular hypertrophy in all types of LVOTO

Valvar aortic stenosis can be managed either by balloon valvuloplasty in the cardiac catheterization laboratory or by surgical valvotomy. The approach will vary from one center to another, but the advantage of open surgical valvotomy is a more precise procedure with less likelihood of moderate-to-severe aortic insufficiency and a longer time to the second intervention. In the best hands, however, interventional cardiac catheterization with a limited aortic valvuloplasty is extremely successful in many patients with minimal aortic regurgitation. The procedure can be repeated when aortic valve stenosis recurs. Whether the approach to aortic valve stenosis is surgical or the use of balloon valvuloplasty, the most important, and in many cases inevitable, complication is aortic insufficiency, but either approach is designed to delay the need for aortic valve replacement.

In neonates with critical aortic stenosis, it is important to assess the size of the aortic valve, mitral valve, and left ventricle to decide whether the left heart is large enough and capable of supporting the systemic circulation. In patients with "left heart hypoplasia" this can often be a difficult decision. In cases where the left side of the heart is felt to be too small, an infant may have a better outcome with an initial **Norwood procedure** followed by univentricular palliation.

Aortic valve replacement
- The Ross operation is the replacement of the aortic valve and proximal ascending aorta with a pulmonary

autograft accompanied by the insertion of a pulmonary or aortic homograft in the right ventricular outflow. In the best hands results are excellent with normal or virtually normal neoaortic valve function. The gradual degeneration or lack of growth of the right-sided homograft results in the need for replacement or insertion of a stented pulmonary valve some years later. The Ross operation can be performed during infancy, although the early and medium-term outcome is not as good as those in children over the age of 5 years. The presence of an ascending aortopathy is a relative contraindication.

• Aortic valve replacement with a prosthetic valve achieves a good outcome in older children and young adults, but repeat operation is often required in the medium term and lifelong treatment with warfarin/coumarin is essential. This has implications for girls as anticoagulation has profound implications for pregnancy later in life. These patients are at risk of bacterial endocarditis. The AHA guidelines suggest endocarditis prophylaxis for all prosthetic heart valves or when prosthetic material has been used for valvar repair. It is best to clarify with the patient's cardiologist whether endocarditis prophylaxis is required. Endocarditis prophylaxis is covered in Appendix D.

Novel techniques

• Percutaneous aortic valve replacement performed in the cardiac catheterization laboratory is being employed in some patients considered too frail for open heart surgery, but is currently reserved for the elderly.

• Fetal aortic valvuloplasty has been used for the management of severe aortic valve stenosis during the second trimester. The rationale is the prevention of fetal hydrops or prevention of the development of hypoplastic left heart syndrome. While the procedure is technically feasible with good immediate results, the postnatal outcome has been disappointing with redevelopment of the original stenosis.

Late complications and long-term outcome
See Chapter 31.

Aortic valve regurgitation
Aortic valve regurgitation (AR) or insufficiency is the term given to retrograde blood flow through the aortic valve into the left ventricle during ventricular diastole. As an isolated condition in childhood it is uncommon and usually found in combination with aortic stenosis, other congenital malformations, or acquired heart disease.

> **Causes of aortic regurgitation**
> • Congenital abnormality of the aortic valve, e.g. bicuspid aortic valve
> • Congenital abnormalities of the other parts of the heart which affect aortic valve function, e.g.:
>   ◦ Perimembranous and doubly committed VSD where non-coronary or right coronary aortic leaflet prolapsed into the defect
>   ◦ Subaortic stenosis
> • Acquired abnormality of the aortic valve, e.g.:
>   ◦ Acute rheumatic fever
>   ◦ Infective endocarditis
>   ◦ Post LVOTO surgery
>   ◦ Post balloon aortic valvuloplasty
> • Dilatation of the aortic root, e.g. Marfan syndrome

The most frequent causes worldwide are rheumatic heart disease (see Chapter 25) and balloon aortic valvuloplasty. There is a well-recognized association with doubly committed subarterial VSD, which can lead to prolapse of the right coronary cusp, and with perimembranous inlet VSD, which can lead to prolapse of the non-coronary cusp.

Presentation and clinical course in childhood
Symptoms depend upon the severity of the regurgitation and tend to occur late. In the vast majority, the AR is chronic. Patients with trivial, mild, or moderate AR are frequently asymptomatic, whereas those with severe AR are breathless, exercise intolerant, and occasionally suffer from syncope or angina.

Acute insufficiency occurs extremely rarely in the pediatric population (e.g. trauma or aortic valve rupture due to bacterial endocarditis). When it does occur in this way, the patient is extremely unwell, presenting with circulatory collapse and acute renal failure.

The clinical findings are:
• Peripheral pulses may be normal in mild regurgitation;
• Collapsing pulses with a wide pulse pressure in moderate or severe insufficiency;
• Hyperdynamic apical impulse displaced laterally and inferiorly in moderate or severe insufficiency;
• Diastolic decrescendo murmur heard above the nipple line but absent in severe acute regurgitation;
• Low-pitched, mid-diastolic rumble at the apex (**Austin–Flint murmur**) due to vibration of the anterior mitral valve leaflet caused by regurgitant jet from the aorta;

• Ejection systolic murmur is frequently heard due to associated LVOTO or simply increased flow across the aortic valve.

Investigations

- **EKG:**
  - Normal in cases of mild AR
  - Left atrial enlargement
  - Left ventricular hypertrophy In more severe disease.
- **CXR:**
  - Often normal in mild disease
  - Cardiomegaly from left heart dilatation
  - Prominence of the ascending aorta in more severe disease.
- **Echocardiography:**
  - Important in assessing mechanism and severity of the AR
  - Anatomy of the aortic valve and other structures
  - Left ventricular function and dilatation assessed with M-mode
  - Serial measurements of ventricular dimensions are important to monitor disease progression
  - Color flow and continuous wave Doppler can assess severity of the AR (mild, moderate, severe) (Figure 11.4).

Management

Medical treatment includes ACE inhibitors and diuretics, which can be used in very symptomatic patients.

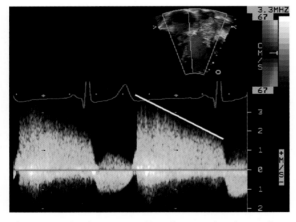

Figure 11.4 Continuous wave Doppler trace showing aortic valve regurgitation. The steeper the gradient of the white line, the more severe the disease. The velocity at end-diastole (at the R wave) reflects the difference between the diastolic blood pressure and the left ventricular end-diastolic pressure which governs flow across the coronary bed.

Surgical treatment is determined by the cause of the AR. For example, when AR is caused by prolapse of the right coronary cusp of the aortic valve in a doubly committed VSD, surgery will require closure of the VSD and perhaps re-suspension of the aortic cusp. If the aortic valve is the problem, this can be replaced with either a mechanical prosthesis or the Ross operation (see above). Timing of surgery is difficult as many of these patients may be asymptomatic. Change and rate of change in ventricular dimensions are important to consider. There is concern that if the left ventricle becomes too dilated, subsequent valve replacement will not always allow complete left ventricular recovery.

Late complications and long-term outcome
See Chapter 31.

Anomalies of left heart inflow

Mitral valve prolapse
Mitral valve prolapse (MVP) is characterized by billowing of one or both mitral valve leaflets into the left atrium during systole. Morphologic features include accumulation of acid mucopolysaccharides, weakening the fibrous core of the valve, and the inequality of chordal support to the free edge of the affected valvar leaflet. This is a common anomaly occurring in approximately 2% of the population. MVP usually occurs in isolation but may be familial, associated with Marfan syndrome or other connective tissue diseases.

MVP is generally asymptomatic in childhood with the diagnosis commonly being made by cardiac auscultation or echocardiography performed for other purposes. Occasionally, patients complain of symptoms: atypical chest pain, palpitations, dyspnea, fatigue, syncope, and anxiety.

Clinical findings
The main auscultatory feature of MVP is a mid-systolic click. There may be one or more clicks, varying in intensity and timing according to left ventricular loading conditions and contractility. The clicks result from sudden tensing of the mitral valve apparatus as the leaflets prolapse into the left atrium during systole. Frequently the mid-systolic click(s) is followed by a late systolic murmur, loudest at the apex and again variable. Occasionally this murmur has a musical or honking quality and rarely is heard across the room.

Investigations

- **EKG:**
  - Usually normal
  - Left-sided "T" wave inversion can occur.
- **CXR:**
  - Usually normal
  - Skeletal manifestations of connective tissue disease, e.g. scoliosis in Marfan syndrome, may be present.
- **Echocardiography:**
  - Establishes the diagnosis
  - Image the prolapsing leaflets with M-mode and 2D
  - Assess associated mitral regurgitation with continuous wave and color Doppler
  - Tendency toward over diagnosis of MVP: those with mild billowing of non-thickened leaflet(s) toward the left atrium with leaflet co-aption on the left ventricular side of the annulus and with minimal or no regurgitation are probably normal.

Management

In most patient studies, MVP is associated with a benign prognosis. However, in a minority of patients it may be associated with progressive mitral regurgitation that occurs in adulthood. Reassurance is a major part of the management of patients with MVP; those who are asymptomatic with milder forms of prolapse should be assured of a benign prognosis and encouraged to have a normal lifestyle. They should be reviewed every 3–5 years. Beta-blockers may be of some benefit in patients who are particularly troubled by symptoms. The very small proportion of patients who develop progressive mitral regurgitation may go on to require mitral valve repair in adult life. Sudden death is rare in adults and virtually unheard of in children.

Left ventricular inflow obstruction

Congenital left ventricular inflow obstruction is extremely rare. Acquired mitral valve stenosis is common in some parts of the world as a consequence of rheumatic fever. Acquired mitral stenosis and rheumatic fever are discussed in Chapter 25. In this chapter we will concentrate on congenital obstructive lesions of left ventricular inflow. These can occur at several levels:

- **Mitral valve:** Isolated congenital mitral valve disease is uncommon in the pediatric population, unlike in adults. It accounts for approximately 4 of every 1000 children with congenital heart disease. The normal functioning of the mitral valve depends upon its various components (annulus, leaflets, tendinous chords, papillary muscles). Any of these component parts can be congenitally malformed, producing a wide range of congenital lesions which affect valvar function. This can cause either valvar stenosis, regurgitation, or both. For example, a "**parachute mitral valve**" is a mitral valve abnormality in which all the tendinous chords may be shortened and thickened, inserting into a single papillary muscle and usually causing mitral stenosis.
- **Supravalvar mitral membrane and ring** (Figure 11.5): A layer of fibrous connective tissue adherent to (membrane) or directly above (ring) the mitral valve causing functional mitral stenosis. The foramen ovale and left atrial appendage lie above the plane of the membrane. It is rarely isolated and often associated with other

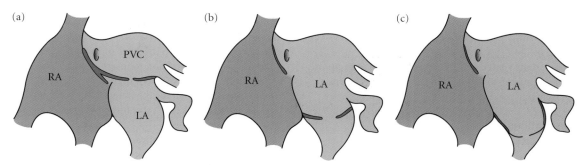

Figure 11.5 Schematic diagram showing morphologic features of cortriatriatum, supramitral ring, and supramitral membrane. (a) Cortriatriatum. The membrane is located above the foramen ovale and left atrial appendage. (b) Supravalvar ring. The ring is inserted below the foramen ovale and left atrial appendage. (c) Supravalvar membrane. As for a supravalvar ring but the membrane is adherent to the mitral valve. LA, left atrium; PVC, pulmonary venous confluence; RA, right atrium.

anomalies such as parachute mitral valve, subaortic stenosis, or coarctation of the aorta.

• **Cortriatriatum** (Figure 11.5): The pulmonary venous confluence is situated above an obstructing membrane in the left atrium. Unlike a supravalvar mitral membrane and ring, the foramen ovale and left atrial appendage are below the plane of the membrane (Figure 11.5). Cortriatriatum is often associated with other defects such as an oval fossa atrial septal defect (ASD) (70–80%).

• **Pulmonary vein stenosis:** Intrinsic narrowing of the individual pulmonary veins is extremely rare and the incidence is not known. Pulmonary vein stenosis can occur in isolation or associated with other forms of congenital heart disease, e.g. hypoplastic left heart syndrome and atrioventricular septal defect (AVSD). The stenosis can be discrete, segmental (tubular hypoplasia), or diffuse. It can be associated with prematurity.

Presentation and clinical course in childhood

Left ventricular inflow obstruction leads to a raised left atrial and pulmonary venous pressure. If severe, there can be pulmonary edema and/or secondary pulmonary arterial hypertension. Timing of presentation and symptoms depend upon the severity of obstruction.

The child with significant obstruction presents with breathlessness, cough, recurrent chest infections, and failure to thrive. Some patients present in adulthood with atrial fibrillation and/or thromboembolic events such as transient ischemic attack or stroke. Other patients with minimal obstruction may be asymptomatic with the anomaly being diagnosed incidentally.

Clinical findings of left ventricular inflow obstruction:
• Diminished peripheral perfusion and weak pulses indicating low systemic output;
• First heart sound may be soft with an additional low frequency, low intensity mid-diastolic murmur (valvar mitral stenosis and supravalvar mitral membrane);
• No murmur (cortriatriatum and pulmonary vein stenosis);
• Active right ventricular heave and accentuated pulmonary component to the second heart sound (pulmonary hypertension).

Investigations
• **EKG:**
  ◦ Left atrial hypertrophy.
  ◦ Right atrial and ventricular hypertrophy with right axis deviation if pulmonary hypertension.
• **CXR:**
  ◦ Cardiomegaly

  ◦ Pulmonary venous congestion
  ◦ Pulmonary trunk prominent with pulmonary hypertension.
• **Echocardiography:**
  ◦ Mainstay of diagnosis
  ◦ Type of left heart inflow obstruction – mitral valve, supravalvar membrane, cortriatriatum, pulmonary vein
  ◦ Morphology of mitral apparatus
  ◦ Mechanism of stenosis – annulus, leaflets, tendinous chords, papillary muscles
  ◦ 3D echocardiography important in ascertaining exact mechanism of stenosis
  ◦ Mitral valve leaflet movement with M-mode
  ◦ Severity of mitral stenosis/regurgitation with pulsed and continuous wave Doppler
  ◦ Echocardiographic assessment of a supramitral membrane is notoriously difficult and frequently missed
  ◦ Evidence of pulmonary hypertension by interrogating tricuspid and pulmonary regurgitant jets using continuous wave Doppler
  ◦ Assess for associated congenital heart disease.
• **Additional imaging:**
  ◦ CT angiography and magnetic resonance scanning to assess the pulmonary venous anatomy
  ◦ MRI helpful for intracardiac anatomy
  ◦ Angiography useful only for the assessment/treatment of pulmonary vein stenosis (Figure 11.6).

Management
The treatment of mitral valve stenosis in children includes medical management with diuretics to help relieve the symptoms of pulmonary venous congestion and to allow the patient to grow. Balloon valvuloplasty has a very limited role because of potential damage to leaflets and chords. Surgical management is also problematic. Although mitral valve replacement is commonplace in the adult population, it is avoided in infants and small children if at all possible because of the likelihood of the need for future reoperation to insert a larger valve. When obstruction is severe and surgery is required, every attempt is made to repair the native valve with particular attention not only to the valve leaflets but also the chords and papillary muscles.

Management of supravalvar mitral membrane involves surgical resection of the membrane and repair of the underlying mitral valve if required. Similarly, management of cortriatriatum, where there is significant obstruction, involves surgical resection of the membrane and repair of any associated defects.

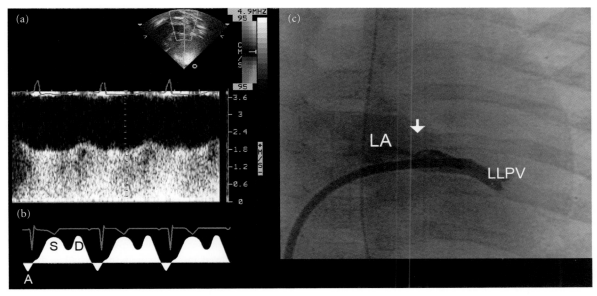

Figure 11.6 Pulmonary vein stenosis. (a) Pulsed wave Doppler showing high velocity continuous flow indicating pulmonary venous obstruction. (b) Normal pulmonary vein Doppler trace for comparison. (c) Angiogram in left lower pulmonary vein (LLPV) showing a discrete stenosis (arrow) at the junction of the left atrium (LA) and pulmonary vein.

Treatment of pulmonary vein stenosis is difficult. Despite surgical and catheter interventions, these patients tend to have progressive stenosis leading to pulmonary hypertension and death. More recently, newer techniques have been used to try and treat this devastating disease, including a "sutureless" surgical technique and cutting balloon dilatation at the time of cardiac catheterization. Optimal management is controversial.

Mitral valve regurgitation

Mitral valve regurgitation (MR) refers to retrograde flow of blood from the left ventricle into the left atrium during ventricular systole; the result is varying degrees of left atrial and ventricular enlargement caused by volume overload. Worldwide, the commonest cause of mitral regurgitation is rheumatic heart disease. Left atrioventricular valve insufficiency is frequently observed in the follow-up of patients who have undergone repair of an AVSD (see Chapter 9). In contrast, congenital mitral insufficiency is extremely rare (2–3% of congenital heart disease presenting in infancy). Abnormalities of virtually any part of the mitral valve and its tensor apparatus, including the free margin of the valve leaflets, chordal apparatus, and papillary muscles have been implicated in the etiology of regurgitation. Such abnormalities include:

- Dysplasia of the valve leaflets;
- Double orifice;
- Deficient leaflet tissue;
- Isolated cleft of the anterior leaflet;
- Poly-valvular disease;
- Ebstein-like displacement of the valve leaflets;

Causes of mitral regurgitation

- Congenital abnormality of the mitral valve apparatus:
  - Leaflets, e.g. isolated cleft
  - Chordae tendinae, e.g. parachute mitral valve
  - Papillary muscle, e.g. parachute mitral valve
- Acquired abnormality of the mitral valve apparatus:
  - Leaflets, e.g. rheumatic fever
  - Chordae tendinae, e.g. infective endocarditis
  - Papillary muscle, e.g. amyloid
  - Annulus dilatation, e.g. dilated cardiomyopathy, anomalous left coronary artery from pulmonary artery (ALCAPA)

• Arcade lesion in which the leaflets are attached directly to the papillary muscles, the chordae being absent.

Presentation and clinical course in childhood

Symptoms depend upon the severity of the regurgitation. Patients with trivial or mild MR are asymptomatic; those with moderate-to-severe MR have signs of heart failure with breathlessness, sweating, fatigue, and failure to thrive. Paroxysmal nocturnal dyspnea may occur in older children.

Clinical findings are:
• Blowing pan-systolic murmur best heard at the apex and radiating to the axilla;
• Diastolic murmur due to increased flow across the mitral valve;
• Signs of pulmonary hypertension if MR is extremely severe.

Investigations
• **EKG:**
  ○ Normal in mild MR
  ○ First-degree heart block if the left atrium is enlarged
  ○ Left atrial and ventricular hypertrophy may be present
  ○ Right ventricular hypertrophy with pulmonary hypertension
  ○ May provide clues as to the cause of the MR
  ○ Pattern of anterolateral infarction suggests ALCAPA (see Chapter 13)
  ○ Superior axis may indicate that the atrioventricular valve regurgitation is due to an AVSD (see Chapter 9).
• **CXR:**
  ○ Normal heart size in mild disease
  ○ Cardiomegaly from left heart dilatation due to volume overload in moderate-to-severe disease
  ○ Pulmonary venous congestion and upper lobe blood diversion may be present.
• **Echocardiography:**
  ○ Mainstay of diagnosis
  ○ Assess mechanism and severity of the MR with 2D color Doppler and 3D echocardiography (mild, moderate, severe)
  ○ Anatomy of the mitral apparatus and other structures can be inspected
  ○ Ensure coronary anatomy is normal with antegrade flow into the left anterior descending aorta excluding ALCAPA
  ○ Left ventricular function assessed using M-mode
  ○ Left ventricle may appear "hyperdynamic" in the presence of severe MR and it is difficult to predict what function would be after mitral valve repair

○ Serial measurements of ventricular dimensions are important to monitor disease progression.

Management
Medical management
Medical treatment comprises diuretics to help relieve symptoms of pulmonary venous congestion. ACE inhibitors are also used, but there is little evidence to support their use, although some children have improvement in exercise performance.

Surgical management
The type of surgical treatment is determined by the mechanism of the MR. In general and wherever possible, the mitral valve is repaired rather than replaced. Replacement is usually with a prosthetic tilting disc valve. A valve diameter of 25 mm or more is needed for a typical adult. Tissue valves can be employed in infants and small children but re-operation within 4 years is usually needed.

Further reading

Cheung MM, Sullivan ID, de Leval MR, Tsang VT, Redington AN. Optimal timing of the Ross procedure in the management of chronic aortic incompetence in the young. *Cardiol Young* 2003;13:253–257.

McElhinney DB, Lock JE, Keane JF, Moran AM, Colan SD. Left heart growth, function, and reintervention after balloon aortic valvuloplasty for neonatal aortic stenosis. *Circulation* 2005;111:451–458.

Mori Y, Nakazawa M, Tomimatsu H, Momma K. Long-term effect of angiotensin-converting enzyme inhibitor in volume overloaded heart during growth: a controlled pilot study. *J Am Coll Cardiol* 2000;36:270–275.

Rhodes LA, Colan SD, Perry SB, Jonas RA, Sanders SP. Predictors of survival in neonates with critical aortic stenosis. *Circulation* 1991;84:2325–2335.

Sadr IM, Tan PE, Kieran MW, Jenkins KJ. Mechanism of pulmonary vein stenosis in infants with normally connected veins. *Am J Cardiol* 2000;86:577–579.

Seale AN, Webber SA, Uemura H, *et al.*; British Congenital Cardiac Association. Pulmonary vein stenosis: the UK, Ireland and Sweden collaborative study. *Heart* 2009;95:1944–1949.

Tworetzky W, Wilkins-Haug L, Jennings RW, *et al.* Balloon dilatation of severe aortic stenosis in the fetus. Potential for prevention of hypoplastic left heart syndrome. Candidate selection, technique, and results of successful intervention. *Circulation* 2004;110:2125–2131.

Yun T, Coles JG, Konstantinov IE, *et al.* Conventional and suture-less techniques for management of the pulmonary veins: Evolution of indications from postrepair pulmonary vein stenosis to primary pulmonary vein anomalies. *J Thorac Cardiovasc Surg* 2005;129:167–174.

12 Aortic malformations, rings, and slings

Alex Gooi

Mater Children's Hospital, Brisbane, QLD, Australia

Aortic coarctation

Aortic coarctation usually refers to an area of narrowing of the thoracic aorta where the arterial duct inserts (Figure 12.1); abdominal coarctation is extremely rare. Additional abnormalities of the aortic arch may be present, including aortic arch hypoplasia and hypoplasia of the isthmus, the part of the aorta between the left subclavian artery and arterial duct. There is a spectrum of anomalies from variable degrees of tubular hypoplasia to more discrete coarctation. It can occur in isolation or be associated with other anomalies, including:
- Ventricular septal defect (VSD) (see Chapter 9);
- Bicuspid aortic valve (see Chapter 11);
- Valvar and subvalvar aortic stenosis (see Chapter 11);
- Ascending aortopathy (see Chapter 11);
- Congenital mitral valve anomalies, e.g. parachute mitral valve;
- Supravalvar mitral membrane or stenosing ring (see Chapter 11);
- Tricuspid atresia (see Chapter 16);
- Double inlet left ventricle (see Chapter 16);
- Transposition of the great arteries (see Chapter 14);
- Double outlet right ventricle with subpulmonary VSD (see Chapter 15)

Incidence

Aortic coarctation accounts for 6–8% of live births with congenital heart disease. A higher incidence is found in stillborn infants, with one autopsy study reporting aortic coarctation in 17% of neonates with congenital heart disease. The overall incidence is about 1 in 12 000. One study reported a ratio of males to females of 1.74:1.

Presentation and clinical symptomatology
- Can be diagnosed during fetal life.
- Neonates and infants can present with:
  - Poor feeding
  - Breathlessness
  - Sweating
  - Lethargy
  - Failure to thrive
  - Varying degrees of heart failure
  - Often significant hepatomegaly.
- In severe neonatal coarctation, closure of the arterial duct during the first few days of life may give rise to:
  - Cardiogenic shock
  - Hypotension
  - Mottled and cool lower body and extremities
  - Peripheral cyanosis
  - Renal failure.
  Clinical examination may show:
- Femoral pulses are usually impalpable or considerably weaker than the brachial pulses;
- Left brachial pulse may be weaker than the right brachial pulse if the origin of the left subclavian artery is at the site of coarctation;
- In severe shock, no pulses are palpable;
- Prominent precordial impulse may be palpable unless myocardial function is poor;
- Gallop rhythm;
- Soft systolic murmur at the left sternal edge;
- Ejection click indicating an associated bicuspid aortic valve;
- Hepatomegaly and pulmonary crepitations indicating heart failure;
- Four-limb blood pressures will reveal a gradient between the upper and lower limbs.

Pediatric Heart Disease: A Practical Guide, First Edition. Piers E. F. Daubeney, Michael L. Rigby, Koichiro Niwa, and Michael A. Gatzoulis.
© 2012 Blackwell Publishing Ltd. Published 2012 by Blackwell Publishing Ltd.

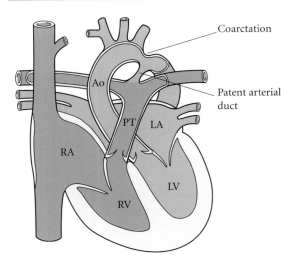

Figure 12.1 Coarctation of the aorta. Coarctation with patent arterial duct, common in neonates. Often patent duct dependent systemic circulation. One of the few pediatric emergencies, with infants presenting with reduced or absent femoral pulses and cardiovascular collapse. Patients require prostaglandin infusion for maintaining patency of the arterial duct until transfer to a cardiothoracic center for prompt coarctation repair. Ao, aorta; LA, left atrium; LV, left ventricle; PT, pulmonary trunk; RA, right atrium; RV, right ventricle. (Adapted from Gatzoulis MA, Swan L, Therrien J, Pantely GA, eds. *Adult Congenital Heart Disease, A Practical Guide*, 2005, with permission from Blackwell Publishing Ltd.)

In older children, aortic coarctation may be diagnosed following discovery of an incidental heart murmur, absence or weakness of the femoral pulses, or systemic hypertension. Weak or absent femoral pulses with a blood pressure gradient between the upper and lower limbs is virtually pathognomonic of aortic coarctation. Late presentation, with the complications of chronic hypertension (subarachnoid hemorrhage, hypertensive encephalopathy or retinopathy), have been reported.

In older children the femoral pulses are absent, diminished, or delayed compared with brachial or radial pulses. The apex beat may be displaced and heaving because of left ventricular hypertrophy. An apical fourth heart sound may be heard with left ventricular diastolic dysfunction. The classical continuous murmur of coarctation is uncommon; it is best heard in the left subclavicular fossa and radiates to the back, peaks late in systole, and continues into early diastole. A continuous murmur can also be caused by significant collateral arteries, which are frequently associated with coarctation in older children.

Investigations

- **EKG:**
  - Normal right ventricular dominance in neonates with extreme right axis deviation
  - Left ventricular hypertrophy in older children.
- **CXR:**
  - Cardiomegaly and pulmonary venous congestion are common in neonates
  - Normal heart size may occur in older children, although left ventricular hypertrophy may cause mild cardiomegaly
  - Two pathognomonic signs, relatively uncommon in the current era are:
    Rib notching, usually bilateral and observed posteriorly in the lower borders of the fourth to eighth ribs, where they are crossed by intercostal arteries
    "3" sign on the left mediastinum, caused by pre- and post-stenotic aortic dilatation.
- **Echocardiography:**
  - Almost always establishes the diagnosis in infancy
  - Can be more challenging in the presence of a widely patent arterial duct
  - Suprasternal cross-sectional echocardiography shows a short narrowed segment just distal to the left subclavian artery caused by a posterior shelf projecting into the aorta
  - The entire aortic arch, head and neck vessels, and aortic valve should be carefully assessed for potential associated anomalies
  - In the absence of an arterial duct, Doppler echocardiography can assess severity of the coarctation
  - Doppler typically shows an extension of antegrade flow and persistent gradient into diastole (the "diastolic tail")
  - Abnormalities of systolic and diastolic function are frequently found, particularly in infancy.

Management
Medical management
The newborn infant with severe coarctation is dependent on the arterial duct to maintain systemic blood flow distal to the site of coarctation. If aortic coarctation is diagnosed or strongly suspected from antenatal screening, it is important to start a prostaglandin E1 infusion at birth. This will maintain patency of the arterial duct. When neonates present with cardiogenic shock (hypotension, low cardiac output, heart failure, acidosis, and impaired

renal function), prostaglandin can be used to dilate the patent arterial duct, allowing clinical improvement and safe transport to a cardiac center. Metabolic derangements should be corrected prior to surgical repair. By the age of 2 weeks in the term infant, prostaglandin has no effect.

Surgical repair
Common techniques of repair include:
- Resection and end-to-end anastomosis;
- Subclavian flap aortoplasty;
- Extended end-to-end repair.

Percutaneous balloon angioplasty is rarely performed in the neonate or small infant because the outcome compares unfavorably with that of surgery. However, it is often the preferred form of treatment for older children and adults, and patients with recurrent coarctation after surgical repair.

Complications of surgery
- **Early:**
  - Bleeding due to leakage from suture lines (rare)
  - Acute hypertension
  - Vocal cord paresis/paralysis
  - Horner syndrome
  - Diaphragmatic paralysis
  - Chylothorax from damage to the thoracic duct
  - Spinal cord injury due to poor collaterals (rare).

- **Late:**
  - Recoarctation
  - Ascending aortopathy and aneurysm formation
  - Hypertension
  - Premature late death from coronary artery disease and stroke.

Late complications and long-term outcome
See Chapter 31.

Key clinical points
- Weak or absent femoral pulses with blood pressure gradient between upper and lower limbs is virtually pathognomonic of aortic coarctation.
- If significant coarctation diagnosed or strongly suspected from antenatal scanning, important to start a prostaglandin E1 infusion at birth prior to transfer to a cardiac center.

Interrupted aortic arch

Interruption of the aorta (IAA) occurs when there is complete anatomic discontinuity between two adjacent segments of the aortic arch (Figure 12.2). It has been classified into three types.

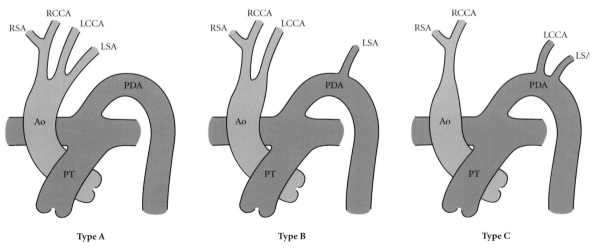

Type A	**Type B**	**Type C**

Figure 12.2 Schematic diagram showing the three subtypes of interrupted aortic arch. Type A: interruption distal to the left subclavian artery. Type B: interruption between left subclavian and left common carotid arteries. Type C: interruption between the brachiocephalic and left common carotid arteries. Ao, aorta; LCCA, left common carotid artery; LSA, left subclavian artery; PDA, patent arterial duct; PT, pulmonary trunk; RCCA, right common carotid artery; RSA, right subclavian artery.

> **Types of interrupted aortic arch**
> • **Type A:** Interruption distal to the left subclavian artery
> • **Type B:** Interruption between the left subclavian and left common carotid arteries (the most common)
> • **Type C:** Interruption between the brachiocephalic and left common carotid arteries (the least common)

It is almost always associated with a VSD but aortic interruption with an intact ventricular septum is encountered.

The VSD can be perimembranous or has a muscular posteroinferior rim. Typically there is posterior deviation of the outlet septum resulting in varying degrees of sub-aortic stenosis. In cases with a doubly committed subar-terial defect there will not be subaortic stenosis.

The aortic valve is frequently bicuspid and aortic valve stenosis may occur. The aortic valve size is often small.

Other associated anomalies are:
• Common arterial trunk (truncus arteriosus) (see Chapter 16);
• Double inlet left ventricle with discordant ventricular–arterial connection (see Chapter 16);
• Complete transposition of the great arteries (see Chapter 14);
• Double outlet right ventricle with subpulmonary VSD (see Chapter 15).

Incidence
The overall incidence of interrupted aortic arch is about 1% of congenital heart defects. The sex incidence is equal. There is a high incidence of chromosome 22q11 deletion (DiGeorge, velocardiofacial, Shprintzen syndromes) in those with type B interruption.

Presentation and clinical symptomatology
As with other duct-dependent obstructive left heart lesions, IAA tends to present soon after birth with acute-onset heart failure and shock simultaneous with arterial duct closure. The symptoms are similar to those previously described for aortic coarctation.

The most specific diagnostic sign is palpation of dif-ferential upper body pulses:
• Weak left arm and femoral pulses with normal right arm and carotid pulses occur in type B IAA;
• If the left carotid pulse is also weak, then type C IAA is suspected;
• If only the femoral pulses are weak, it is impossible to distinguish between type A IAA and aortic coarctation.

Auscultative findings are usually unhelpful.

Investigations
• **EKG:**
  ○ May be normal
  ○ Typically right ventricular dominance and hypertro-phy present
  ○ QT interval is occasionally prolonged secondary to hypocalcemia of DiGeorge syndrome.
• **CXR:**
  ○ Cardiomegaly and increased pulmonary vascular markings with pulmonary venous congestion in infants
  ○ Narrow mediastinum may suggest absent thymus gland, a feature of DiGeorge syndrome.
• **Echocardiography:** Diagnostic method of choice as it allows imaging of the aorta, the site of interruption, the anatomy of the great arteries, and other associated defects.

Management
Medical management
• Stabilization of the infant is as for duct-dependent aortic coarctation (see above).
• Chromosomes analysis, especially fluorescent *in situ* hybridization (FISH) test to look for 22q11 deletion.
• Hypocalcemia should be anticipated and treated.
• Assays of T-cell number and function should be sent as abnormalities in T-cell function can occur in DiGeorge syndrome. Before results are known, irradiated blood should be used to avoid the possibility of transfused lym-phocytes causing graft-versus-host disease.

Surgical repair
• One-stage repair with direct end-to-end or end-to-side anastomosis of the distal arch to the ascending aorta.
• Standard closure of the VSD.
• Resection of the subaortic stenosis where present.
• Interposed Dacron graft to restore continuity of the arch if direct anastomosis is not possible.
• In those unsuitable for biventricular repair because of extreme hypoplasia of the aortic valve and ascending aorta, management is similar to the hypoplastic left heart syndrome with initial palliation being a Norwood opera-tion or Damus–Kaye–Stansell procedure (see Chapter 16).

Complications
• **Early:**
  ○ Bleeding due to leakage from suture lines
  ○ Vocal cord paresis/paralysis
  ○ Horner syndrome
  ○ Diaphragmatic paralysis
  ○ Chylothorax from damage to the thoracic duct.

- **Late:**
  - Aortic arch stenosis/recoarctation
  - Subaortic stenosis
  - Aortic valve stenosis.

Key clinical points

- High incidence of chromosome 22q11 deletion (DiGeorge, Velocardiofacial, Shprintzen syndromes) in those with type B interruption.
- Before 22q11 deletion status is clarified, irradiated blood should be used to avoid the possibility of transfused lymphocytes causing graft-versus-host disease.

Vascular ring

Vascular ring comprises a variety of vascular malformations in which there is encirclement of the trachea and esophagus by vascular structures, causing tracheal and/or esophageal compression often associated with tracheomalacia.

Common examples of vascular ring

- **Double aortic arch:** Most commonly both arches are patent, the right being larger than the left, with a left arterial duct and left descending aorta. Occasionally, there is anatomic continuity but luminal atresia of one arch, usually the left. Atresia can be between the left common carotid artery and the left subclavian artery, or distal to the left subclavian artery. A double aortic arch can be associated with other congenital heart defects such as tetralogy of Fallot, VSD, aortic coarctation, patent arterial duct and common arterial trunk.
- **Aberrant subclavian artery with an ipsilateral duct:** A vascular ring is formed when the anomalous subclavian artery arises distally and there is a duct on the same side (Figure 12.3). If the duct arises from the subclavian artery itself, the ring is usually loose. If the duct arises from an aortic diverticulum (diverticulum of Kommerel), the ring will be tight. Right aortic arch with an aberrant left subclavian artery is far more likely to produce a clinically important ring than a left aortic arch with an aberrant right subclavian artery.

Presentation and clinical symptomatology

Symptoms vary with the severity of compression by the abnormal vessel on the trachea, bronchus or esophagus. Patients present with:

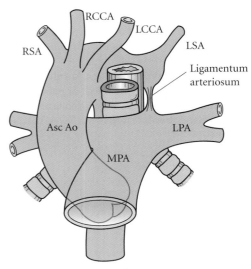

Figure 12.3 Vascular ring right aortic arch with aberrant left subclavian artery arising from an aortic diverticulum (diverticulum of Kommerel) forming a vascular ring. Note the encircling of the trachea and esophagus by the ring. Asc Ao, ascending aorta; LCCA, left common carotid artery; LPA, left pulmonary artery; LSA, left subclavian artery; MPA, main pulmonary artery; RCCA, right common carotid artery; RSA right subclavian artery.

- Stridor (inspiratory or biphasic);
- Wheezing;
- Cough exacerbated by crying, exertion, and upper respiratory chest infection;
- Dysphagia (quite rare);
- May be history of recurrent chest infection.

  Patients with a double aortic arch tend to develop symptoms earlier, usually in the first few months of life.

Investigations

- **Barium esophagraphy:**
  - Non-invasive and useful screening tool
  - In patients with stridor, posterior indentation of the esophagus can be considered diagnostic
  - Does not allow precise anatomic diagnosis.
- **Echocardiography:** usually provides an accurate diagnosis but additional imaging is often required.
- **High-resolution CT angiography with 3D reconstruction:** preferred diagnostic tool in most cardiac centers.
- **Cardiac MRI or angiography:** alternative to CT angiography.

Management

Surgical intervention is indicated whenever there is significant airway narrowing and/or dysphagia. Almost always it can be performed through a left lateral thoracotomy. In double aortic arch, the smaller or atretic of the two arches should be divided. In patients with a right aortic arch, aberrant left subclavian artery, and left duct, division of the duct usually relieves the airway obstruction.

Complications

- Chylothorax
- Aortoesophageal fistula
- Vocal cord paresis/paralysis
- Prolonged postoperative ventilation because of tracheomalacia

Pulmonary artery sling

In this rare anomaly, there is anomalous origin of the left pulmonary artery from the right pulmonary artery (Figure 12.4). It then passes over the right main bronchus and courses posterior to the trachea to reach the hilum of the left lung. It usually occurs in isolation but can be associated with other congenital cardiac anomalies such as:

- VSD (see Chapter 9);
- ASD (see Chapter 9);
- Patent arterial duct (see Chapter 9);
- Aortic coarctation (see Chapter 12);
- Tetralogy of Fallot with right aortic arch (see Chapter 15);

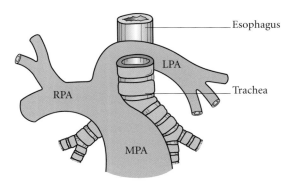

Figure 12.4 Pulmonary artery sling. Anomalous origin of the left pulmonary artery (LPA) from the right pulmonary artery (RPA). It then passes over the right main bronchus and courses posterior to the trachea to reach the hilum of the left lung thereby creating a "sling". MPA, main pulmonary artery.

- Double inlet left ventricle (see Chapter 16);
- Persistent left superior vena cava;
- Common arterial trunk with an interrupted aortic arch (see Chapter 16).

There is a high incidence of associated tracheobronchial abnormalities, including tracheobronchomalacia, hypoplasia of the distal trachea, stenosis of the left main bronchus, and direct origin of the right epiarterial bronchus from the trachea.

Presentation and clinical symptomatology

Compression of the right main bronchus and distal end of the trachea causes predominantly expiratory stridor, wheezing, and cough. Symptoms may begin in the neonatal period and severe airway obstruction may lead to death in the first few months of life. In other cases milder symptoms persist for many years and patients are thought to have asthma.

Investigations

- **CXR:**
  - May demonstrate hyperinflation of right lung with mediastinal shift to the left
  - In severe right main bronchus obstruction the right lung may be atelectatic.
- **Barium esophagraphy:**
  - Useful non-invasive study
  - In the lateral view an anterior indentation of the esophagus by the aberrant left pulmonary artery.
- **Echocardiography:**
  - Usually diagnostic
  - Anomalous origin of the left from the right pulmonary artery is easy to demonstrate.
- **CT angiography/MRI:** Demonstrate the anatomy and extent of any serious abnormalities of the airways.
- **Cardiac catheterization and angiography:** Usually unnecessary in the current era.

Management

This involves surgical repair with cardiopulmonary bypass to reimplant the left pulmonary artery into the pulmonary trunk anterior to the trachea. Associated airway abnormalities rarely require correction at the time of surgery.

Complications

Prolonged postoperative ventilation because of tracheomalacia or other airway abnormality is sometimes required. Late origin stenosis of the left pulmonary artery requiring treatment by balloon angioplasty or stenting is occasionally required.

Aorto-left ventricular tunnel

An extremely rare defect with a male-to-female frequency of 2:1, aorto-left ventricular tunnel comprises an endothelialized channel connecting the ascending aorta above the right coronary sinus to the left ventricle. The hemodynamic effect is that of severe aortic regurgitation; aorto-left ventricular tunnel should be included in the differential diagnosis of any neonate, infant or child with severe aortic regurgitation.

It usually occurs in isolation but associated cardiac defects can occur: bicuspid aortic valve with aortic stenosis or regurgitation, patent arterial duct, VSD, and pulmonary stenosis.

Presentation and clinical symptomatology

Symptoms and signs depend on the size of the tunnel and the severity of aortic regurgitation. Congestive cardiac failure can occur in early life but the clinical presentation is extremely variable, occurring at any time from birth to adult life.

A wide pulse pressure and loud systolic and diastolic to-and-fro murmurs at the base of the heart are frequent findings.

Investigations
- **EKG:**
  - Left ventricular hypertrophy
  - Left-sided T wave inversion may be present.
- **CXR:** Cardiomegaly.
- **Echocardiography:**
  - Will establish the diagnosis
  - Severity of aortic insufficiency.

Management

Early surgical intervention will prevent progressive damage to the aortic valve or deformity of the aortic root. In selected cases, interventional cardiac catheterization with occlusion of the tunnel is an alternative option in experienced hands.

Key clinical points
- In any neonate, infant or child with severe aortic regurgitation, aorto-left ventricular tunnel should be included in the differential diagnosis.
- Early diagnosis and intervention can prevent dilation of the aortic root and distortion of the aortic valve leaflets

---

Aneurysm of the sinuses of Valsalva

This rare defect may be congenital or acquired. Congenital aneurysms result from a weakness in the sinus, which produces a downward prolapse. The dilated sinus may bulge into an atrium or ventricle and may rupture. It is rare in infancy and childhood. The right coronary aortic sinus is the most commonly affected, the least frequent being the left coronary sinus.

Aneurysms of the right coronary sinus usually prolapse into the right ventricle or right atrium. An aneurysm of the non-coronary sinus will rupture into the right atrium and the left coronary sinus into the left ventricle. Rupture into the right heart chambers is most frequent.

Aneurysms may be acquired through bacterial endocarditis. However, endocarditis can also occur on a congenital aneurysm. It can be difficult to distinguish between the two, although congenital aneurysms are frequently associated with a VSD. Some cases are examples of aortic valve prolapse associated with a doubly committed or perimembranous VSD in which the aortic sinus has completely occluded the defect.

Presentation and clinical symptomatology

An aneurysm of an aortic sinus rarely causes angina or even myocardial infarction from compression of a coronary artery.

Rupture of an aneurysm may produce central chest pain and sudden dyspnea from a large left-to-right shunt and aortic regurgitation. The sudden onset of a low diastolic pressure may result in acute renal failure.

Investigations
- **EKG:**
  - Left or biventricular hypertrophy
  - Left-sided T wave inversion.
- **Echocardiography:**
  - Dilatation of the aortic root
  - Severe aortic insufficiency with left ventricular volume overload
  - Color flow mapping can assess the severity of aortic regurgitation
  - Transesophageal echocardiography – demonstrates the anatomy in more detail and is perhaps superior in some individuals.

Management

Aneurysms can be repaired through an incision in the ascending aorta, through the right ventricle or the right atrium. Resuspension of the aortic valve leaflets may be required to reduce aortic regurgitation.

It is debatable whether an incidental finding of an aneurysm in an asymptomatic patient requires repair.

Small defects in an aortic sinus have been closed by interventional cardiac catheterization in selected patients.

Complications

• Recurrence of the aneurysm.
• Worsening of aortic regurgitation following surgery.

Further reading

Anderson RH, Baker EJ, Macartney FJ, Shinebourne EA, Rigby ML, Tynan MJ, eds. *Paediatric Cardiology*, 2nd edn. Edinburgh: Churchill Livingstone, 2002.

Garson A Jr, Bricker JT, Fisher DJ, Neish SR. *The Science and Practice of Paediatric Cardiology*, 2nd edn. Philadelphia: Williams & Wilkins, 1998.

13 Coronary artery lesions

Alex Gooi

Mater Children's Hospital, Brisbane, QLD, Australia

Normal coronary arterial anatomy

The right coronary artery (RCA) arises from the right sinus of Valsalva. It enters the atrioventricular groove, courses backward and inferiorly, and usually terminates in the posterior interventricular groove. It gives rise to infundibular, sinus, and atrioventricular nodal branches. In about 50% of people, there is a separate origin of the infundibular branch.

The left coronary artery (LCA) arises from the left sinus of Valsalva and emerges perpendicularly for a few millimeters before bifurcating into a left anterior descending (LAD) and a circumflex (LCx) branch. The former traverses the anterior interventricular groove, while the latter courses around the left atrioventricular groove.

These three principal arteries each provide tributaries to the atrial and ventricular myocardium. The ventricular myocardium is perfused only during diastole.

Anomalous left coronary artery from the pulmonary artery

The LCA originates typically from the pulmonary trunk, although origin from the right pulmonary artery is encountered (Figure 13.1).

Incidence
This is an extremely rare anomaly, accounting for 1 in 250–400 of all cases of congenital heart disease. The male-to-female incidence is documented at 2.3:1.

Pathophysiology
Anomalous left coronary artery from the pulmonary artery (ALCAPA) is rarely diagnosed during antenatal screening because the favorable fetal physiology includes:

- Similar pressures in the main pulmonary artery and aorta;
- Relatively high oxygen content of blood in the pulmonary artery.

At birth, although the first breath and expansion of the lungs causes an immediate fall in pulmonary vascular resistance, the pulmonary arterial pressure remains sufficiently elevated for adequate left ventricular myocardial perfusion from the LCA during the first 2 months of life. Typically in the third month, the continuing fall in pulmonary vascular resistance results in reduced perfusion pressure into the anomalous coronary artery. Eventually the flow reverses so that the LCA drains into the pulmonary trunk, leading to coronary artery steal. This results in early left ventricular ischemia and infarction with angina, ventricular dysfunction, and heart failure.

Collateral connections between the RCA and LCA systems develop and, because the left ventricular myocardium is then effectively perfused from the RCA, significant ischemia may be prevented. However, even in this group left ventricular myocardial perfusion may not be sufficient to prevent left ventricular dysfunction, myocardial fibrosis, and mitral insufficiency secondary to papillary muscle dysfunction presenting in later childhood or early adult life.

ALCAPA should be considered in the differential diagnosis of childhood dilated cardiomyopathy.

Presentation and clinical symptomatology
Symptoms of congestive heart failure are:
- Tachypnea;
- Sweating;
- Poor feeding;
- Lethargy;
- Failure to thrive after 2 months of age.

Angina can be brought on by the stress of feeding or defecation; the infant suddenly appears to be in severe

Pediatric Heart Disease: A Practical Guide, First Edition. Piers E. F. Daubeney, Michael L. Rigby, Koichiro Niwa, and Michael A. Gatzoulis.
© 2012 Blackwell Publishing Ltd. Published 2012 by Blackwell Publishing Ltd.

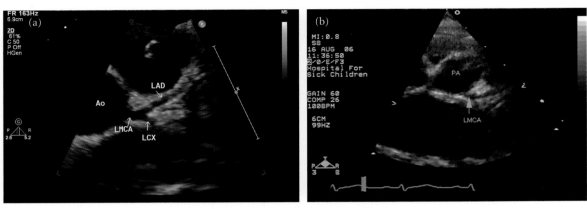

Figure 13.1 (a) Echocardiogram in the parasternal short axis view showing normal origin of the left main coronary artery (LMCA) and its branches from the aorta. (b) Parasternal short axis view showing anomalous origin of the left main coronary artery (LMCA) from the pulmonary artery (PA), as seen in ALCAPA. Ao, aortic root; LAD, left anterior descending; LCX, left circumflex; LMCA, left main coronary artery; PA, pulmonary artery; RV, right ventricle.

distress, grunting or crying in short gasps, and is dyspneic, gray, and sweaty. Such irritable episodes have often been attributed to infantile colic, delaying the diagnosis and allowing progressive myocardial ischemia.

Physical examination often reveals:
• Overactive precordium;
• Inferior/lateral displacement of the cardiac apex which has a dyskinetic quality;
• Fourth heart sound gallop rhythm;
• Apical pan-systolic murmur of mitral regurgitation and apical diastolic rumble may be heard.
A child who has escaped myocardial ischemia because of early collateralization in infancy may present on a routine examination with an unexplained heart murmur, mild cardiomegaly, and/ or an abnormal EKG.

In rare instances, myocardial ischemia may first present in childhood, adolescence or young adult life, with typical angina pectoris, syncope, arrhythmias, or even sudden or near-miss death.

Investigations

• **EKG** may show (Figure 13.2):
   ○ Sinus tachycardia
   ○ Pathologic Q waves
   ○ Abnormalities of the QRS and ST–T segments compatible with anterior, anteroseptal, or anterolateral infarction
   ○ Rarely, premature ventricular contractions or ventricular tachycardia.

• **CXR** in infants with heart failure commonly shows:
   ○ Cardiomegaly
   ○ Left atrial enlargement
   ○ Pulmonary venous congestion.
• **Echocardiography:**
   ○ 2D and color flow mapping are often diagnostic and almost always replace the need for cardiac catheterization, angiography, or other imaging
   ○ Identifies the abnormal origin of the LCA arising from the main pulmonary artery
   ○ Caution: the transverse sinus of the pericardium may be confused with a normal origin of the LCA, leading to a false-negative diagnosis
   ○ Color flow and Doppler mapping enhances the diagnostic accuracy by demonstrating retrograde flow in the LCA and into the pulmonary trunk during diastole. This retrograde flow is dependent on the development of collaterals between the LCA and RCA systems, and may be absent if collateralization has not occurred (as with early presentation)
   ○ Abnormal dilatation of the proximal RCA, when present, reflects development of extensive collateralization between the RCA and LCA systems in patients presenting later in childhood
   ○ Left ventricular dilatation and dysfunction, dilated cardiomyopathy, functional or ischemic mitral insufficiency, and myocardial fibrosis are frequently observed.
• **Cardiac catheterization and angiography:**
   ○ Performed if echocardiography is not diagnostic
   ○ Aortography or selective right coronary arteriography usually shows early filling of an enlarged RCA

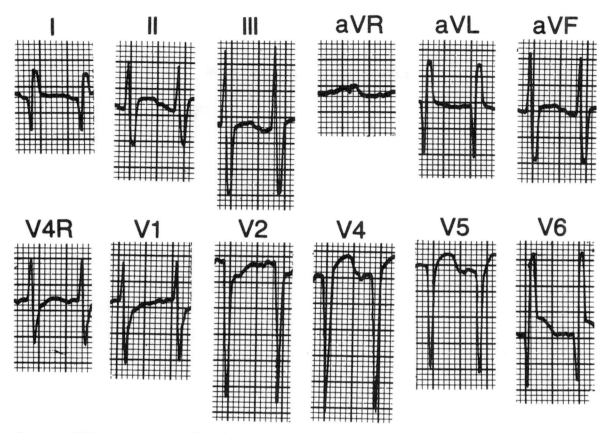

Figure 13.2 EKG in anomalous origin of the left coronary from the pulmonary artery (ALCAPA). This is a highly abnormal EKG with pathologic Q waves and ST segment elevation, particularly in the precordial leads V4–6, and reciprocal changes in V4R, V1–2.

system with delayed passage via collateralization into the LCA and eventual reflux of contrast into the pulmonary arterial system

  ○ If collateralization is poor, the pulmonary trunk does not opacify; pulmonary angiography may opacify the LCA system.
• **CT angiography/MRI with 3D reconstruction:** May aid diagnosis and is replacing coronary angiography.

Management
Medical management
• Initial management is both supportive and temporary. Treatment of congestive heart failure requires careful and balanced use of diuretics, afterload reducing agents, and inotropic drugs.
• Aggressive afterload reduction will lead to hypotension, which can reduce RCA perfusion, leading to decreased LCA blood flow.

• Inotropic agents, on the other hand, may significantly increase myocardial oxygen consumption, which may result in worsening ischemia in the presence of reduced myocardial perfusion.
• Excessive oxygen may also be deleterious. Oxygen reduces pulmonary vascular resistance, thereby increasing steal from the LCA.

Surgical repair
Current surgical procedures are aimed at establishing revascularization by creating a two coronary artery system. There can then be normalization of the left ventricular systolic function and improved long-term survival. Common techniques include:
• **Direct reimplantation:** Experience gained in reimplanting coronary arteries during the arterial switch procedure for complete transposition of the great arteries has made this approach the most popular.

• **Takeuchi procedure:** Creation of an aortopulmonary window and an intrapulmonary tunnel extending from the anomalous ostium to the window.

• **Bypass grafting** using carotid and internal mammary arteries and then the saphenous vein is now performed infrequently.

• **Ligation of the LCA at its origin** from the main pulmonary artery is an original technique, performed without the use of cardiopulmonary bypass. The long-term results were not optimal since myocardial perfusion remained solely dependent on extensive collateralization from the RCA, and the patient remained at risk of ischemic episodes and sudden death. This technique has been abandoned.

• **Simultaneous mitral valve repair**, in the presence of significant incompetence, is often unnecessary because spontaneous improvement of mitral valve function often occurs following surgical revascularization.

• **Heart transplantation**: In the small group of patients with profoundly impaired cardiac function from extensive myocardial damage, heart transplantation may be a more desirable option.

Key clinical points

• In ALCAPA, echocardiography demonstrates the LCA arising from the pulmonary trunk.

• Color flow Doppler in the vessel usually shows flow from the LCA to the pulmonary artery once outside the neonatal period.

• The transverse sinus of the pericardium may be confused with normal origin of the LCA, leading to a false-negative diagnosis.

• Consider a diagnosis of ALCAPA in all cases of childhood dilated cardiomyopathy.

Coronary artery fistula

A coronary artery fistula is a congenital or acquired anomaly characterized by communications between branches of the coronary arteries and another large vessel or cardiac chamber (Figure 13.3). Fistulae vary from simple direct connections to complex, worm-like aneurysmal cavities in which blood may stagnate, clot, and calcify.

The majority of congenital coronary artery fistulae arise from the RCA or LAD; the left circumflex coronary artery is rarely involved. The fistula can drain into any of the following: superior vena cava, coronary sinus, right

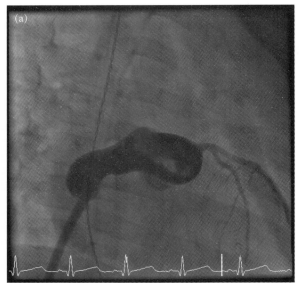

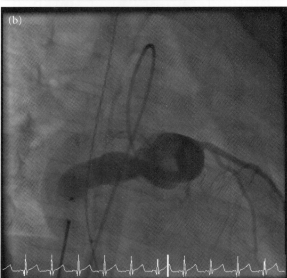

Figure 13.3 Large left coronary artery fistula to the right atrium. (a) Angiogram shows the LCA and fistula following introduction of a long femoral venous sheath into the exit of the fistula into the right atrium. (b) Coil occlusion of the fistula. Repeat angiography shows no remaining shunt.

atrium, right ventricle, pulmonary artery, pulmonary vein, left atrium, or left ventricle.

The acquired causes of coronary fistulae, which are rare in childhood, include atherosclerosis, Takayasu arteritis (see Chapter 27), and trauma.

A left-to-right shunt exists in more than 90% of cases. The largest shunts tend to occur in those draining to the right heart because of the greater pressure gradients.

Coronary fistulae associated with pulmonary or aortic atresia with intact ventricular septum are discussed in Chapters 15 and 16 respectively.

Incidence
Angiographic series reveal an incidence of 0.3–0.8%.

Presentation and clinical symptomatology
Clinical presentation is dependent on the severity of the left-to-right shunt.
- **Infancy:** Symptoms of congestive heart failure may occur although the majority is symptom-free.
- **Older children or adolescents:**
  - Usually asymptomatic
  - Presenting physical finding that brings them to the cardiologist is a continuous murmur over the precordium; the murmur may resemble that of an arterial duct, except that the murmur is often heard maximally in unusual locations, and may peak in diastole rather than during systolic ejection.
- **Other rare modes of presentation:** Include exercise intolerance, dyspnea, angina, arrhythmia, endocarditis, stroke, myocardial ischemia, or myocardial infarction.

Investigations
- **Echocardiography with color flow mapping:**
  - Demonstrates site of origin, course, and site of entry of the fistula
  - Guided by color flow map, pulsed and continuous wave Doppler can confirm the nature of the disturbed flow at the site of entry.
- **Cardiac catheterization with aortography/selective coronary angiography** (see Figure 13.3):
  - Identifies the size and anatomic features of the fistula
  - Relation of the coronary artery fistula to other structures, and their origin and course may not always be apparent.
- **CT angiography or MRI with 3D reconstruction:** Can be used as an adjunct to coronary angiography.

Management
Medical management
- Antiplatelet therapy recommended, especially in patients with distal coronary artery fistulae and abnormally dilated coronary arteries.
- Endocarditis prophylaxis is not now recommended, although bacterial endocarditis is a known complication.

Surgical/interventional closure
- Main indications for closure are congestive heart failure, myocardial ischemia, or the perceived risk of myocardial ischemia in the future when the fistula is large.
- Surgery and direct epicardial or endocardial ligation was a traditional method of closure of a coronary fistula.
- Transcatheter closure has been performed and is now recognized as an effective and safe treatment (see Figure 13.3). A variety of devices, including controlled-release patent ductus arteriosus coils, ductal occluders, or vascular plugs can be used. The various techniques employed are the exclusive domain of the specialist interventional cardiologist in congenital heart disease.

Complications
- If left untreated, coronary fistulae can result in complications such as fistulous "steal" from the neighboring myocardium, with ischemia, atherosclerotic changes at points of stress, thrombosis and embolization, rupture, and endocarditis.
- After closure, long-term follow-up is essential because of the possibility of recanalization, persistent dilatation of the coronary artery and ostium, thrombus formation, calcification, and myocardial ischemia.

Aberrant course with myocardial ischemia

A single coronary artery or both coronary arteries can arise from the right sinus of Valsalva, with the left branch coursing between the aorta and pulmonary trunk and subject to compression (Figure 13.4). Sudden unexplained death in adolescents and young adults, especially during heavy exertion, has been reported. An intramural course can further complicate this anomaly and may well be the most important cause of ischemia.

In contrast, when a single coronary arises from the left sinus of Valsalva, or both coronaries arise from separate orifices in that sinus, with the RCA coursing between the aorta and subpulmonary infundibulum, compression can occur with or without an intramural course, but sudden death is unusual, probably because of the relatively low perfusion pressure required for the right ventricle (Figure 13.4).

A myocardial bridge refers to an intramyocardial course of a segment of a proximal coronary artery, rarely

(a)

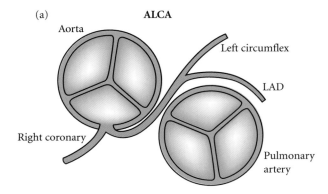

(b)

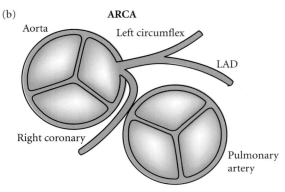

Figure 13.4 Schematic diagram of anomalous course of the coronary arteries. (a) Anomalous course of the left coronary artery (ALCA). Left coronary artery arising from the right sinus and coursing between the aorta and pulmonary trunk. (b) Anomalous course of the right coronary artery (ARCA). Right coronary artery arising from the left sinus and coursing between the aorta and pulmonary trunk. LAD, left anterior descending branch.

resulting in compression and myocardial ischemia with risk of sudden death.

A coronary artery may originate from an artery other than the aorta, such as an intercostal or internal thoracic artery. If subject to compression along its course, it may result in sudden unexplained death during heavy exertion.

Stenosis or atresia of the coronary arteries

Stenosis or atresia of the main stem of the left coronary artery

This very rare anomaly results from failure of canalization or involution of the proximal LCA. The perfusion of left ventricular myocardium then depends on collateral blood flow from the RCA. The diagnosis should be considered in cases of unexplained neonatal myocardial ischemia or infarction.

Pulmonary atresia with intact ventricular septum (see Chapter 15)

Right ventricular-to-coronary connections "fistulae" can occur particularly where there is right ventricular hypoplasia and a hypertensive right ventriculum. The coronary artery with fistulous connection is then exposed to suprasystemic right ventricular pressures and can respond by developing coronary artery stenoses, interruptions, ectasia, or atresia. This is termed "right ventricular dependence" and is discussed further in Chapter 15.

Further reading

Anderson RH, Baker EJ, Macartney FJ, Shinebourne EA, Rigby ML, Tynan MJ, eds. *Paediatric Cardiology*, 2nd edn. London: Churchill Livingstone Harcourt Publishers Limited, 2002.

Chetlin MD, de Castro CM, McAllister HA. Sudden death as a complication of anomalous left coronary origin from the anterior sinus of Valsalva, a not so minor congenital anomaly. *Circulation* 1974;50:780–787.

Garson A Jr, Bricker JT, Fisher DJ, Neish SR. *The Science And Practice Of Paediatric Cardiology*, 2nd edn. Philadelphia: Williams & Wilkins, 1998.

Gowda RM, Vasavada BC, Khan IA. Coronary artery fistulas: Clinical and therapeutic considerations. *Int J Cardiol* 2006; 107:7–10.

Neufeld HN, Schneeweis A, eds. Coronary artery disease in infants and children. Philadelphia: Lea & Febiger, 1983, p. 1.

Weber HS. Anomalous left coronary artery from the pulmonary artery. *e Medicine*, Feb 2006.

14 Transposition and transposition complexes

Georgios Giannakoulas[1,2] and Michael A. Gatzoulis[2,3]

[1]Ahepa Hospital, Aristole University, Thessaloniki, Greece
[2]Royal Brompton Hospital, London, UK
[3]National Heart and Lung Institute, Imperial College, London, UK

Transposition of the great arteries

In complete transposition of the great arteries (TGA), there is atrioventricular (AV) concordance and ventricular–arterial (VA) discordance, i.e. the right atrium connects to the morphologic right ventricle, which gives rise to the aorta, and the left atrium connects to the morphologic left ventricle, which gives rise to the pulmonary artery (Figure 14.1). Consequently, the pulmonary and systemic circulations are connected in parallel rather than the normal in series connection (Figure 14.2). This situation is incompatible with life unless a communication between the two circulations exists, either with an atrial septal defect (ASD), a ventricular septal defect (VSD), or at the great arterial level (patent ductus arteriosus [PDA]). Complete TGA is also known as d-TGA; the "d-" refers to the dextroposition of the bulboventricular loop, i.e. the position of the right ventricle (RV), which is on the right side. The most common relationship of the great arteries is an anterior and rightward position of the aorta relative to the pulmonary artery (95% of cases). Many other arrangements have been recognized, the most common being an anterior but leftward position of the aorta. In rare cases the aorta is the posterior vessel.

Common associated lesions are:
- VSD – almost 50% of cases;
- Left ventricular outflow tract obstruction (LVOTO) – up to 25%;
- Coarctation of the aorta – about 5%.

In approximately one-third of patients with TGA, the coronary artery anatomy is abnormal, with the left circumflex artery arising from the right coronary artery (22%), a single right coronary artery (9.5%), a single left coronary artery (3%), or inverted origin of the coronary arteries (3%) representing the most common variants. The most important variation from a management perspective occurs when one coronary artery takes an intramural course between the aorta and pulmonary artery (3% of all cases).

Incidence and etiology

TGA is the most common form of cyanotic congenital heart disease presenting in the neonatal period. Of all forms of cyanotic congenital heart disease, only tetralogy of Fallot is more common. TGA represents approximately 5–7% of all congenital heart disease and has a birth incidence of 20–30 in 100 000 live births, with a male preponderance of approximately 2:1. There has been a small number of reports of possible genetic associations but in the great majority of cases, TGA is not currently known to be associated with any specific single gene defects. There has been some suggestion that TGA in human fetuses may be related to maternal intrauterine hormonal imbalance. There is also a higher than expected incidence of TGA in infants of diabetic mothers.

Clinical features
Presentation
The clinical course and manifestations depend on the extent of cardiac or extracardiac mixing and the presence of associated anatomic lesions. Neonates with TGA and intact ventricular septum present with prominent and progressive cyanosis within the first 24 h of life. In the case of TGA with VSD, infants may not initially manifest symptoms of heart disease, although mild cyanosis (particularly when crying) is often noted. Symptoms and

Pediatric Heart Disease: A Practical Guide, First Edition. Piers E. F. Daubeney, Michael L. Rigby, Koichiro Niwa, and Michael A. Gatzoulis.
© 2012 Blackwell Publishing Ltd. Published 2012 by Blackwell Publishing Ltd.

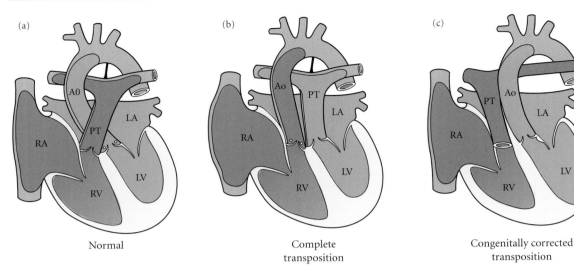

Normal

Complete
transposition

Congenitally corrected
transposition

Figure 14.1 (a) A structurally normal heart with normal spiraling of the great arteries. (b) Transposition of the great arteries (discordant ventricular-arterial connection). Note the parallel great arteries with the aorta to the right. (c) Congenitally corrected transposition (discordant atrioventricular and ventricular-arterial connections). Again note the parallel great vessels but with the aorta to the left. Ao, aorta; LA, left atrium; LV, left ventricle; PT, pulmonary trunk; RA, right atrium; RV, right ventricle. (Adapted from Gatzoulis MA, Swan L, Therrien J, Pantely GA, eds. *Adult Congenital Heart Disease, A Practical Guide*, 2005, with permission from Blackwell Publishing Ltd.)

(a)

	RA	LA	
Body			Lungs
	RV	LV	

(b)

	RA	LA	
Body			Lungs
	RV	LV	

Figure 14.2 (a) Normal circulation where the systemic and pulmonary blood flows are in series. (b) Circulation in transposition of the great arteries (TGA) where the systemic and pulmonary blood flows are in parallel. The red color denotes oxygenated blood, blue deoxygenated. Clearly this is a lethal circuit unless there are mixing points at atrial (ASD or patent foramen ovale), ventricular (VSD) or great vessel sites (PDA). LA, left atrium; LV, left ventricle; RA, right atrium; RV, right ventricle.

signs of congestive heart failure (tachypnea, tachycardia, diaphoresis, and failure to gain weight) may become evident over the first 3–6 weeks as pulmonary blood flow increases. Infants with TGA, VSD, and LVOTO may present with extreme cyanosis at birth, proportional to the degree of left ventricular (subpulmonary) outflow tract obstruction. The clinical scenario may be similar to that of an infant with tetralogy of Fallot. Finally, children with TGA and a large VSD may survive into adulthood without any intervention and present with late pulmonary hypertension.

Physical examination

Newborns with TGA usually have good somatic growth and no dysmorphic features. Physical findings at presentation depend solely on the presence of associated lesions. Newborns are typically pink at birth but become progressively cyanotic as the duct closes. When the ventricular septum is intact, infants usually become cyanotic in the first day of life.

The remainder of the cardiac examination reveals a murmurless heart in the absence of associated lesions. S2 is single and loud because of the relationship of the great arteries, the aortic valve being anterior behind the sternum. Patients with a previous atrial switch procedure usually have a right ventricular lift, a normal S1, a single loud S2, and a pan-systolic murmur from tricuspid regurgitation, if present. Patients with an arterial switch have in general a normal physical examination. A diastolic murmur from neoaortic valve regurgitation and systolic ejection murmur from right ventricular outflow tract obstruction (RVOTO) may be present.

Investigations

- **EKG:**
  - Newborns with TGA have evidence of right axis deviation and right ventricular hypertrophy
  - Atrial switch: Sinus bradycardia or junctional rhythm with evidence of right-axis deviation and right ventricular hypertrophy
  - Arterial switch: EKG is typically normal, but care should be taken to exclude signs of myocardial ischemia and right ventricular hypertrophy suggesting pulmonary outflow obstruction
  - Rastelli operation: Right bundle branch block pattern and risk of late development of complete heart block.
- **CXR:**
  - May appear normal in newborns with TGA and an intact ventricular septum, although a narrow vascular pedicle is more common after the first week of life
  - With a VSD, cardiomegaly usually occurs with increased pulmonary arterial vascular markings
  - Following the atrial switch, a narrow vascular pedicle with an oblong cardiac silhouette ("egg on its side") is typically seen on the posteroanterior film
  - For the arterial switch, normal heart size.
- **Echocardiography:**
  - The bifurcating pulmonary artery arises posteriorly from the left ventricle in the parasternal long-axis view, where the two great arteries are seen running in parallel
  - The parasternal short-axis view shows the aorta usually arising anteriorly and to the right of the pulmonary artery in cross-section. The coronary artery anatomy needs to be ascertained
  - Most associated anatomic lesions, including ASD, VSD, and PDA, are diagnosed readily by echocardiography
  - Following the atrial switch, parallel great arteries are the hallmark of TGA. Qualitative assessment of systemic right ventricular function, the degree of tricuspid regurgitation, and the presence or absence of subpulmonary left ventricular obstruction (dynamic or fixed) are all to be assessed and recorded. Assessment of baffle leak or obstruction is best done using color and Doppler flow

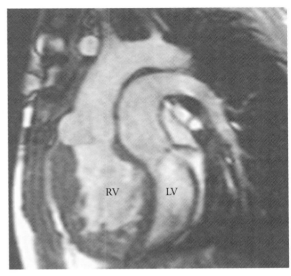

Figure 14.3 Cardiac MRI showing complete transposition of the great arteries (ventricular–arterial discordance). The aorta arises from a hypertrophied systemic right ventricle (RV) and ascends anteriorly and to the right. The pulmonary artery arises from a squashed banana-shaped left ventricle (LV) and ascends posteriorly and to the left. The great vessels are parallel. (Adapted from Gatzoulis MA, Swan L, Therrien J, Pantely GA, eds. *Adult Congenital Heart Disease, A Practical Guide*, 2005, with permission from Blackwell Publishing Ltd.)

  - After arterial switch, neoaortic valve regurgitation, supra-neopulmonary valve stenosis, branch pulmonary artery stenosis, and segmental wall motion abnormalities from ischemia due to coronary ostial stenosis should be sought
  - In patients with the Rastelli operation, left ventricular-to-aorta tunnel obstruction, right ventricular-to-pulmonary artery conduit degeneration (stenosis/regurgitation) as well as residual VSDs must be sought.
- **MRI:** An invaluable imaging modality for the older patient with TGA (Figure 14.3). It provides quantitative assessment of right and left ventricular function and dimensions:
  - In atrial switch, assessment of atrial baffles (assessment of systemic and pulmonary venous inflow channels for baffle stenosis and baffle leaks)
  - In arterial switch patients, exclusion of supravalvar or branch pulmonary artery stenosis
  - In Rastelli patients, assessment of conduit stenosis and gradient, and ventricular mass measurements, which in turn may guide future medical therapy.

Management

Although TGA was first described over two centuries ago, no treatment was available until the middle of the 20th century, prior to the development of surgical atrial septectomy (1950s) and balloon atrial septostomy (1960s). These palliative therapies were followed by physiologic repair procedures (atrial switch operations – Mustard or Senning) and anatomic repair (arterial switch operation). Today, the survival rate for infants with TGA exceeds 95%.

Initial treatment consists of maintaining ductal patency with intravenous prostaglandin E1 infusion to ensure mixing of blood. For the sick neonate, metabolic acidosis should be corrected with fluid replacement and bicarbonate administration. Mechanical ventilation may be necessary if pulmonary edema develops in concert with severe hypoxemia. Cardiac catheterization, depending on the degree of restriction at the atrial septum and the timing of operative repair, is indicated for balloon atrial septostomy. Balloon atrial septostomy is used to enhance the atrial level shunt and to improve mixing. After the procedure, most infants can be weaned off intravenous prostaglandin and will maintain a systemic arterial oxygen saturation of between 50% and 80%. In the previous era of atrial switch repair, atrial septostomy allowed adequate oxygenation for growth until such time as the atrial switch operation was performed – often beyond 6 months of age.

- **Atrial switch (Mustard or Senning procedure):** Blood is redirected at the atrial level using a baffle made of Dacron or pericardium (Mustard operation) or atrial flaps (Senning operation), achieving physiologic correction. Deoxygenated blood from the vena cavae is diverted through the mitral valve into the subpulmonary morphologic left ventricle and the pulmonary venous return is re-routed via the tricuspid valve into the subaortic morphologic right ventricle. By virtue of this repair, the morphologic right ventricle supports the systemic circulation.

- **Arterial switch (Jatene procedure):** Blood is redirected at the great artery level by switching the aorta and pulmonary arteries such that the morphologic left ventricle becomes the subaortic ventricle and supports the systemic circulation, and the morphologic right ventricle becomes the subpulmonary ventricle. Coronary arteries are detached from the aortic wall along with a "button" which is sutured into the "neoaorta." In the current era, most infants undergo definitive repair with the arterial switch within the first month of life, as the left ventricle may not be able to deliver the systemic pressure thereafter (if left for too long connected to the low-pressure, low-resistance pulmonary circulation).

- **Rastelli procedure** (for patients with large VSDs and pulmonary or subpulmonary stenosis): Blood is redirected at the ventricular level with the aorta tunneled to the left ventricle via the VSD and a valved conduit placed from the right ventricle to the pulmonary artery. By virtue of this procedure, the left ventricle supports the systemic circulation. With the Rastelli-type procedure, it may be preferable to wait until the infant grows larger because of the need for a right ventricle–pulmonary artery conduit and the obvious advantage of using a larger conduit in a larger patient.

Late complications and long-term outcome

- Complications following **atrial switch** procedures:
  - Significant systemic (tricuspid) AV valve regurgitation (40%). Occasionally the tricuspid valve apparatus may be intrinsically abnormal or may have been damaged at the time of prior VSD repair or by endocarditis
  - Systemic right ventricular dysfunction (40%)
  - Superior or inferior vena cava pathway obstruction
  - Pulmonary venous obstruction (rare)
  - Atrial baffle leak
  - Pulmonary hypertension
  - Symptomatic bradycardia (sinus node dysfunction or AV node block, 50%)
  - Atrial re-entrant tachycardia (20% by age 20 years)
  - Sudden cardiac death (most frequent cause of death, usually due to ventricular tachycardia)
  - Endocarditis.
- Complications following the **arterial switch** procedure:
  - RVOTO (supravalvar or branch pulmonary artery, relatively common)
  - Neoaortic valve regurgitation
  - Myocardial ischemia
  - Endocarditis.
- Complications following the **Rastelli** procedure:
  - Right ventricle-to-pulmonary artery conduit stenosis (inevitable with time and somatic growth)
  - Significant subaortic obstruction (across the VSD and aorta-to-left ventricular tunnel)
  - Residual VSD
  - Right or left ventricular dysfunction
  - Atrial and ventricular tachycardia
  - Sudden cardiac death
  - Complete heart block
  - Endocarditis.

Without surgical intervention, the survival rates of patients with TGA are very poor. Most patients will die in the first few months of life, with around 90% of patients dying in infancy. Patients with isolated TGA and no associated lesions have the worst outcome – only 30% survive beyond the first month of life. Patients with a large VSD have a somewhat better outcome, but less than 50% will survive the first year of life. The subset of patients with coexistent LVOTO and VSD has the best outcome, with approximately 50% surviving to 3 years of age. These patients may occasionally be seen as cyanosed adults with "balanced" circulation despite no previous surgical intervention.

- **Atrial switch:**
  - Following atrial baffle surgery, most patients reaching adulthood will be in NYHA class I–II
  - Progressive systemic right ventricular dysfunction and systemic (tricuspid) AV valve regurgitation are common
  - Symptoms of congestive heart failure occur in about 10% of patients
  - Atrial flutter/fibrillation
  - Progressive sinus node dysfunction.
- **Arterial switch:**
  - Supra neopulmonary artery and branch pulmonary artery stenosis
  - Ostial coronary artery disease
  - Progressive neoaortic valve regurgitation.
- **Rastelli:**
  - Progressive right ventricular-to-pulmonary artery conduit obstruction can cause exercise intolerance or right ventricular angina
  - Left ventricular tunnel obstruction can present as dyspnea or syncope.

The Senning group has a better survival rate at 5, 10, and 15 years than the Mustard group (95% versus 86%, 94% versus 82%, and 94% versus 77% respectively). For the arterial switch the cumulative survival at 5 and 10 years is 93%, and at 15 years is 86%. Finally, for the Rastelli operation mortality at 5, 10, 15, and 20 years is 93%, 82%, 80%, 68%, and 52% respectively.

Congenitally corrected transposition of the great arteries

In congenitally corrected transposition of the great arteries (ccTGA), the connections of both atria to ventricles and both ventricles to the great arteries are discordant (AV and ventricular–arterial or double discordance) (see Figure 14.1). This is occasionally referred to as l-TGA. Systemic venous blood passes from the right atrium through a mitral valve to the left ventricle and then to the right-sided posteriorly located pulmonary artery. Pulmonary venous blood passes from the left atrium through a tricuspid valve to the right ventricle and then to an anterior, left-sided aorta (see Figure 14.1). The circulation is thus "physiologically" corrected but it is the morphologic right ventricle supporting the systemic circulation.

Associated anomalies are very common and include:
- Approximately 20% of patients have **dextrocardia**.
- **VSD:** This is a common associated cardiac malformation (60–80%). The defect is usually large and perimembranous but can occur in any position along the ventricular septum.
- **LVOTO:** Pulmonary outflow tract stenosis occurs in approximately 40% of patients and is typically associated with a VSD. It may result from an aneurysm of the interventricular septum or may be associated with fibrous tissue tags or a discrete ring of tissue in the subvalvular area.
- **Abnormal left-sided (tricuspid) valve** in up to 90% of patients: Dysplasia (malformed or imperforate leaflets), apical displacement of the septal leaflet ("Ebstein-like"), or straddling and overriding of an inlet VSD.
- **Conduction system abnormalities:** The sinus node is normal but the AV node and bundle of His have an unusual location and course. There appear to be dual AV nodes in some patients. The second anomalous AV node and bundle are usually anterior, and the long penetrating bundle is vulnerable to fibrosis with advancing age. Thus, there is an increasing incidence of AV block with increasing age (about 2% per year), which is higher in patients with a VSD or following tricuspid valve surgery.
- **Coronary anatomy:** The coronary arteries usually have a mirror-image distribution.
- Less common conditions (1–10%) are ASD or PDA, coarctation of the aorta, interruption of the aortic arch, aortic or subaortic stenosis, double outlet right ventricle, and right AV (mitral) valve abnormalities.

Incidence and etiology
ccTGA is a rare condition, accounting for less than 1% of all congenital heart disease. As with almost all forms of congenital heart disease, the causes are thought to be multifactorial. There is a slight male predominance. Recently, an autosomal recessive mechanism of transmission was suggested in some families. Interestingly, it has been found that TGA was the most common recurrent

defect in families with ccTGA, suggesting a genetic link between these two entities.

Clinical features

ccTGA is one of the most common anomalies associated with dextrocardia (apex pointing to the right).

Presentation

Symptoms in early life reflect associated cardiac anomalies:
• Patients with no associated defects are pink and often remain asymptomatic until late adulthood. The diagnosis may be suspected by a CXR or EKG performed for another reason; otherwise dyspnea and exercise intolerance from systemic ventricular failure and significant left AV valve regurgitation will usually manifest themselves at some stage in adulthood. Patients may also present with palpitations from supraventricular arrhythmias or complete heart block.
• Patients with a VSD and pulmonary outflow tract obstruction will either present in congestive heart failure (if VSD is large) or cyanosis (if LVOTO is severe) and may need to undergo surgery early on.

Physical examination

The physical findings depend on the associated anomalies:
• In patients with large left-to-right shunts, the precordium is hyperdynamic.
• Individuals with pulmonary stenosis tend to have a relatively quiet precordium, and cyanosis is prominent.
• A single loud and often palpable S2 is commonly present at the left sternal border and is related to the anterior and leftward position of the aorta.
• The murmur of left AV valve (tricuspid) regurgitation may be mistaken for the typical pan-systolic murmur of VSD since it is often maximal at the fourth intercostal space near the sternum rather than at the apex, reflecting the side-by-side orientation of the ventricles in ccTGA with the ventricular septum in the sagittal plane.
• Although the murmur of pulmonary stenosis is often heard well in the pulmonary area, it may be loudest lower on the left side or in the aortic area, because of the inferior and posteriorly displaced pulmonary valve.
• If complete heart block is present, there are cannon A waves with an S1 of variable intensity.

Investigations

• **EKG:**
  ◦ Varying degrees of AV block are common
  ◦ The presence of Q waves in leads V1–2 combined with an absent Q wave in leads V5–6 is typical and reflects the initial right-to-left septal depolarization

occurring in the setting of inversion of the right and left bundles
  ◦ Wolff–Parkinson–White syndrome is present in 2–4% of patients.
• **CXR:**
  ◦ With mesocardia or dextrocardia, the diagnosis may be suspected
  ◦ Because of the unusual position of the great vessels, the pulmonary trunk is inconspicuous and an abnormal bulge along the left side of the cardiac contour reflects the left-sided ascending aorta rising to the aortic knuckle. The ventricular border on the left may also appear more vertical than usual.
• **Echocardiography:** Usually not straightforward, particularly when dextrocardia or mesocardia are present:
  ◦ Initially, multiple subcostal planes should be used to verify atrial and ventricular connections, and atrial and ventricular morphology. Atrial situs is usually normal and atrial morphology is determined by the systemic and pulmonary venous return and the atrial appendages
  ◦ Multiple, non-conventional planes from subcostal, parasternal short-axis and suprasternal notch coronal views may be needed. Ventricular morphology is usually best defined from the subcostal and apical four-chamber views and the parasternal short-axis views
  ◦ The septum is usually oriented in a straight antero-posterior direction
  ◦ The systemic right ventricle is on the patient's left; it is heavily trabeculated and has a prominent moderator band with muscular and tricuspid valve attachments to the interventricular septum
  ◦ The tricuspid valve mural leaflet is often significantly displaced toward the right ventricular apex
  ◦ Mitral–pulmonary valve fibrous continuity usually can be determined from a four-chamber view. The ventricular–arterial connections and spatial relationships of the great arteries are best defined using multiple subcostal, apical, and parasternal views. There can be multiple levels of outflow obstruction in the left (pulmonary) ventricle.

Initial investigations

• **EKG:** Q wave in leads V1–2 combined with an absent Q wave in leads V5–6
• **CXR:** Pulmonary trunk is inconspicuous and an abnormal bulge along the left side of the cardiac contour reflects the left-sided ascending aorta rising to the aortic knuckle
• Other imaging if suitable, e.g. transthoracic echo, MRI or CT

Management
Medical management

Medical management of congestive heart failure in infants and children secondary to a large VSD or severe tricuspid regurgitation may entail use of diuretics, digitalis, beta-blockers, and/or ACE inhibitor therapy. They may lead to temporary relief of symptoms but have little impact on survival and late outcome.

Surgical repair

- **Physiologic repair:** This procedure consists of VSD patch closure, left ventricular-to-pulmonary artery valved conduit insertion with or without systemic tricuspid valve replacement. Patients having undergone physiologic repair continue to have a morphologic right ventricle supporting the systemic circulation.
- **Double switch operation – anatomic repair:** This procedure consists of the arterial switch procedure combined with an atrial switch procedure (Mustard or Senning; see above). It is considered for patients with severe tricuspid regurgitation and systemic ventricular dysfunction. Its purpose is to achieve anatomic correction by incorporating the left ventricle into the systemic circulation and the right ventricle into the pulmonary circulation. First the left ventricle must be appropriately "trained" with pulmonary arterial banding.

Complete AV block may require pacemaker implantation for symptoms, progressive or profound bradycardia, poor exercise heart rate response, or cardiac enlargement.

Late complications and long-term outcome

- **Right ventricular dysfunction or congestive heart failure:** Due to systemic AV valve regurgitation, other associated lesions, open heart surgery, heart block, and arrhythmia.
- **Systemic AV valve regurgitation:** Usually progressing with age. Can be the cause and/or the effect of right ventricular dysfunction. May increase after VSD repair.
- **Heart block:** Increasing incidence of pacemaker requirement with age, after open heart surgery or in the presence of a VSD.
- **Arrhythmia:** Increasing incidence with age, more commonly of atrial origin.
- **Sudden cardiac death** (relatively uncommon): Usually associated with ventricular dysfunction, hemodynamic abnormalities, and arrhythmia.
- **Conduit stenosis,** inevitable with longer follow-up: Approximately 50% need replacement in 10 years.

- **Mitral/aortic regurgitation** (less common).
- **Endocarditis** (more common with residual VSD, tricuspid valve abnormalities, Blalock–Taussig shunt).

A minority of patients with ccTGA (and no associated lesions) may remain asymptomatic, and survive to the seventh or eighth decade. Failure of the systemic right ventricle is much more common, and usually associated with intrinsic abnormalities of the systemic (tricuspid) valve.

Isolated ventricular inversion

Isolated ventricular inversion (AV discordance with ventricular–arterial concordance) is an extremely rare form of cyanotic congenital heart disease. The malformation is characterized by an anatomic right atrium connecting to a morphologic left ventricle through a mitral valve. The anatomic left atrium, in turn, connects to the morphologic right ventricle through the tricuspid valve. In contrast to ccTGA, the connections at the ventricular–arterial level are concordant.

Partial anomalous pulmonary venous connection, complete AV septal defect (AVSD), interruption of the inferior vena cava, PDA, left atrial isomerism, tricuspid and supravalvar stenosis, and aortic coarctation have all been described in association with ventricular inversion. This anomaly results in parallel circulation similar to that of TGA; hence, most cases present with cyanosis and/or congestive cardiac failure in infancy. Without reparative surgery, survival beyond infancy is rare. In the current era, isolated ventricular inversion forms one of the remaining indications for an atrial switch (Mustard or Senning), although technically this is more challenging.

Further reading

Transposition

Jatene AD, Fontes VF, Paulista PP, *et al.* Anatomic correction of transposition of the great arteries. *J Thorac Cardiovasc Surg* 1976;72:364–370.

Kirklin JW, Barrett-Boyes BG. Complete transposition of the great arteries. In: *Cardiac Surgery*, 2nd edn. White Plains, New York: Churchill Livingstone; 1993, pp. 1383–1467.

Kreutzer C, De Vive J, Oppido G, *et al.* Twenty-five-year experience with Rastelli repair for transposition of the great arteries. *J Thorac Cardiovasc Surg* 2000;120:211–223.

Mustard WT. Successful two-stage correction of transposition of the great vessels. *Surgery* 1964;55:469–472.

Rashkind WJ, Miller WW. Creation of an atrial septal defect without thoracotomy. A palliative approach to complete transposition of the great arteries. *JAMA* 1966;196:991–992.

Rastelli GC, McGoon DC, Wallace RB. Anatomic correction of transposition of the great arteries with ventricular septal defect and sub-pulmonary stenosis. *J Thorac Cardiovasc Surg* 1969;58:545–552.

Sarris GE, Chatzis AC, Giannopoulos NM, et al. The arterial switch operation in Europe for transposition of the great arteries: A multi-institutional study from the European congenital heart surgeons association. *J Thorac Cardiovasc Surg* 2006;132:633–639.

Senning A. Surgical correction of transposition of the great vessels. *Surgery* 1959;45:966–980.

Wernovsky G, Sanders SP. Coronary artery anatomy and transposition of the great arteries. *Coronary Artery Dis* 1993;4: 148–157.

Congenitally corrected transposition

Connelly MS, Liu PP, Williams WG, et al. Congenitally corrected transposition of the great arteries in the adult: functional status and complications. *J Am Coll Cardiol* 1996;27:1238–1243.

Freedom RM, Dyck JD. Congenitally corrected transposition of the great arteries. In: Emmanouilides GC, Riemenschneider TA, Allen HD, Gutgesell HD, eds. *Moss and Adams Heart Disease in Infants, Children and Adolescents*, 5th edn, Vol II. Baltimore: Williams and Wilkins, 1995, pp. 1225–1245.

Graham TP Jr, Bernard YD, Mellen BG, et al. Long-term outcome in congenitally corrected transposition of the great arteries: a multi-institutional study. *J Am Coll Cardiol* 2000;36: 255–261.

Lundstrom U, Bull C, Wyse RKH, Somerville J. The natural and "unnatural" history of congenitally corrected transposition. *Am J Cardiol* 1990;65:1222–1229.

Termignon JL, Leca F, Vouhe PR, et al. "Classic" repair of congenitally corrected transposition and ventricular septal defect. *Ann Thorac Surg* 1996;62:199–206.

Webb CL. Congenitally corrected transposition of the great arteries: clinical features, diagnosis, and progression. *Prog Pediatr Cardiol* 1999;10:17–30.

Yagihara T, Kishimoto H, Isobe F, et al. Double switch operation in cardiac anomalies with atrioventricular and ventriculoarterial discordance. *J Thorac Cardiovasc Surg* 1994;107:351–358.

15 Abnormalities of right ventricular outflow

Michael L. Rigby

Royal Brompton Hospital, London, UK

Tetralogy of Fallot

Tetralogy of Fallot is best considered a malformation resulting from anterior and cephalad deviation of the outlet (infundibular) septum; this is in essence what creates all the anatomic features (Figure 15.1). The outlet septum is malaligned from the remainder of the ventricular septum, producing a large **ventricular septal defect (VSD)**. The anterior deviation causes **the aorta to override** the septum so that it takes a biventricular origin; and finally the proximity of the outlet septum to the parietal wall of the right ventricle produces **infundibular pulmonary stenosis**.

> **Features of tetralogy of Fallot**
> • Outlet VSD
> • Overriding of the aorta
> • Infundibular pulmonary stenosis
> • Right ventricular hypertrophy

During fetal life pulmonary stenosis reduces pulmonary blood flow, resulting in relative hypoplasia of the pulmonary arteries; the right-to-left shunting across the VSD, by giving rise to an increased aortic flow volume, causes the ascending aorta to be larger than normal, providing a possible explanation for the late risk of aortic insufficiency in adults.

The large VSD and overriding aorta allow equal systolic pressures in the aorta and right and left ventricles. The right ventricular pressure overload gives rise to hypertophy. Postnatally, when the infundibular stenosis is mild,

there will be a predominantly left-to-right shunt across the VSD and a mildly elevated pulmonary artery pressure. The excessive pulmonary blood flow will result in left atrial and ventricular volume loading. These are the features of the so-called "pink tetralogy," which is very occasionally associated with congestive heart failure. As the severity of infundibular pulmonary stenosis increases, so pulmonary blood flow decreases and right-to-left shunting across the VSD gives rise to increasingly severe central cyanosis.

In the extreme form, complete infundibular obstruction or pulmonary valve atresia occurs. Pulmonary atresia with VSD is dealt with later in this chapter. Pulmonary stenosis may be not only infundibular but also valvar and supravalvar. There are varying degrees of hypoplasia of the infundibular septum and pulmonary arteries.

The VSD may be perimembranous or have a muscular posteroinferior rim separating the anterior leaflet of the tricuspid valve from the aortic valve. There is a close cousin of tetralogy in which the VSD is described as "doubly committed and subarterial" because of complete absence of the infundibular septum and fibrous continuity between the pulmonary and aortic valves.

Additional important associated anomalies which may change the clinical presentation and modify the surgical management include:
• Left atrial isomerism (visceral heterotaxy);
• Secundum atrial septal defect (ASD);
• Partial anomalous pulmonary venous connection;
• Atrioventricular septal defect (AVSD);
• Straddling tricuspid valve;
• Muscular ventricular septal defect(s);
• Double outlet right ventricle;
• Aortic valve stenosis;

Pediatric Heart Disease: A Practical Guide, First Edition. Piers E. F. Daubeney, Michael L. Rigby, Koichiro Niwa, and Michael A. Gatzoulis.
© 2012 Blackwell Publishing Ltd. Published 2012 by Blackwell Publishing Ltd.

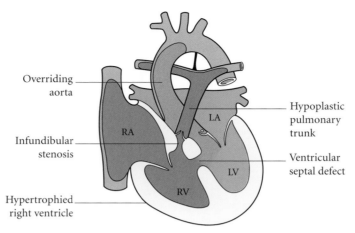

Figure 15.1 Tetralogy of Fallot. Tetralogy (from the Greek) means four components, namely: infundibular stenosis (subvalvar pulmonary stenosis), ventricular septal defect, aortic overriding (of the ventricular septum) and secondary right ventricular hypertrophy. The pulmonary valve is usually dysplastic and stenotic too, and occasionally the pulmonary trunk (as per drawing) or distal pulmonary arteries can be hypoplastic or stenotic. LA, left atrium; LV, left ventricle; RA, right atrium; RV, right ventricle. (Adapted from Gatzoulis MA, Swan L, Therrien J, Pantely GA, eds. *Adult Congenital Heart Disease, A Practical Guide*, 2005, with permission from Blackwell Publishing Ltd.)

- Anomalous origin of the left anterior descending coronary artery from the right coronary artery;
- Right aortic arch;
- Right aortic arch with left patent arterial duct from the aberrant left subclavian artery (vascular ring);
- Unilateral absence of right or left pulmonary artery;
- Systemic pulmonary collaterals;
- Peripheral pulmonary artery stenosis;
- Absent pulmonary valve syndrome;
- Wolff–Parkinson–White syndrome.

Incidence and etiology

With a frequency of about 1 in 1800 live births, tetralogy of Fallot accounts for 10% of all congenital heart disease and is the most common malformation to cause cyanosis. There is a well-recognized association with chromosomal abnormalities and syndromes, including 22q deletion, Down syndrome, and Cornelia de Lange syndrome.

Clinical features

- **At birth:** Some infants are markedly cyanosed because of severe pulmonary stenosis, but the majority display mild cyanosis or are acyanotic. Heart failure in the latter is observed occasionally.
- **Cardinal physical signs:**
  - Varying degrees of cyanosis
  - Single second heart sound
  - Ejection systolic murmur of pulmonary stenosis at the mid and upper left sternal edge.
- **Less constant features** include:
  - Right ventricular impulse
  - Systolic thrill
  - Aortic ejection click
  - Finger clubbing in late infancy
  - Occasionally a continuous murmur from a PDA or aortopulmonary collaterals.
- **Acyanotic ("pink") tetralogy:** A pan-systolic murmur or long ejection murmur is heard widely over the precordium, and the pulmonary component of the second heart sound may be audible.
- **Older patients:** Central cyanosis with pronounced finger clubbing is common, while exertional dyspnea, polycythemia, and squatting become more marked with increasing age.
- **Hypercyanotic spells:**
  - Approximately 40% will develop increasingly severe hypercyanotic spells during the first year of life. These are mild at first, but become progressively more severe
  - Characterized by paroxysms of rapid breathing with irritability and an obvious gray/blue coloration with a shorter murmur which may disappear completely
  - A severe spell may lead to limpness, convulsions, stroke or even death

∘ There is no relationship between the degree of resting cyanosis and the likelihood of a spell.

Investigations
- **EKG:** Right ventricular hypertrophy and right axis deviation.
- **CXR:**
  ∘ Normal heart size, uptilted apex ("boot-shaped heart"), pulmonary artery bay (concave pulmonary artery segment), normal-to-oligemic lung fields, and right aortic arch (in 25%)
  ∘ Pulmonary plethora and mild cardiac enlargement occur in "pink" tetralogy.
- **Echocardiography:**
  ∘ Establishes the diagnosis in almost every case and the only imaging modality usually required
  ∘ Typical findings are an outlet VSD with overriding aorta and infundibular pulmonary stenosis
  ∘ Valvar and supravalvar pulmonary stenosis are common, together with varying degrees of proximal pulmonary artery hypoplasia
  ∘ It is important for the cardiologist to exclude anomalous origin of the left anterior descending coronary artery from the right coronary artery.
- **MRI:** While not required in most patients, it is used when the echocardiographic examination is incomplete or extreme pulmonary artery hypoplasia is suspected.
- **Cardiac catheterization and angiography:** An alternative to MRI when more detailed hemodynamic information is required and when information is required about systemic-to-pulmonary artery collaterals, peripheral pulmonary arteries, or coronary arteries. It is probably superior to MRI in infants and small children.
- **CT angiography:** Rarely used in diagnosis; it can provide useful information about pulmonary artery size and anatomy, coronary arrangement, and aortic arch and head and neck vessels.

Management
Medical management
- Intravenous prostaglandin E to maintain ductal patency and pulmonary blood flow in those newborn infants with severe cyanosis.
- Identify any associated chromosomal abnormalities or syndromes.
- Educate the parents in how to identify hypercyanotic spells.
- The acute management of spells is important (see below).

- Recurrent hypercyanotic spells are an absolute indication for surgery but patients with a history of recent onset of mild spells should be prescribed oral propranolol while awaiting surgical repair or palliation.

Management of a cyanotic "spell"
- Place infant in the "knee–chest" position
- Oxygen via a face mask
- Intramuscular morphine sulfate (0.1 mg /kg)
- Intravenous propranolol (0.025 mg/kg)
- Intravenous vasoconstrictors such as phenylephrine (0.02 mg/kg)
- Treatment of acidosis
- Recurrent hypercyanotic spells are an absolute indication for surgery

(For hypercyanotic spell resuscitation guidelines see Appendix A.)

Surgical management
Surgical management will inevitably vary from center to center. For an individual institution the emphasis should be on low operative mortality (< 2%) and morbidity, short hospital stay (5–9 days), and good medium- and long-term outcomes. Surgical and medical teams should pursue those management strategies producing the best outcomes in their own institution!
- **Systemic artery-to-pulmonary artery shunt procedures (modified Blalock–Taussig shunt or "central" shunt)** are recommended for neonates with duct-dependent pulmonary blood flow, for those with severe hypercyanotic spells that cannot be managed by conventional medical treatment, and for infants younger than 3–4 months in whom there is severe central cyanosis or a systemic arterial oxygen saturation persistently below 75–80% at rest. These palliative operations are also employed when the pulmonary arteries are considered too small for surgical repair.
- **Radical repair carried out under cardiopulmonary bypass** is usually performed between the ages of 3 and 18 months, and there is now a trend to earlier operation even in infants who are symptom-free. The procedure includes patch closure of the VSD and resection of infundibular myocardium, often with pericardial or synthetic patch enlargement of the infundibulum. In approximately 65% of patients the patch to the infundibulum is extended across the pulmonary valve "annulus" into the

pulmonary trunk. This inevitably gives rise to virtually free pulmonary insufficiency, which is almost always well tolerated during childhood and early adolescence. Well-recognized but avoidable early complications include complete heart block and a residual VSD. Right bundle branch block on the EKG occurs in the majority.

• **Other treatment strategies** occasionally employed during early infancy include balloon dilatation of the right ventricular outflow tract and balloon pulmonary valvuloplasty or the placement of a valved conduit from the right ventricle to the bifurcation of the pulmonary arteries when there is severe pulmonary artery hypoplasia.

Late complications and long-term outcome

• **Pulmonary insufficiency** is the most important consequence of surgical repair and is the major cause of late complications. Right ventricular volume loading and dilatation eventually result in impaired exercise performance, cardiac arrhythmias, and increased risk of sudden death. Pulmonary valve replacement with a homograft valve and with reduction of the dilated right ventricular outflow tract is commonly performed during adolescence and early adult life to reduce the risk of late complications.

• **Peripheral pulmonary artery stenosis** is well recognized and increases the severity of pulmonary regurgitation. Treatment by percutaneous balloon angioplasty with or without stenting can be helpful.

• **Paroxysmal tachyarrhythmias** such as atrial flutter, atrial fibrillation or ventricular tachycardia, although often responsive to antiarrhythmic drugs, are best managed by radiofrequency ablation in the electrophysiology laboratory. However, some patients will still require an implantable cardiac defibrillator to minimize the risks of late sudden death.

Absent pulmonary valve syndrome

This rare condition, usually associated with tetralogy, is best considered as a separate entity because of the presence of severe pulmonary regurgitation, huge central pulmonary arteries, bronchial compression, bronchomalacia, and obstructive emphysema. Most cases do not have an arterial duct and the morphogenesis has been attributed to its congenital absence or premature closure. Mild examples are occasionally encountered and cases can also occur with tricuspid atresia, VSD, double outlet right ventricle, or an otherwise normal heart.

Important morphologic features are:
• Anatomic features of tetralogy of Fallot (outlet VSD, overriding of the aorta, and pulmonary stenosis);
• Virtual absence of pulmonary valve leaflets, which instead are represented by a rudimentary ridge;
• Dilated and hypertrophied right ventricle;
• Aneurysmal dilatation of the pulmonary trunk and right and left pulmonary arteries causing varying degrees of bronchial compression;
• Compression of intrapulmonary bronchi by abnormally branching pulmonary arteries in the more severe cases;
• Peripheral pulmonary artery stenosis in some;
• Unusual morphologic variants include anomalous origin of the right pulmonary artery from the ascending aorta, a normal sized right or left pulmonary artery, and an additional muscular VSD.

Clinical features

• Presentation during the neonatal period is common and some infants will be ventilator dependent because of respiratory failure, some will have tachypnea, while others remain symptom-free.

• Most striking features are an active precordium with loud systolic and early diastolic "to-and-fro" murmurs, normal peripheral pulses (effectively excluding the presence of aortic regurgitation), and a single second heart sound. This is a complex condition for which physical examination provides the diagnosis!

• In most cases there is a predominantly left-to-right shunt across the VSD and cyanosis is absent or very mild. Mild-to-severe congestive heart failure with pronounced liver enlargement can occur in the latter.

• Moderate-to-severe hypoxia, although less common, occurs in cases with more severe pulmonary stenosis or because of severe proximal or distal bronchial compression.

Investigations

• **EKG:** Right atrial and right ventricular hypertrophy with right axis deviation.
• **CXR:**
  ○ Cardiomegaly, pulmonary plethora, and large central pulmonary arteries are often observed
  ○ Normal pulmonary blood flow because of moderate pulmonary stenosis
  ○ Heart size is normal.
• **Echocardiography:** An outlet VSD with overriding of the aorta is found, but in contrast to the typical case of tetralogy, there is dilatation of the proximal pulmonary

arteries, rudimentary pulmonary valve leaflets, and only mild infundibular pulmonary stenosis.

• **Cardiac catheterization and angiography with bronchography and bronchoscopy:** Should always be performed before surgery.

• **MRI and pulmonary CT:** Can also be helpful in precise diagnosis. CT is particularly helpful in the diagnosis of compression of intrapulmonary bronchi.

Management

• In the majority, surgical treatment involves homograft pulmonary valve replacement, reduction of the pulmonary arteries, and closure of the VSD.

• Less than 20% of cases will require surgery during the neonatal period or early infancy.

• Early operation with a further reduction in the size of the central pulmonary arteries is reserved for those with severe symptoms or requiring ventilatory support.

• Surgical repair for infants and children with mild symptoms should be delayed.

Late complications and long-term outcome

• Because of compression of the intrapulmonary bronchi, severe peripheral pulmonary artery stenosis or obstructive emphysema, a significant number of infants will not survive any attempt at surgical repair.

• Some survivors require prolonged ventilation until growth of the lungs allows improvement in the severity of bronchomalacia.

• While some survivors progress without any respiratory symptoms, others continue to manifest symptoms of bronchial compression.

Pulmonary atresia with ventricular septal defect

The term "pulmonary atresia" refers to incomplete development of the pulmonary valve and/or pulmonary arteries; as a result blood cannot enter the pulmonary trunk directly from the right or left ventricle.

Working classification of pulmonary atresia with ventricular septal defect (Figure 15.2)

• Infundibular atresia

• Pulmonary valve atresia

• Atresia of the pulmonary trunk

• Atresia of the right and /or left pulmonary arteries

• Non-confluent pulmonary arteries

With absence or severe hypoplasia of the pulmonary trunk there is no potential connection of the ventricular mass to the pulmonary artery. Because only the aorta arises from a ventricle, the ventricular–arterial connection is described as "single outlet." The aorta may arise entirely from the right or left ventricle; alternatively there is aortic overriding of the ventricular septum.

Pulmonary atresia with VSD occurs in a variety of congenital heart malformations including:

• Tetralogy of Fallot;

• Double outlet right ventricle;

• Complete transposition;

• Discordant atrioventricular (AV) connection;

• Right atrial isomerism with biventricular AV connection.

With the exception of tetralogy, pulmonary blood supply in these cases is almost always dependent on flow through the arterial duct and rarely on systemic pulmonary collaterals.

Tetralogy of Fallot with pulmonary atresia

By far the most common variant of pulmonary atresia with VSD occurs in the setting of tetralogy of Fallot. The anteriorly deviated infundibular septum often fuses with the parietal wall of the right ventricle. Alternatively, the subpulmonary infundibulum may remain patent but with pulmonary valve atresia.

When infundibular atresia develops early in gestation, the pulmonary arteries themselves regress, often becoming severely hypoplastic or "absent"; the arterial duct fails to develop and pulmonary blood flow is derived from systemic-to-pulmonary collateral arteries.

With later development of pulmonary atresia in the fetus, pulmonary blood flow is duct-dependent and the pulmonary arteries do not regress completely, often remaining only mildly hypoplastic.

Thus, at birth, pulmonary blood flow is almost always dependent upon either an arterial duct or systemic-to-pulmonary collateral arteries.

Systemic-to-pulmonary collateral arteries

There is enormous variability in the morphology, distribution, and size of collateral arteries so that it is often said that every case is unique. The name invariably used to describe them, "MAPCAs" or "major aortopulmonary collateral arteries," is inappropriate because they originate not only from the thoracic descending aorta but also from the subclavian and even carotid arteries. There can be anything from one to six, each supplying different lung segments.

(a)

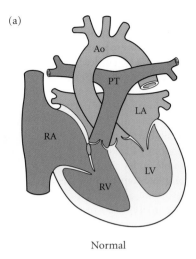

Normal

(b)

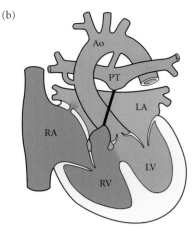

Pulmonary atresia with VSD
and confluent pulmonary arteries
and blood supply from PDA

(c)

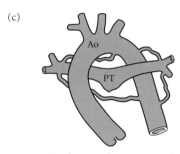

Confluent pulmonary arteries
with blood supply from systemic
to pulmonary arterial collaterals

(d)

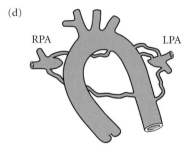

Non-confluent pulmonary arteries
with blood supply from systemic
to pulmonary arterial collaterals

Figure 15.2 (a) Normal pulmonary arterial anatomy. (b–d) Three common patterns of pulmonary arterial anatomy in patients with tetralogy of Fallot with pulmonary atresia. (b) Unifocal circulation with all the intrapulmonary arteries connected to unobstructed, confluent pulmonary arteries with blood supply from a patent duct. This is the most common pattern (85% of cases). (c) Multifocal circulation with confluent, but hypoplastic, pulmonary arteries and blood supply from systemic-to-pulmonary arterial collaterals.

(d) Multifocal circulation with blood flow from systemic-to-pulmonary arterial collaterals, but the pulmonary arteries are non-confluent. Ao, aorta; LA, left atrium; LPA, left pulmonary artery; LV, left ventricle; PDA, patent ductus arteriosus; PT, pulmonary trunk; RA, right atrium; RPA, right pulmonary artery; RV, right ventricle; VSD, ventricular septal defect. (Adapted from Gatzoulis MA, Swan L, Therrien J, Pantely GA, eds. *Adult Congenital Heart Disease, A Practical Guide*, 2005, with permission from Blackwell Publishing Ltd.)

Central pulmonary arteries are usually found when there are collateral arteries. They vary in size from a tiny "seagull" to mildly hypoplastic, although not infrequently they are absent. Central pulmonary arteries are connected to some but not all the collaterals, usually at the hilum or within lobar segments. Stenosis of collaterals at their origin or peripherally within the lung is common.

Occasionally large collaterals cause excessive pulmonary blood flow and heart failure. Moderate-to-severe cyanosis due to small collaterals or balanced systemic-to-pulmonary blood flow with mild-to-moderate cyanosis in infancy are more frequent.

Alternative sources of pulmonary blood flow other than a PDA or collateral arteries are sometimes encountered and include:

- Coronary artery-to-pulmonary artery fistula;
- Aortopulmonary window;
- Patent fifth aortic arch;
- Acquired hypoplastic collateral arteries.

Clinical features

- Most patients are cyanosed at birth and the second heart sound is single. In the majority there is no heart murmur.
- With duct-dependent pulmonary blood flow, cyanosis becomes intense as the duct closes and the systemic arterial oxygen saturation will fall to below 60%.
- When pulmonary blood flow is provided by systemic pulmonary collaterals, the severity of cyanosis and hypoxia is extremely variable and depends on the amount of pulmonary blood flow. Severe cyanosis during early life is unusual but small collaterals with multiple stenoses result in severe hypoxia with no response to prostaglandin E, which can be a clue to diagnosis. Symptoms of heart failure due to excessive pulmonary blood flow through large collaterals can also occur. Many infants have a systemic arterial oxygen saturation ranging from 75% to 90% and are symptom-free. Continuous murmurs audible over the back and precordium, although not present at birth, will become obvious a few weeks later. In some instances, mild cyanosis is not detected immediately, and patients present much later with mild effort intolerance, finger clubbing, and continuous murmurs.

Investigations

- **EKG:** Right axis deviation with right ventricular hypertrophy is the typical finding, although in cases with systemic-to-pulmonary collaterals it is not unusual for there to be left ventricular hypertrophy.
- **CXR:** The heart size appears small or normal with an uptilted apex, pulmonary artery bay, right aortic arch in 25%, and normal-to-diminished pulmonary vascular markings in the majority.
- **Echocardiogram:**
  - The typical findings are an outlet VSD with overriding aorta.
  - It is important to distinguish between an arterial duct and collaterals arising from the descending aorta, as the source of pulmonary blood flow.
  - For cases with duct-dependent pulmonary blood flow, surgical management is usually based on echocardiographic imaging alone.
- **Cardiac catheterization/MRI/CT angiography.**
The ideal management of some patients with pulmonary atresia depends upon detailed information about sys-temic pulmonary collaterals and central pulmonary arteries. Particularly important questions are:
- Which lung segments are supplied by collaterals alone?
- Which have a dual supply involving true central pulmonary arteries as well?

Where possible any sites of connection between collaterals and central pulmonary arteries should be determined and the direct measurement of the distal pressure in large collaterals should be made. In some patients it will not be possible to define any central pulmonary arteries, while peripheral pulmonary artery stenosis and hypoplasia is relatively common. Pulmonary venous wedge angiography may outline central pulmonary arteries not identified by other imaging techniques.

In general, cardiac catheterization and angiography provides the most precise hemodynamic and anatomic information, but MRI and CT angiography are being used with increasing frequency. In practical terms, a pragmatic approach with individualized imaging protocols for each patient is the most appropriate. Whatever investigation is being used, it is important to be aware of the other potential sources of pulmonary blood flow outlined above.

Management
Medical management

- Prostaglandin E and correction of any metabolic acidosis when neonatal hypoxia is associated with duct-dependent pulmonary blood flow.
- Exclusion of chromosomal abnormality, particularly 22q deletion.
- Stenting of the arterial duct is sometimes employed as an alternative to a systemic artery-to-pulmonary artery shunt procedure.
- Embolization of systemic pulmonary collaterals during cardiac catheterization is sometimes undertaken as part of a staged approach to surgical management.

Surgical management

Most infants with a duct-dependent pulmonary circulation have sufficiently large pulmonary arteries to permit radical repair with insertion of right ventricular-to-pulmonary artery conduit and closure of the VSD. An alternative approach preferred by many is an initial systemic artery-to-pulmonary artery shunt with repair 6–18 months later.

A small subset of patients with an imperforate pulmonary valve can be managed either by surgical repair using a transannular patch or by initial radiofrequency-assisted balloon pulmonary valvuloplasty with or without stenting of the right ventricular outflow tract as a prelude to later repair. The latter approach is useful when the pulmonary arteries are moderately hypoplastic, because anterograde blood flow may promote growth.

With such variability in the anatomy of the systemic pulmonary collaterals and the size of central pulmonary arteries, patients without a duct-dependent pulmonary circulation are often managed with individualized protocols. Extreme variation in surgical management can occur from one center to another.

It should also be stressed that some patients with balanced systemic and pulmonary blood flows may remain well for the first two decades of life without any intervention. Arguably, even in the current era, there are significant numbers of patients made worse by radical and innovative surgery.

The principles of surgical treatment are to connect systemic pulmonary collateral arteries to central pulmonary arteries and then to insert a right ventricular-to-pulmonary conduit. When there are no central pulmonary arteries or they are extremely hypoplastic, a prosthetic tube is connected from hilum to hilum. While it may be possible to perform a single operation during infancy, bilateral unifocalization procedures with insertion of a modified Blalock–Taussig shunt may be performed separately, with completion of the repair at a second or third stage. The presence of severe peripheral pulmonary artery stenosis and hypoplasia may prevent complete closure of the VSD. Once continuity between the right ventricle and pulmonary arteries has been established, balloon pulmonary angioplasty with or without stenting can be used to improve pulmonary blood flow to some affected lung segments.

Late complications and long-term outcome

Late complications are the consequence of pulmonary insufficiency and right ventricular dysfunction or hypertension. The latter is particularly frequent following radical repair in patients with systemic pulmonary collaterals and peripheral pulmonary stenosis. Premature death and late morbidity is due to:
- Ventricular and atrial arrhythmias;
- Right ventricular failure ;
- Cerebral abscess in patients with a residual VSD and right-to-left shunt.

Double outlet right ventricle

In hearts with a double outlet right ventricle (DORV) the aorta and pulmonary artery both arise predominantly from the morphologically right ventricle. The classification, clinical presentation, and surgical treatment are dependent upon the relationship of the VSD (perimembranous or with muscular posterior rim) to the arterial trunks. When the aorta or pulmonary trunk overrides the ventricular septum, more than 50% of the corresponding valve must take origin from the right ventricle for this to be termed "DORV."

Most examples are found in hearts with a concordant AV connection, but all types of atrial arrangement or AV connection have been described.

Although the ascending aorta and the pulmonary trunk may have a normal spiraling relationship, more frequently they are parallel with the aorta to the right. When there is a discordant AV connection, the aortic valve is usually to the left of the pulmonary valve, but a left-sided aorta (L-malposition) is occasionally found with a concordant AV connection. To recognize the latter is of surgical importance because the right coronary artery arises from the right anterior aortic sinus and passes across the anterior aspect of the pulmonary trunk at the ventricular–arterial junction.

Classification of DORV based on the location of the VSD
- Subaortic VSD
- Subpulmonary VSD
- Doubly-committed subarterial VSD
- Uncommitted VSD
- Intact ventricular septum (rare) (Figure 15.3)

The **most common variants** are:
- **Subaortic VSD, aortic valve to the right of the pulmonary valve, infundibular pulmonary stenosis ("tetralogy type").** The clinical features and management are the same as those of tetralogy.
- **Subaortic VSD with normally related or side-by-side great arteries, aortic valve to the right of the pulmonary valve, and without pulmonary stenosis.** This condition is a very close cousin of an isolated large VSD, and the clinical course and management are similar.
- **Subpulmonary VSD with parallel great arteries and aorta, and aortic valve to the right of the pulmonary valve ("Taussig–Bing anomaly").** A very close cousin of complete transposition with large VSD, this has a similar clinical presentation and management. It is not unusual for coarctation of the aorta to modify and complicate the clinical course.

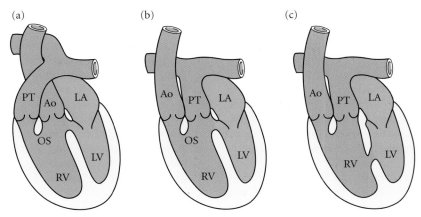

Figure 15.3 (a–c) Three types of double outlet right ventricle. In each type there may be variable degrees of pulmonary or aortic stenosis depending on the deviation of the outlet septum: (a) subaortic ventricular septal defect (VSD) has pulmonary stenosis; (b)subpulmonary VSD (Taussig–Bing) has neither aortic nor pulmonary stenosis; (c) non-committed VSD has aortic stenosis. Ao, aorta; LA, left atrium; LV, left ventricle; OS, outlet septum; PT, pulmonary trunk; RV, right ventricle.

• **Subpulmonary VSD with muscular subpulmonary stenosis and anterior right-sided aortic valve and aorta.** A close cousin of transposition with pulmonary stenosis and VSD, the clinical course and management are similar.

Less common but well-recognized variants are:
• **Concordant AV connection, mitral stenosis, hypoplastic left ventricle, and restrictive subaortic VSD.** In some cases only a univentricular repair will be possible, providing the presence of mitral stenosis and an intact atrial septum has not caused the pulmonary vascular to be raised.
• **Discordant AV connection with subpulmonary VSD and aortic valve anterior and to the left of the pulmonary valve.** DORV is present in about 20% of hearts with a discordant AV connection.
• **Concordant AV connection, subaortic VSD, muscular subpulmonary stenosis, and "L-malposition" or left-sided aortic valve ("Lincoln–Danielson heart").** The course of the right coronary artery across the junction of the right ventricle and pulmonary trunk dictates the use of an external conduit for the relief of pulmonary stenosis.
• **Right atrial isomerism, biventricular AV connection, complete AVSD, and pulmonary atresia or muscular subpulmonary stenosis.** In such hearts it is not unusual for the aorta to be in an anterior position and for a biventricular repair to be impossible to achieve. Commonly, there is extracardiac total anomalous pulmonary venous connection which is obstructed in the majority (see Chapter 17).

Additional important associated anomalies, which may modify the clinical presentation and surgical management, include:
• Right atrial isomerism (often with obstructed extracardiac total anomalous pulmonary venous connection);
• AVSD;
• Mitral stenosis and hypoplastic left heart;
• Criss-cross heart;
• Discordant AV connection;
• Straddling mitral or tricuspid valve;
• Additional muscular VSD(s);
• Muscular subpulmonary stenosis;
• Pulmonary atresia;
• Pulmonary artery hypoplasia;
• Restrictive (small) VSD;
• Muscular subaortic stenosis;
• Coarctation of the aorta;
• Aortic interruption.

Incidence and etiology

There are no specific etiologic factors.

The diagnosis is uncommon with a prevalence of 3–6 per 1000 live births.

Clinical features

There is a wide variation in the clinical presentation, which is not surprising given the anatomic heterogeneity. In almost every case there is systemic arterial desaturation, but cyanosis varies from very mild to severe.

Without pulmonary stenosis, cyanosis is mild, heart failure begins to develop during the second month of life, and characteristically there is a palpable cardiac impulse, loud P2, and short ejection systolic murmur at the left sternal border, although it is not unusual for there to be no murmur at all.

With pulmonary stenosis, cyanosis becomes more severe with increasing age. Although some cases with severe stenosis present with profound arterial oxygen desaturation shortly after birth and require prostaglandins to maintain ductal patency, many remain symptom-free in early infancy. Typically there is a single second heart sound and an ejection systolic murmur at the upper left sternal edge. In the "tetralogy-type," the clinical course is that described earlier in the chapter.

Older patients without pulmonary stenosis may present in later childhood with pulmonary vascular disease, cyanosis, and clubbing. For those with pulmonary stenosis, cyanosis and clubbing are also late features but the P2 is inaudible.

Investigations

• **EKG:** Right ventricular hypertrophy and right axis deviation are the usual findings.
• **CXR:** Without pulmonary stenosis, cardiac enlargement and pulmonary plethora are found. When there is pulmonary stenosis, a normal heart size and pulmonary vascularity are the usual findings.
• **Echocardiography:** The investigation of choice to establish the diagnosis.
• **Other investigations:** Cardiac catheterization, MRI or CT angiography can be used if additional information is needed.

Management

Medical management
• Intravenous prostaglandin E to maintain ductal patency in the newborn with severe hypoxia.
• Exclude a chromosomal abnormality.
• Tetralogy type is managed in the same way as usual cases of tetralogy.
• Diuretics if there is heart failure prior to surgery.
• Balloon atrial septostomy for cases with subpulmonary VSD, all cases with restrictive VSD, and hearts with mitral stenosis.

Surgical management
Surgical management varies from one center to another. The emphasis should always be to use surgical strategies producing the best results in one's own institution.
• **Banding of the pulmonary trunk** can be used as initial palliation for cases without pulmonary stenosis and at the time of repair of associated coarctation of the aorta.
• **Systemic-to-pulmonary artery shunt procedures** are sometimes employed as an initial palliation for infants with severe cyanosis associated with pulmonary stenosis or pulmonary atresia.
• **Atrial septectomy ("Blalock–Hanlon")** may be the initial palliation for infants with mitral stenosis or subpulmonary VSD.
• **Bidirectional Glenn operation/total cavopulmonary connection (Fontan)** is reserved for those patients considered unsuitable for biventricular repair, including those with hearts with hypoplastic left ventricle or straddling AV valves.
• **Closure of subaortic VSD ± relief of pulmonary stenosis** for "tetralogy" type of DORV.
   • **Closure of VSD with insertion of right ventricle-to-pulmonary artery conduit ("Rastelli operation")** is employed for hearts with subaortic VSD and L-malposition of the aorta; with subpulmonary VSD and pulmonary stenosis, the aorta is connected to the morphologically left ventricle. When there is a discordant AV connection, this latter approach is combined with a Mustard or Senning procedure (see Chapter 14).
• **Arterial switch operation and closure of VSD** is the operation of choice for most cases with subpulmonary VSD without pulmonary stenosis. This approach can be combined with an atrial redirection procedure (Mustard or Senning) when there is a discordant AV connection.
• **Intraventricular tunnel repair** is the operation sometimes chosen when there is a subpulmonary VSD without pulmonary stenosis but side-by-side great arteries with right-sided aortic valve. The other indication is in some hearts with a non-committed or a doubly-committed VSD.

Late complications and long-term outcome

Late complications depend on the type of DORV and surgical repair employed. The need for a revision operation during adolescence or early adult life is not unusual.

Late sequelae include:
• **Atrial or ventricular arrhythmias and complete heart block** are potential lifelong complications.

• **Aortic insufficiency**, usually mild, is common to most groups.
• **Pulmonary arterial stenosis** is particularly prevalent following conduit procedures or the arterial switch operation.
• **Pulmonary insufficiency** is common following surgical relief of pulmonary stenosis in the "Fallot" type.

Double outlet left ventricle

Because double outlet left ventricle (DOLV) is so rare and morphological features so variable, it is difficult to make generalizations about the pathophysiology or clinical features. The most important aspect is the presence or absence of pulmonary stenosis which, in the same way as in DORV, is a major determinant of clinical presentation and natural history. The VSD is rarely subpulmonary. The most frequent variants are:
• DOLV with concordant AV connection, subaortic or doubly-committed VSD, and posterior right-sided aorta;
• DOLV with discordant AV connection, subaortic or doubly-committed VSD, muscular subpulmonary stenosis, and anterior left-sided aorta.

Pulmonary atresia with intact ventricular septum

Pulmonary atresia with intact ventricular septum is an uncommon and complex condition of variable severity, and characterized by pulmonary valve atresia, right ventricular hypertrophy and fibrosis, tricuspid valve dysplasia, and coronary artery abnormalities (Figure 15.4). Atrial situs and cardiac connections are almost always normal, while typically the pulmonary arteries are supplied by an arterial duct and are only mildly hypoplastic. The diagnosis is often made prenatally when progression from severe pulmonary valve stenosis to valve atresia may occur during the third trimester.

The most striking feature is severe hypertrophy of the right ventricle with variable degrees of cavity hypoplasia resulting from the muscular overgrowth. Muscular obliteration of the apex and infundibulum may occur and in the most extreme form results in a diminutive right ventricle. The smaller the right ventricular cavity, the more likely is tricuspid valve hypoplasia and ventricular–coronary connections or "fistulae". There may be muscular or membranous pulmonary atresia. Occasionally Ebstein malformation and/or an imperforate tricuspid

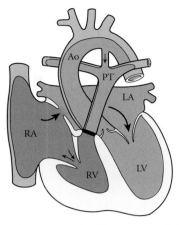

Figure 15.4 Pulmonary atresia with intact ventricular septum. There is a hypoplastic tricuspid valve with muscular overgrowth of the right ventricle, causing cavity hypoplasia. There is (in this case) membranous pulmonary atresia with retrograde pulmonary blood supply from the arterial duct. Ao, aorta; LA, left atrium; LV, left ventricle; PT, pulmonary trunk; RA, right atrium; RV, right ventricle.

valve are found. Coronary fistulae may be associated with coronary arterial stenosis or atresia, giving rise to a so-called "right ventricular-dependent coronary circulation."

Tricuspid insufficiency is a common finding, but the most severe regurgitation is found in a small subset of patients who have a dilated and thin-walled right ventricle.

Left ventricular myocardial abnormalities may occur, particularly in cases with a severely hypertensive and diminuitive right ventricle. Rarely there is a small muscular VSD or systemic pulmonary collateral arteries from the descending aorta.

Clinical features
• Antenatal diagnosis is common in the current era.
• Cyanosis is present at birth and increases abruptly as the arterial duct closes.
• There is a slightly prominent left ventricular impulse, single second heart sound, soft pan-systolic murmur of tricuspid regurgitation at the lower left sternal edge and less frequently, a soft continuous murmur under the left clavicle.
• For the small group with severe tricuspid regurgitation and right ventricular dilatation, cyanosis, an active precordium, hepatomegaly, loud pan-systolic murmur, and thrill are the striking findings. Lung hypoplasia as a result

of severe cardiomegaly may predispose to respiratory failure.

Investigations

- **EKG:**
  ◦ For the commonest group of infants with moderate-to-severe right ventricular hypoplasia, the EKG demonstrates a mean frontal QRS axis of 30–90 degrees, right atrial enlargement, paucity of right ventricular forces, dominant S wave in the right precordial leads, and pure R wave in leads V5 and V6
  ◦ For those with a near normal-sized right ventricle, right axis deviation and right ventricular dominance with a tall or pure R wave in leads V4R and V1 and dominant S wave in V5 and V6 are the typical findings.
- **CXR:**
  ◦ Most cases demonstrate mild-to-moderate cardiomegaly with a prominent, bulging right atrium and pulmonary oligemia
  ◦ Severe cardiac enlargement is characteristic of those with severe tricuspid insufficiency, the "wall-to-wall heart."
- **Echocardiogram:**
  ◦ Exquisite detail may already be available from antenatal studies, but postnatal cross-sectional echocardiography is the definitive investigation in making a precise diagnosis and management plan, particularly regarding suitability for biventricular or univentricular repair
  ◦ Such a decision depends on the size of the tricuspid valve and right ventricle together with the nature of the infundibulum (membranous versus muscular pulmonary atresia)
  ◦ Imaging of the interatrial septum and determination of the size of the ASD is important because maintenance of cardiac output depends on an obligatory right-to-left shunt through the ASD
  ◦ It is important to distinguish critical pulmonary valve stenosis from pulmonary valve atresia by subcostal and parasternal imaging and Doppler interrogation of the right ventricular outflow as the treatment will be different (balloon versus radiofrequency perforation)
  ◦ Tricuspid insufficiency is a usual finding in all but cases with severe right ventricular hypoplasia
  ◦ Doppler estimates reveal a right ventricular systolic pressure greater than systemic levels
  ◦ Factors favoring biventricular repair:
    Patent subpulmonary infundibulum (tripartite or bipartite right ventricle)

Membranous pulmonary atresia
Tricuspid valve annulus diameter Z score > −4
Absence of ventricular–coronary connections.
- **Cardiac catheterization/angiography:**
  ◦ All the cardiac chambers can be accessed by femoral venous catheterization
  ◦ The right ventricular systolic pressure is greater than systemic pressure while the end-diastolic and right atrial pressures are high
  ◦ Patients considered candidates for biventricular repair are likely to undergo radiofrequency-assisted balloon pulmonary valvuloplasty
  ◦ When an eventual total cavopulmonary anastomosis is the only option, balloon atrial septostomy should be performed
  ◦ Infants with severe hypoplasia of the right ventricle and tricuspid valve are likely to have major ventriculo-coronary connections and are at risk of coronary ostial atresia or stenosis. The latter is a major incremental risk factor for early death and should be documented by angiography before palliative surgery is considered.

Treatment

Cyanosis at birth that increases abruptly with closure of the arterial duct requires the administration of intravenous prostaglandin E. Subsequent management depends on the size of the right ventricle and tricuspid valve.

When biventricular repair is considered the best option, cardiac catheterization with radiofrequency-assisted balloon pulmonary valvuloplasty achieves excellent results in the best hands, but surgical pulmonary valvotomy or RVOT enlargement is an alternative approach favored by some. Up to 50% of infants will require an additional systemic-to-pulmonary artery shunt because of early persistent cyanosis caused by right-to-left atrial shunting.

When there is a hypoplastic and hypertensive right ventricle, balloon atrial septostomy followed by a systemic-to-pulmonary artery shunt is the preferred treatment. Subsequently, a bidirectional Glenn procedure followed by total cavopulmonary connection will be undertaken. Where there are extreme and extensive right ventricular-to-coronary connections with stenosis and/or atresia of the coronary arteries, heart transplantation or palliative care may be the only realistic options.

The so-called "one and a half ventricle repair" refers to the combination of pulmonary valvuloplasty or valvotomy with a bidirectional cavopulmonary anastomosis (Glenn) for cases with moderate right ventricular and tricuspid valve hypoplasia in whom there is uncertainty about suitability for a biventricular circulation. This would be the definitive procedure but initially the infant would undergo a systemic-to-pulmonary shunt and/or RVOT reconstruction (catheter or surgical).

Late complications and long-term outcome

Complications and outcome relate to right ventricular scarring and fibrosis, pulmonary regurgitation, and tricuspid insufficiency. As a consequence there is a risk of atrial and ventricular arrhythmias and often a need for pulmonary valve replacement.

For patients undergoing total cavopulmonary connection, there is risk of the usual complications associated with such surgery (atrial arrhythmias, myocardial dysfunction, thromboembolic events, protein-losing enteropathy). Acquired coronary artery lesions associated with ventricular–coronary connections may predispose to ventricular dysfunction.

Further reading

Anderson RH, Baker EJ, Penny DJ, Redington AN, Rigby ML, Wernovsky G (eds). *Paediatric Cardiology,* Third Edition. Philadelphia: Churchill Livingstone/Elsevier, 2010.

Daubeney PEF. Pulmonary atresia with intact ventricular septum. In: Gatzoulis MA, Webb GD, Daubeney PEF (eds). *Diagnosis and Management of Congenital Heart Disease.* London: Churchill Livingstone, 2003, pp. 339–347.

16 Common mixing situations

Michael L. Rigby

Royal Brompton Hospital, London, UK

When applied to congenital heart disease, the term "common mixing" refers to those malformations in which there is complete mixing of systemic and pulmonary venous blood. Unless associated with pulmonary venous obstruction or significant pulmonary stenosis or pulmonary atresia, such malformations cause mild central cyanosis in early infancy.

Total anomalous pulmonary venous connection

All the pulmonary veins drain by abnormal routes directly or indirectly to the right atrium. The most common types of total anomalous pulmonary venous connection (TAPVC) are:
- Supracardiac;
- Infracardiac;
- Cardiac to coronary sinus;
- Cardiac direct to right atrium (Figure 16.1).

Most cases of supracardiac drainage are to the superior caval vein via a vertical vein to the innominate. The pulmonary veins may drain directly to the right atrium or enter via the coronary sinus. Infracardiac drainage is via a descending vein to the hepatic portal vein and ductus venosus.

The pulmonary venous drainage to the right atrium results in a volume-loaded, dilated right ventricle and increased pulmonary blood flow with enlargement of the pulmonary arteries, unless there is obstruction to pulmonary venous return. Survival depends upon the presence of an interatrial communication to permit a right-to-left shunt. In contrast to the right-sided chambers, the left atrium and ventricle are usually small and squashed, but always large enough to permit an adequate cardiac output. Obstruction to pulmonary venous return most frequently involves the infracardiac type, occurring in the liver or at the ductus venosus. In the supracardiac type, obstruction may occur where the vertical vein passes between the left main bronchus and left pulmonary artery. One or more pulmonary veins may be small, giving the potential for late pulmonary venous obstruction after surgical repair in all types.

Hearts with right atrial isomerism by definition have anomalous pulmonary venous connection. In about half the cases, the anomalous connection is extracardiac and will be obstructed in the majority.

Apart from the obligatory atrial septal defect (ASD) and a few cases with a patent arterial duct or ventricular septal defect (VSD), associated congenital heart disease is uncommon, but includes coarctation, atrioventricular septal defect (AVSD), and hearts with a univentricular atrioventricular (AV) connection.

Incidence and etiology
This is an uncommon condition with an incidence of less than 1% of all congenital heart disease and a prevalence of 7 per 100 000 live births. There are no specific etiologic factors and familial cases are rare. Eighty percent of the infracardiac type occurs in males.

Clinical features
With obstructed pulmonary venous return
- Severe central cyanosis and respiratory distress with marked subcostal and intercostal recession soon after birth.
- A loud single second heart sound (simultaneous A2 and P2) and no murmurs are the usual findings; in cases of infracardiac drainage, there is often severe hepatomegaly.
- **EKG:** Can be normal but right ventricular hypertrophy (RVH) is often present.
- **CXR:** Pulmonary venous congestion and pulmonary edema with a miliary or reticular pattern and a small heart.

Pediatric Heart Disease: A Practical Guide, First Edition. Piers E. F. Daubeney, Michael L. Rigby, Koichiro Niwa, and Michael A. Gatzoulis.
© 2012 Blackwell Publishing Ltd. Published 2012 by Blackwell Publishing Ltd.

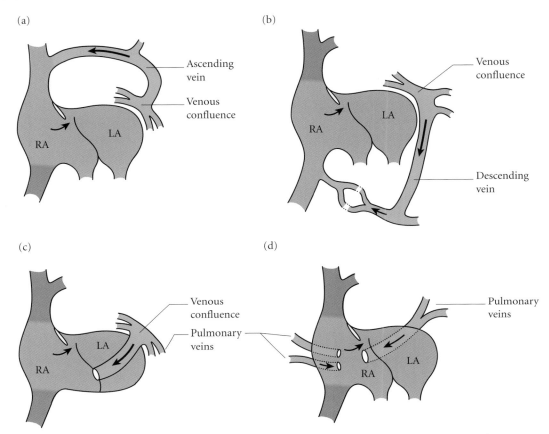

Figure 16.1 Types of total anomalous pulmonary venous connection. (a) Supracardiac; (b) infracardiac; (c) cardiac to coronary sinus; (d) cardiac direct to right atrium. The arrows show the direction of flow of blood. LA, left atrium; RA, right atrium.

A **small ("restrictive") interatrial communication**, by limiting the right-to-left shunt, causes symptoms of heart failure and low cardiac output early in infancy; tachypnea, pallor, and hepatomegaly are often quite striking.

Without obstructed pulmonary venous return
• Unless the interatrial defect is too small, the nonobstructed type may not cause any significant symptoms for the first 2 or 3 months of life; arterial oxygen desaturation is often so mild that cyanosis may not always be clinically evident. Often there is mild cyanosis on crying, minimal tachypnea and subcostal recession, mild failure to thrive, tachycardia, and a prominent right ventricular precordial impulse.
• There is wide but often variable splitting of the second heart sound, an accentuated P2, and third and fourth heart sounds may be present, with an ejection systolic murmur at the upper left sternal edge and sometimes a soft diastolic tricuspid flow murmur at the lower left sternal edge.
• A frequent mode of presentation is with a chest infection. Recurrent chest infection diagnosed as "asthma" is another mode of presentation; a few children are symptom-free and present after 1 year of age.
• **EKG:** Right axis deviation, right atrial enlargement, and RVH.
• **CXR:** At least moderate cardiomegaly with a dilated right atrium and markedly increased pulmonary vascular markings. After the age of 3–4 months, the supracardiac type has a "snowman" cardiac silhouette.

Investigations
• **Echocardiography:** Almost always establishes the exact diagnosis and identifies the site of pulmonary

venous obstruction where the normal phasic Doppler flow pattern becomes continuous.
- **MRI:**
  - Sometimes hypoplasia of one or more pulmonary veins is not suspected on clinical grounds or identified by echocardiography.
  - Requires general anesthesia in children younger than 7 years.
- **CT angiography:**
  - Provides excellent anatomic information about the pulmonary venous connection and caliber of the pulmonary veins
  - Exposes the subject to radiation
  - Rarely needed in the newborn period as most, if not all, information can be obtained with 2D echocardiography
  - Particularly useful in evaluating postoperative pulmonary vein stenosis.
- **Cardiac catheterization:**
  - Rarely performed in the newborn period since the emergence of cross-sectional echocardiography as a diagnostic tool
  - Useful in imaging postoperative pulmonary vein stenosis and as a means of performing balloon dilatation of such stenosis (see below).

Key features of TAPVC on echocardiography

- Dilated right atrium and ventricle.
- Small (squashed) left atrium and ventricle.
- Failure to demonstrate the pulmonary veins connecting to the left atrium
- Pulmonary venous confluence posterior to the left atrium from which arises a large vertical vein ascending on the left, a dilated coronary sinus or a large descending vein passing through the diaphragm posteriorly and to the left. In the latter, dilated veins are seen in the liver because of obstructed pulmonary venous return.
- Always a right-to-left shunt across an ASD in the oval fossa. Be aware that a small interatrial communication, by limiting flow to the left atrium, can lead to severe symptoms!

Management
Medical management
- **Intubation and ventilation** for neonates with severe respiratory distress and hypoxia due to pulmonary venous obstruction or a restrictive ASD. Prostaglandins are likely to make the symptoms worse.

- **Balloon or blade atrial septostomy** can be performed in an emergency for the infant with a restrictive ASD and severe symptoms, but is rarely used in treatment.
- **Diuretics** for mild-to-moderate heart failure prior to surgical repair.

Surgical repair
Surgical repair under cardiopulmonary bypass is required in every patient. The exact procedure depends on the type of anomalous drainage:
- **Emergency repair** for neonates and infants with severe symptoms;
- **Elective repair** aged 2–4 months for infants without pulmonary venous obstruction and with mild symptoms.

Late complications and long-term outcome
In the current era more than 85% of infants will survive surgical repair. The major causes of early death are pulmonary venous obstruction and pulmonary hypertensive crises.

Late pulmonary vein stenosis is usually due to unrecognized stenosis in the early postoperative period. Treatment algorithms include cutting balloon-assisted pulmonary venous angioplasty or surgical revision using a sutureless technique. Stenting of pulmonary veins results in almost inevitable death.

Atrial arrhythmias such as flutter, fibrillation, or ectopic atrial tachycardia are unusual in childhood or early adolescence, but are more likely after the second decade.

Partial anomalous pulmonary venous connection

Some of the pulmonary veins drain directly to the right atrium, superior caval vein, inferior caval vein, coronary sinus or innominate vein. If all the pulmonary veins from one lung drain anomalously but from the contralateral lung connect to the left atrium, the condition is called "hemi-anomalous" drainage. The most frequent associated anomaly is an ASD but partial anomalous pulmonary venous connection (PAPVC) is an integral part of a superior sinus venosus ASD (see Chapter 9) and the scimitar syndrome (see Chapter 17). The hemodynamics are very similar to those of an ASD with an increased pulmonary blood flow and right atrial and ventricular volume loading.

Clinical features
- Most children are symptom-free.
- There is wide splitting of the second heart sound, which is fixed if there is an associated ASD, a soft ejection systolic murmur at the upper left sternal edge, and a soft mid-diastolic flow murmur at the lower left sternal edge.

Investigations
- **EKG:** Usually right axis deviation and "partial" right bundle branch block.
- **CXR:** Cardiomegaly with a large right atrium and increased pulmonary vascular markings.
- **Other imaging:** The diagnosis should always be considered when there is unexplained right heart dilatation on an echocardiogram; the connection of the pulmonary veins cannot always be determined so that additional imaging from cardiac catheterization and angiography, CT angiography or MRI might be needed.

Management
- When only one of four pulmonary veins has an anomalous connection, common practice is not to undertake surgical repair.
- Surgical treatment under cardiopulmonary bypass, usually after the age of 5 years, is undertaken if more than one pulmonary vein drains anomalously or if there is right heart volume overload seen on the echocardiogram.

Late complications and long-term outcome
From the published literature there appears to be a significant risk of superior caval vein obstruction after repair of an anomalous pulmonary vein to the superior caval vein. The risk is greatest when surgery is performed at a young age.

In the scimitar syndrome (see Chapter 17), repair carries a significant risk of right pulmonary vein stenosis so that surgery should not be recommended lightly in these patients.

There is a late risk of atrial arrhythmia in adult life in both patients who have and who have not undergone surgery.

Hearts with univentricular atrioventricular connection

This group of cardiac anomalies has in common that the atria are connected to only one ventricle, rather than a biventricular AV connection of the type found in most hearts. The term "univentricular AV connection" used to describe these anomalies was coined by Robert Anderson, but the nomenclature remains contentious.

Types of univentricular AV connection
- Absent right
- Absent left
- Double inlet

With absence of the right or left AV connection, a sulcus or recess filled with fibrofatty tissue interposes between the muscular floor of the corresponding atrium and the ventricular myocardium. The contralateral atrium is connected to a ventricle via a single AV valve.

In double inlet ventricle, each atrium is connected to the same ventricle either via separate left and right AV valves or, less frequently, via a common valve. When there are two AV valves, various "modes" of connection may be encountered, such as an imperforate, stenotic, overriding, or straddling valve. An overriding valve orifice is committed to both ventricles. A straddling valve usually overrides the ventricular septum but also has tensor apparatus in each. A right or left AV valve or common valve can therefore override and straddle the ventricular septum. Providing more than 50% of both valves or more than 75% of a common valve are committed to one ventricle, the connection is described as double inlet. Rarely, the left or right AV valve in hearts with absent connection may straddle the ventricular septum; the AV connection is then described as "uniatrial and biventricular."

Although most hearts with a univentricular AV connection will have the usual atrial arrangement of situs solitus, any arrangement (solitus, inversus, right or left isomerism) can be found.

With regard to the morphology of the main ventricular chamber, there are only three possibilities.

Ventricular morphology in hearts with univentricular AV connection
- Dominant left ventricle with anterosuperior rudimentary right ventricle
- Dominant right ventricle with posteroinferior rudimentary left ventricle
- Solitary indeterminate ventricle

With the exception of a solitary indeterminate ventricle, there is almost always a VSD. A left ventricle has fine apical trabeculations, whereas a morphologic right ventricle has coarse trabeculations. In a solitary indeterminate ventricle, the trabeculations are extremely coarse with extensive muscle bundles.

This complex group of anomalies is often diagnosed during fetal life. Conventional postnatal imaging by echocardiography, MRI or angiography will usually allow ventricular morphology to be determined. Importantly:
• When the outlet of the small and rudimentary ventricle is anterior, there is a dominant left ventricle;
• When the outlet of the small and rudimentary ventricle is posterior and inferior, there is a dominant right ventricle.

Any type of ventricular–arterial (VA) connection (concordant, discordant, single outlet, double outlet ventricle) can occur. A combination of muscular and valvar pulmonary stenosis or atresia is present in fewer than half the cases.

Finally, the similarities in this group of heart malformations mean the clinical presentation together with the medical and surgical management will be almost the same.

Tricuspid atresia and absent right atrioventricular connection

Most cases of tricuspid atresia are characterized by absence of the right AV connection (Figure 16.2). Usually

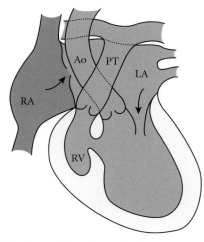

Figure 16.2 Absent right atrioventricular connection. The arrows show the direction of flow of blood. Ao, aorta; LA, left atrium, LV, left ventricle; PT, pulmonary trunk; RA, right atrium; RV, right ventricle.

the left atrium connects to the left ventricle and the VA connection is concordant or discordant. An interatrial communication to allow egress of blood from the right atrium to the left is essential for survival. The rudimentary right ventricle is anterior and right-sided while a muscular VSD will vary from large to extremely small. Cases are encountered without a VSD or with multiple defects.

Morphologic variants that present the usual clinical profile of classical tricuspid atresia are:
• Imperforate tricuspid valve with concordant AV connection;
• Imperforate right AV valve with double inlet ventricle;
• Absent right AV connection with left atrium connected to the morphologic right ventricle; in morphologic terms this is an example of "mitral atresia";
• Absent right AV connection with solitary indeterminate ventricle;
• Absent right AV connection with straddling left AV valve;
• Absent left AV connection with situs inversus.

The **more common variants** of tricuspid atresia are:
• **Concordant VA connection with pulmonary stenosis or atresia:** This is the commonest type. The site of pulmonary stenosis is usually a small ("restrictive") VSD which obstructs blood flow to the rudimentary right ventricle and pulmonary trunk. The defect often becomes progressively smaller, leading to increasingly severe cyanosis during infancy. Hypercyanotic spells of the type described in tetralogy of Fallot can occur. Patients with mild-to-moderate pulmonary stenosis will have balanced systemic and pulmonary blood flows with milder cyanosis and minimal symptoms. Severe pulmonary stenosis or atresia, usually associated with extreme right ventricular hypoplasia and very small VSD, causes severe cyanosis.
• **Concordant VA connection and large VSD:** Characterized by mild cyanosis after birth. Symptoms of heart failure develop during the second month.
• **Discordant VA connection with restrictive VSD, hypoplastic aorta, and coarctation:** The typical neonatal presentation is with mild cyanosis, absent femoral pulses, heart failure, low cardiac output, and sometimes cardiogenic shock. Prostaglandin E will maintain ductal patency and systemic blood flow.
• **Discordant VA connection and moderate-to-large VSD:** Infants are mildly cyanosed and develop heart failure after a few weeks. The VSD may become relatively smaller with growth and particularly following banding of the pulmonary trunk.

• **Discordant VA connection, large VSD, and muscular subpulmonary stenosis:** Pulmonary stenosis results in more severe cyanosis, which is occasionally so severe that a duct-dependent pulmonary circulation exists.

Mitral atresia and absent left atrioventricular connection (with normal ascending aorta)

Hearts with an absent left AV connection (Figure 16.3) include those with mitral atresia, but the former term is preferable. Common to most patients is the pulmonary venous return received by the left atrium, and the only egress of blood is through an ASD that is essential for survival. A restrictive defect causes left atrial hypertension, pulmonary edema, and a raised pulmonary artery pressure.

Morphologic variants are:
• **Right atrium connects to the right ventricle:** This is the most common variant. The left ventricle is posterior and left sided, and usually there is a large VSD. The VA connection is concordant or double outlet from the right ventricle.
• **Right atrium connects to the left ventricle:** This is also encountered quite frequently. The rudimentary right ventricle is anterior and left sided; there is usually a discordant VA connection with an anterior and left-sided aortic valve. This variant is in fact an example of tricuspid atresia so the term "mitral atresia" should not be used. It

is noteworthy that the ventricular mass is very similar to that found in a double inlet left ventricle with a left-sided rudimentary right ventricle.
• **Associated anomalies** that are sometimes encountered include pulmonary stenosis, subaortic stenosis, and coarctation of the aorta.
• **Unusual morphologic variants** giving rise to a similar clinical profile include:
  ◦ Imperforate left AV valve with concordant or discordant AV connection
  ◦ Double inlet ventricle with imperforate left AV valve
  ◦ Absent left AV connection and straddling right AV valve
  ◦ Absent left AV connection and solitary indeterminate ventricle
  ◦ Absent right AV connection and situs inversus.

Double inlet ventricle

Each atrium is connected to the same ventricle, usually via separate right and left AV valves, but sometimes via a common valve (Figure 16.4). The most frequent type is double inlet left ventricle (80% of cases). A solitary indeterminate ventricle accounts for only 2% of cases, with a dominant right ventricle found in all others.

Morphologic variants are:
• **Double inlet left ventricle with discordant VA connection:** There are two common variants. In one, the rudimentary right ventricle is right sided and anterior;

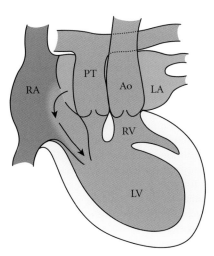

Figure 16.3 Absent left atrioventricular connection. The arrows show the direction of flow of blood. Ao, aorta; LA, left atrium, LV, left ventricle; PT, pulmonary trunk; RA, right atrium; RV, right ventricle

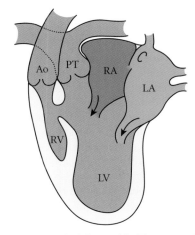

Figure 16.4 Double inlet left ventricle. The arrows show the direction of flow of blood. Ao, aorta; LA, left atrium, LV, left ventricle; PT, pulmonary trunk; RA, right atrium; RV, right ventricle.

the ventricular mass is then almost identical to that found in tricuspid atresia. In the other, the rudimentary right ventricle is left sided and anterior. Both of these can be associated with a restrictive VSD (subaortic stenosis) predisposing to coarctation or even interruption of the aortic arch. Alternatively, muscular subpulmonary stenosis with a large VSD may occur.

• **Double inlet left ventricle with concordant VA connection with or without muscular subpulmonary stenosis ("the Holmes heart"):** Relatively rare.

• **Atrial isomerism and/or a common AV valve:** Uncommon but even less frequent in hearts with double inlet left ventricle.

• **Double inlet right ventricle:** With the usual atrial arrangement, separate right and left AV valves are typical. Double outlet right ventricle, anterior right-sided aortic valve, and muscular subpulmonary stenosis or atresia are the common associations. When there is right atrial isomerism, there is almost always a common AV valve, pulmonary stenosis or atresia, and often an extracardiac total anomalous pulmonary venous connection (see Chapter 17).

• **Double inlet indeterminate ventricle:** Rarest type. Atrial isomerism and a common AV valve are the usual findings.

This list of variants described is not exhaustive. Double inlet ventricle is described in association with any atrial arrangement, ventricular morphology, or VA connection.

"Mode" of connection is the term used to describe the morphology of the valves that guard the AV junction. Abnormalities include imperforate, stenotic, prolapsing, overriding or straddling valves.

Clinical features

These depend on the associated lesions, in particular the presence or absence of pulmonary stenosis or atresia and coarctation of the aorta.

• Typically, coarctation is associated with a discordant ventricular connection and a restrictive VSD; infants present soon after birth with low cardiac output, heart failure, and even cardiogenic shock because of a duct-dependent systemic circulation.

• Most infants without coarctation or pulmonary stenosis are well at birth with mild central cyanosis, developing symptoms of heart failure after a few weeks. Both A2 and P2 are accentuated and there may be a short systolic murmur at the mid-left sternal edge.

• The more severe the pulmonary stenosis, the greater the degree of cyanosis. There will be a single second heart sound and variable ejection systolic murmur at the upper left sternal edge. Some neonates present with profound neonatal cyanosis when the arterial duct is closing.

• In cases of absent left AV connection with a small ASD, neonatal respiratory distress, moderate-to-severe hypoxia, loud P2, and hepatomegaly with pulmonary edema on CXR is the usual clinical picture.

• It is important to be aware that the infant or child with tricuspid atresia also requires an ASD to permit right-to-left shunting and maintain cardiac output. The defect can become extremely small, causing a generalized gray coloration with moderate central cyanosis, hypotension, and marked hepatomegaly. This may be a medical emergency requiring the creation of an ASD by an experienced interventional cardiologist or cardiac surgeon.

Investigations

• **EKG:**
  ○ **Tricuspid atresia\:** The classical findings are a superior mean frontal QRS axis (0 to −90 degrees), left ventricular hypertrophy (LVH), and right atrial enlargement. The axis is more likely to be inferior when the VA connection is discordant
  ○ **Absent left AV connection:** Right axis deviation, right ventricular dominant pattern, and left atrial enlargement are typical.
  ○ **Double inlet ventricle:** There are no diagnostic features. Similar QRS complexes with prominent R and S waves across all the precordial leads are sometimes found. A pattern of LVH occurs commonly. Q waves in V1 and V2 are not unusual but may be absent from all precordial leads. Other inconsistent findings include varying degrees of heart block and a superior axis. The P wave axis and morphology of the P waves is abnormal in atrial isomerism.

• **CXR:** This reflects the amount of pulmonary blood flow:
  ○ Without pulmonary stenosis, cardiomegaly and pulmonary plethora are found
  ○ With pulmonary stenosis or atresia, a normal heart size and normal-to-reduced pulmonary vascular markings are found
  ○ With a left-sided rudimentary right ventricle, a left-sided ascending aorta may be obvious and dextrocardia is sometimes present
  ○ Occasionally dextrocardia is found with situs solitus, tricuspid atresia, and pulmonary stenosis
  ○ With a restrictive ASD in absent left AV connection, pulmonary venous congestion and pulmonary edema can be expected.

• **Echocardiogram:** Expert echocardiography provides the initial diagnosis in the majority of infants and children. The features requiring documentation include:
  ○ Atrial situs
  ○ Type and mode of AV connection
  ○ VA connection
  ○ Presence and severity of pulmonary stenosis or atresia
  ○ Size of the ASD
  ○ Ventricular morphology
  ○ Size of the VSD
  ○ Ventricular dysfunction or hypertrophy
  ○ AV valve regurgitation.
• **Further imaging:** Rarely required in early clinical decision-making, although the direct measurement of pulmonary artery pressure and pulmonary vascular resistance at cardiac catheterization is sometimes needed
• **Cardiac catheterization and angiography:** Often performed after initial palliative surgery before more definitive operations; the major role is measurement of pulmonary artery and ventricular end-diastolic pressures together with imaging of the pulmonary arteries. Alternative techniques include CT angiography and MRI.

Management
Medical management
• **Severe hypoxia:**
  ○ Prostaglandin E to maintain ductal patency and provide adequate pulmonary blood flow
  ○ Correction of metabolic acidosis
  ○ Balloon atrial septostomy for severely restrictive ASD in absent left or right AV connection.
• **Heart failure:**
  ○ Prostaglandin E for severe subaortic stenosis, aortic coarctation or aortic interruption to maintain ductal patency and systemic blood flow
  ○ Diuretics for symptoms of heart failure.

Surgical repair
The principles of surgical management are to avoid excessive pulmonary blood flow and ventricular volume loading, to maintain a low pulmonary artery pressure and pulmonary vascular resistance, and to avoid ventricular hypertrophy. The latter might result from excessive pressure loading, when there is a discordant VA connection and restrictive VSD. Chapter 34 gives an overview of surgical strategy.

• **Initial palliation;** Patients will usually have either a systemic-to-pulmonary artery shunt procedure or banding of the pulmonary artery as palliation in early infancy. In a few cases with moderate pulmonary stenosis, balanced systemic and pulmonary blood flows will have caused mild-to-moderate cyanosis and hypoxia so that surgical palliation in the first few months of life is not needed
• **Damus–Kaye–Stansel operation:** The anastomosis of the proximal pulmonary trunk to the ascending aorta to provide unobstructed systemic blood flow when there is a discordant VA connection and restrictive VSD. Pulmonary blood flow is maintained by a systemic-to-pulmonary shunt. **Direct enlargement of the VSD** is an alternative operation preferred by a few surgeons as it can avoid complete heart block.
• **Bidirectional Glenn operation (superior cavopulmonary anastomosis):** Usually performed after the age of 4 months and before 1 year, the superior caval vein is disconnected from the right atrium and anastomosed to the right pulmonary artery. For children with right and left superior caval veins and absence of the bridging innominate vein, the **bilateral bidirectional cavopulmonary anastomosis** is performed.
• **Completion of total cavopulmonary connection (TCPC):** Performed 1–3 years following the bidirectional Glenn, the inferior caval vein is disconnected from the right atrium with the hepatic veins intact and connected to the underside of the right pulmonary artery via an extracardiac prosthetic conduit of 18–22 mm in diameter. A total cavopulmonary connection can be performed as a one-stage procedure in low-risk cases.
• **"Fenestrated" total cavopulmonary connection.** This modification refers to the creation of a 4–6-mm window between the external conduit and the atria. While used routinely in some centers, others reserve this approach for higher risk cases. The fenestration allows right-to-left shunting and, although the patient will be cyanosed, the early postoperative course may be easier. In many instances the fenestration closes spontaneously within a year, but if necessary can be occluded using a transcatheter approach from the femoral vein.
• **Kawashima operation:** This modification is used exclusively for patients with left atrial isomerism, absence of the inferior caval vein, and connection of the azygos vein to the superior caval vein; it refers to the anastomosis of the superior caval vein to the right or left pulmonary artery. Because all but the hepatic venous return is directed into the pulmonary arteries, patients will have minimal systemic arterial desaturation and cyanosis.

Complications and long-term outcome

The natural history of hearts with a "single" ventricle is for the development of ventricular dysfunction, AV valve regurgitation, severe cyanosis, pulmonary vascular disease, and atrial and ventricular arrhythmias in adolescence or early adult life. Life expectancy is improved by surgery in many cases.

• **Early complications:** The most troublesome early complications of the bidirectional Glenn operation and total cavopulmonary connection are recurrent pleural and pericardial effusions, low cardiac output, and atrial arrhythmias.

• **Late complications of TCPC:**
  ◦ Ventricular dysfunction
  ◦ AV valve regurgitation
  ◦ Conduit stenosis
  ◦ Right pulmonary vein occlusion or stenosis
  ◦ Cyanosis due to pulmonary arteriovenous fistulae or systemic venous collaterals to the left atrium
  ◦ Atrial arrhythmias (flutter, fibrillation, re-entrant tachycardia, and ectopic tachycardia)
  ◦ AV conduction abnormalities
  ◦ Thrombus formation with pulmonary and systemic emboli
  ◦ Protein-losing enteropthy and hypoproteinemia
  ◦ Premature death (survival beyond the age of 45 years is unlikely)
  ◦ Hearts with a dominant right ventricle, atrial isomerism, and absent left AV connection have the worst prognosis.

Hypoplastic left heart syndrome

Hypoplastic left heart syndrome (HLHS) comprises a group of closely related anomalies characterized by hypoplasia of the left ventricle, severe stenosis or atresia of the mitral and aortic valves, and variable hypoplasia of the ascending aorta and arch. When there is mitral atresia and no interatrial defect, escape of blood from the left atrium may be via a levoatrial cardinal vein which joins the innominate vein, allowing flow to the superior caval vein and right atrium (Figure 16.5).

Clinical features

In the current era the diagnosis is often made during pregnancy by antenatal fetal ultrasound scanning. Most of these infants will be delivered close to a specialized pediatric cardiology center and commenced on intravenous prostaglandin E immediately following delivery.

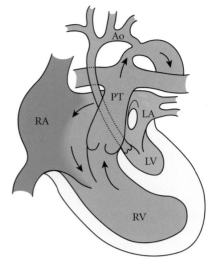

Figure 16.5 Hypoplastic left heart. The arrows show the direction of flow of blood. Ao, aorta; LA, left atrium, LV, left ventricle; PT, pulmonary trunk; RA, right atrium; RV, right ventricle.

Without prior diagnosis, infants almost always become critically ill within a few hours of birth as the arterial duct begins to close. The characteristic findings are:
• Mild cyanosis, pallor, and mottling;
• Tachypnea, often with respiratory distress and tachycardia;
• Poor peripheral pulses and vasoconstriction;
• Loud single S2 (P2 only) and no murmur;
• Marked hepatomegaly.

Investigations

• **EKG:** Right axis deviation, RVH, and sometimes right atrial enlargement.
• **CXR:** Moderate cardiomegaly, pulmonary venous congestion, and pulmonary edema.
• **Echocardiogram:**
  ◦ Usually provides a complete diagnosis
  ◦ Characteristic findings are extreme hypoplasia of the left ventricle (often with obvious endocardial fibrosis), miniaturized or atretic mitral and aortic valves, and hypoplasia of the ascending aorta and arch
  ◦ The ventricular septum is usually intact but a VSD is associated with less extreme aortic hypoplasia
  ◦ Poor prognostic features often considered a contraindication to surgical palliation are a very small ASD, right ventricular dysfunction, and moderate tricuspid insufficiency.

Management
Medical management
Intravenous prostaglandin E should be given early, even when the diagnosis is only suspected and correction of the metabolic acidosis are essential.

Surgical management
Early parental counseling about the severity of the abnormality and need for at least three major operations with cardiopulmonary bypass during the first 2 years of life is an important aspect of care. Some infants are unsuitable for operation while some parents, being aware of the early and medium-term outcomes, prefer their infant not to undergo complex, high-risk surgery.
• **Norwood operation** (Figure 16.6). Performed following the correction of any metabolic acidosis. Pulmonary blood flow is via a systemic-to-pulmonary artery shunt (3.5 mm) or small conduit from the right ventricle to the pulmonary trunk (Sano modification).
• **A hybrid procedure**, with stenting of the arterial duct and banding of the left and right pulmonary arteries, is an alternative to the Norwood.
• **Following neonatal palliation**, the surgical strategy is similar to that for hearts with univentricular AV connection.
• **Bidirectional Glenn operation (cavopulmonary anastomosis)** is undertaken at 3–6 months.

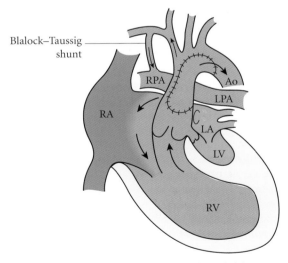

Figure 16.6 Norwood procedure for hypoplastic left heart. The arrows show the direction of flow of blood. Ao, aorta; LA, left atrium; LPA, left pulmonary artery; LV, left ventricle; RA, right atrium; RPA, right pulmonary artery; RV, right ventricle.

• **Completion of TCPC** is from age 18 months to 3 years.
   Heart transplantation is an alternative to other surgical strategies in a small minority of cases only and is not a realistic option for most infants.

Complications and long-term outcome
• **Early outcome:**
  ◦ Surgical management carries up to a 20% combined early mortality in the best hands
  ◦ Early complications include too much or too little pulmonary blood flow, myocardial ischemia and ventricular dysfunction, progressive tricuspid and neoaortic valve insufficiency, and re-coarctation of the aorta.
• **Late outcome:**
  ◦ Late complications are the same as those observed in a heart with univentricular AV connection (see above)
  ◦ Congenital or acquired neurologic problems are surprisingly frequent
  ◦ The outcome of late heart transplantation for the failing TCPC is disappointing.

Common arterial trunk (truncus arteriosus)

Truncus arteriosus is an uncommon malformation associated with deletion of chromosome 22q11 in 50% of cases. A single arterial trunk takes origin from the ventricles, overrides the ventricular septum and, in its proximal part, gives rise to coronary arteries, the ascending aorta, and pulmonary arteries. According to the way the pulmonary arteries arise from the common trunk, three types are described (Figure 16.7).

Types of common arterial trunk
• **Type 1:** A short main pulmonary artery arises from the left posterior aspect
• **Type 2:** The right and left pulmonary arteries arise separately but close together from the posterior aspect
• **Type 3:** The right and left pulmonary arteries arise from the lateral aspects and are widely separated

---

   Other variable features are:
• The truncal valve frequently has three cusps but bicuspid and quadricuspid valves are not unusual. Dysplastic leaflets are common and may be associated with stenosis and or insufficiency.

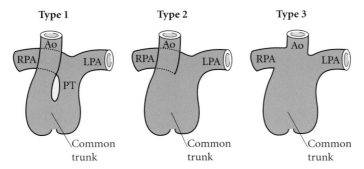

Figure 16.7 Classification of types of common arterial trunk. Ao, aorta; LPA, left pulmonary artery; PT, pulmonary trunk; RPA, right pulmonary artery.

• The common trunk overrides the ventricular septum and usually has a balanced origin from each ventricle, although it may arise exclusively from one or other ventricle.

• There is a large outlet VSD which usually has a muscular posterior rim but may be perimembranous. Rarely the defect is small and restrictive.

• A right aortic arch is present in approaching half the cases. Aortic interruption is a common association but coarctation and an arterial duct are both rare.

• The pulmonary arteries are often enlarged because of the high pulmonary blood flow. Unusual abnormalities are pulmonary artery stenosis, anomalous origin of the right pulmonary artery from the ascending aorta, or absence of the right or left pulmonary artery.

• Very rarely there is a complete AVSD or other congenital heart malformation.

Clinical features

Commonly infants present with mild central cyanosis and the signs and symptoms of heart failure at a few weeks of age. Typically, examination, reveals tachypnea, tachycardia, an active precordium, wide pulse pressure, and "bounding" peripheral pulses. On auscultation there is a loud ejection click, single second heart sound, and ejection systolic murmur at the upper left sternal edge.

In one-third of cases, obvious splitting of the second heart sound is audible. It is not unusual to hear an early diastolic murmur of aortic insufficiency; a continuous murmur caused by pulmonary stenosis is exceptional. The presence of pulmonary stenosis or pulmonary vascular disease causes more obvious cyanosis and in the latter, there may be no heart murmur.

Investigations

• **EKG:**
  ○ A normal mean frontal QRS axis (+50 to +120 degrees), biventricular hypertrophy, and T wave inversion in V5 and V6 are the typical findings
  ○ Isolated RVH or LVH and a superior axis are sometimes present.

• **CXR:**
  ○ In the typical case there is moderate cardiomegaly, a dilated ascending aorta, absence of the usual pulmonary trunk, and pulmonary plethora with or without edema
  ○ There may be left deviation of the trachea caused by a right aortic arch.

• **Echocardiography:**
  ○ A large common trunk overrides the ventricular septum giving rise to the pulmonary arteries posteriorly
  ○ RVH is often striking and the left ventricle is dilated
  ○ Dysplastic truncal valve leaflets with insufficiency and/or stenosis occur in over 25%

• **Other investigations**: these are not usually needed for precise diagnosis.

Management
Medical management
Treatment is focused on the management of heart failure prior to surgical repair. It is particularly important to avoid supplemental oxygen, which can promote torrential pulmonary blood flow at the expense of aortic flow and systemic output.

Surgical management
Repair is undertaken in early infancy from age 1 to 4 months by closing the VSD, disconnecting the pulmonary

arteries from the common trunk, establishing a connection from the right ventricle to the proximal pulmonary arteries, and, if necessary, repairing any associated lesions. With pulmonary stenosis, early repair can often be avoided. Surgery to the neoaortic (truncal) valve is not usually needed at the first operation. There are two surgical techniques in common usage:
• **Repair with right ventricular–to-pulmonary artery homograft conduit;**
• **Repair with direct anastomosis of the pulmonary trunk to the right ventricular outflow tract.**

Late complications and long-term outcome
• Some patients develop progressively more severe aortic insufficiency and require valve replacement during childhood or adolescence.

• Replacement of the homograft conduit is always needed from 4–8 years after the first repair.
• In some older patients, pulmonary insufficiency can be managed with percutaneous insertion of a stented valve.
• Late atrial and ventricular arrhythmias with risk of sudden death are a potential life-long problem.

Further reading

Anderson RH, Crupi G, Parenzan L (eds). *Double Inlet Ventricle.* Tunbridge Wells: Castle House, 1987.
Cor univentriculare. *Herz* 1979;4(2).
Hutter D, Redington AN. Principles of management, and outcomes for patients with functionally univentricular hearts. In: Anderson RH, Baker EJ, Penny DJ, Redington AN, Rigby ML, Wernovsky G (eds). *Paediatric Cardiology.* London: Churchill Livingstone/Elsevier, 2010, pp. 687–696.

17 Heterotaxy, scimitar, and arteriovenous malformations

Michael L. Rigby

Royal Brompton Hospital, London, UK

Atrial isomerism

There is a group of patients in whom it may be difficult or impossible to assign visceral situs because the abdominal viscera are not lateralized (see also Chapter 3). Such patients have been described as having **visceral heterotaxia**. The liver is more symmetrical than normal and the bowel is not fixed in the normal way. At the same time the thoracic contents have partial symmetry with both major bronchi, each having the appearance of a right or left main stem bronchus. Both lungs are frequently trilobed in patients with bilateral right main bronchi and bilobed when there are symmetrical left main bronchi. When there is incomplete lateralization within the abdomen and thorax, the atrial appendages are also not clearly lateralized, and in many of these patients both appendages have the appearance of a morphologically right or left appendage; thus the designation by some authors of left or right **atrial isomerism** to characterize these hearts, which some describe as the **syndrome of visceroatrial heterotaxia** (Figure 17.1).

Associated anomalies include:
• Splenic anomalies, including asplenia in right isomerism or polysplenia in left isomerism, are found in at least 85% of cases;
• Varying degrees of malrotation of the gastrointestinal tract;
• An annular or short pancreas;
• Extrahepatic biliary atresia.

For the pediatric cardiologist it is the presence of atrial isomerism and its association with complex congenital heart disease that is the major concern.

The most consistent marker of atrial morphology is the **appendage**. The morphologically right appendage is a blunt triangle with a broad base, whereas the morphologically left appendage is a narrow, hooked, and crenellated structure. On the basis of atrial appendage morphology there are four possible types of atrial arrangement or "situs" (Figures 17.1 and 6.4; see also Chapter 3).

Types of atrial arrangement or "situs"

• Situs solitus or normal (usual) atrial relationship
• Situs inversus or mirror image of normal atrial relationship
• Right isomerism or bilateral morphologically right atria
• Left isomerism or bilateral morphologically left atria

Investigations

Without resorting to direct anatomic inspection of the atrial appendages, cross-sectional echocardiography (particularly transesophageal studies) or MRI can provide the diagnosis, but the EKG and chest and abdominal radiograph can provide some clues to atrial arrangement.

Standard surface EKG
• Normal atrial arrangement (assuming normal position of the sinoatrial node):
  ○ Positive P wave in leads 1, 2, 3, aVL, and aVF
  ○ Negative P wave in aVR.
• Mirror-image atrial arrangement:
  ○ Positive P wave deflection in leads 1, 2, 3, aVR, and aVF
  ○ Negative in aVL.

Pediatric Heart Disease: A Practical Guide, First Edition. Piers E. F. Daubeney, Michael L. Rigby, Koichiro Niwa, and Michael A. Gatzoulis.
© 2012 Blackwell Publishing Ltd. Published 2012 by Blackwell Publishing Ltd.

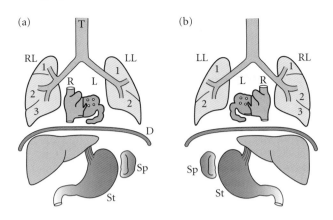
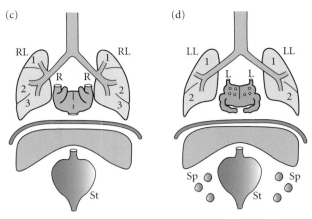

Figure 17.1 Right and left atrial isomerism (asplenia and polysplenia syndromes, respectively). Atrial, bronchial, and abdominal arrangements. (a) Usual or situs solitus; (b) mirror image or situs inversus; (c) right atrial isomerism or asplenia syndrome; (d) left atrial isomerism or polysplenia syndrome.

L, morphologic left atrium; LL, left lung; R, morphologic right atrium; RL, right lung; Sp, spleen; St, stomach; T, trachea. (Adapted from Gatzoulis MA, Swan L, Therrien J, Pantely GA, eds. *Adult Congenital Heart Disease, A Practical Guide*, 2005, with permission from Blackwell Publishing Ltd.)

- Right isomerism:
  ∘ Usually two sinus nodes.
- Left isomerism:
  ∘ Sinus node absent, although histologic studies have identified a rudimentary node close to the atrioventricular junction in some cases
  ∘ Normal sinus rhythm is unusual
  ∘ Left and superior P wave axis frequently found.

Atrial position can be deduced from the position of the abdominal organs, assuming the morphologically right atrium is on the same side as the liver and the morphologically left atrium on the same side as the stomach and spleen. These criteria, however, are unreliable. Certainly, a midline horizontal liver is frequently found with atrial isomerism but, for example, with left isomerism the stomach is often on the left. A discordant relationship between cardiac position and the side of the stomach bubble is always suggestive of atrial isomerism.

Chest X-ray

A very useful indirect method of determining atrial arrangement is the appearance of the tracheobronchial tree imaged with the plain CXR or high kilovoltage filtered films. Atrial arrangement is almost always reflected by bronchial morphology.

> **Normal image atrial arrangement**
> - Morphologically left main bronchus twice as long as right
> - Morphologically left bronchus beneath artery to the lower lobes (hyparterial)
> - Morphologically right bronchus above the corresponding artery (eparterial)

Where there is mirror-image atrial arrangement, the same holds except that the morphologic left bronchus will be right-sided and *vice versa*. Thus, when the bronchi are asymmetrical there will be normal or mirror-image arrangement of the atria with the morphologically left atrium on the side of the longer bronchus.

> **Atrial isomerism and visceral symmetry**
> - Bronchi are also symmetrical
> - Bilateral long hyparterial bronchi are indicative of left isomerism
> - Bilateral short eparterial bronchi are indicative of right isomerism

Very occasionally there is a discordant relationship between bronchial arrangement and atrial situs, and similarly there can be a discordant relationship between abdominal situs and atrial situs. Nevertheless, the determination of atrial arrangement from echocardiographic sections of the abdominal great vessels (see Chapter 6) is the most reliable everyday clinical guide (see Figure 6.4).

Systemic and pulmonary venous connections

In patients with **right isomerism**:
• Atrial septum is often severely deficient, sometimes just a muscular strand;
• Common atrioventricular junction in majority of cases;
• Bilateral superior caval veins found in most cases, each draining directly to the atrial roof;
• Bridging innominate vein is often absent;
• Occasional hypoplasia of one superior caval vein and absent coronary sinus;
• Inferior caval vein almost always drains directly to the atrium mass, sometimes bilaterally but usually unilaterally with connection either to the right-or left-sided atrium;
• Pulmonary veins are always connected in anomalous fashion when there is right isomerism, even when they drain directly to the atria;
• In more than half the cases, however, there is an extracardiac total anomalous pulmonary venous connection either to one of the superior caval veins or to the inferior caval vein;
• With extracardiac drainage pulmonary venous obstruction is common;
• When the pulmonary veins drain directly to the atria they usually connect to the midpoint of what is effectively a common atrial chamber. It is unusual for all the pulmonary veins to drain to one or other of the atria.

In patients with **left atrial isomerism**:
• The atrial septum is usually better formed, but a common atrium can be encountered, often with bilateral connection of the pulmonary veins;
• Usually the atrial septum is intact or there is an atrioventricular septal defect (AVSD) present;
• Bilateral superior caval veins are found just as frequently as in right isomerism;
• Coronary sinus is present in the majority and often drains one of the superior caval veins;
• The major venous anomaly found in hearts with left isomerism is interruption of the abdominal inferior caval vein with continuation through an azygous vein to the right or left superior caval vein;
• Most commonly the hepatic veins drain through a common intrahepatic segment directly to one or both of the left atria (see Chapter 6);
• Pulmonary veins connect to the atrial chambers in normal fashion, but the veins can be connected so that two of them drain to each of the atrial components or alternatively all four veins drain to the same atrium which can be right- or left-sided.

Atrioventricular junction, ventricles, and ventricular–arterial connections

Functionally normal hearts can occasionally exist in the presence of isomerism of the atrial appendages and not all patients exhibit complex combinations. Those with left isomerism can have relatively simple combinations of lesions such as an ostium primum defect, ventricular septal defect (VSD), or tetralogy of Fallot. It is well-known, however, that the combinations of lesions found in atrial isomerism are often the most complex, so each patient must be treated on an individual basis with strict adherence to sequential segmental diagnosis (see Chapter 3).

A common **atrioventricular junction** is frequently encountered either as part of an AVSD with a biventricular atrioventricular connection or in hearts with a double-inlet ventricle when the majority of the atrioventricular junction is committed to one ventricle. In most examples of an AVSD there is a common valve orifice (complete form), but separate left and right valve orifices can occur. Separate atrioventricular junctions guarded by the mitral and tricuspid valves are also encountered, but the absence of the left or right atrioventricular connection is unusual.

Ventricular relationships are interesting in hearts with atrial isomerism because in almost half the cases the morphologically right ventricle is to the left, so that the ventricular mass assumes the appearance of hearts with a discordant atrioventricular connection (so-called "left-hand pattern topology"). Abnormalities of the ventricular outflow tracts are much more frequent in the setting of right isomerism, but can also be found with left isomerism. In right isomerism, a double outlet right ventricle with bilateral infundibuli or discordant ventricular–arterial connections is the most common. These connections themselves are then further complicated by pulmonary stenosis or atresia. With pulmonary atresia, bilateral arterial ducts can be found sometimes with non-confluent pulmonary arteries, but systemic-to-pulmonary artery collaterals are rare. The presence of obstructed extracardiac total anomalous pulmonary venous connection can result in acute pulmonary edema following a palliative systemic-to-pulmonary artery shunt. The ventricular outflow tracts are often normally arranged in hearts with left isomerism, although aortic stenosis, coarctation, and the hypoplastic left heart syndrome are well-described.

Clinical implications

The association of atrial isomerism with complex abnormalities of systemic, pulmonary, and hepatic venous connections, unusual forms of AVSD or univentricular atrioventricular connection, abnormal ventricular and great artery relationships, and pulmonary artery abnormalities, presents a considerable diagnostic challenge to the pediatric cardiologist and a difficult problem for the cardiac surgeon. The full evaluation of cardiac anatomy and hemodynamics requires detailed investigation by echocardiography, cardiac catheterization and angiography, and other imaging techniques such as MRI and CT angiography might be required. In some cases complete biventricular or univentricular repair may be impossible, particularly when there is an obstructed extracardiac total anomalous pulmonary venous connection associated with pulmonary atresia or significant atrioventricular valve regurgitation in AVSDs.

Scimitar syndrome

The clinical presentation is extremely variable and to some extent this is a reflection of the morphologic variability in the condition. The right pulmonary artery and lung can vary from being virtually normal to severely hypoplastic, and the lungs may also have the so-called horseshoe arrangement. In some instances the anomalous right pulmonary vein may be stenosed at its junction with the hepatic vein or inferior caval vein. Stenosis of

the left pulmonary veins is encountered in some patients. The systemic-to-pulmonary collaterals may be solitary or multiple, and small or large, so the pulmonary blood flow to affected lung segments will be very variable.

Apart from a secundum atrial septal defect (ASD), congenital cardiac malformations are unusual in scimitar syndrome, although patients are encountered with a perimembranous or muscular VSD.

Features of classical scimitar syndrome (hypogenetic right lung)

- Normal atrial situs
- Dextroposition (i.e. the cardiac silhouette is placed primarily in the right hemithorax)
- Hypoplasia of the right pulmonary artery
- Underdevelopment of the right lung
- Anomalous connection of the right pulmonary veins to the inferior caval vein near to the junction with the right atrium (scimitar vein; Figure 17.2)
- Anomalous systemic arterial supply to the right lung from the descending aorta
- Abnormal bronchial supply to the right lung with sequestration frequently present

---

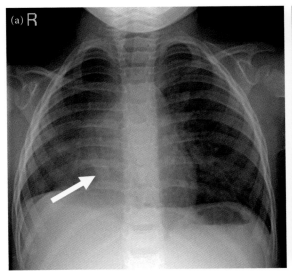 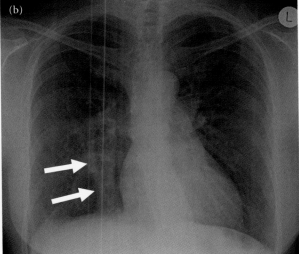

Figure 17.2 Chest X-rays from two patients with scimitar syndrome. (a) CXR shows a scimitar vein associated with a hypoplastic right lung (arrow). The right hemithorax is small, the peripheral pulmonary vessels are attenuated, and the mediastinum is shifted to the right. A curved, vertical, band-like shadow projected over the right heart border is the anomalous ("scimitar") pulmonary vein (arrowed) passing toward the inferior caval vein–right atrium junction. (b) CXR shows a scimitar vein (arrows) draining part of the right lung and passing toward the inferior caval vein–right atrium junction.

Unusual forms of the scimitar syndrome include normal pulmonary venous drainage from the abnormal right lung or a left-sided scimitar syndrome with hypoplasia of the left pulmonary artery and lung, anomalous connection of a left pulmonary vein, and an abnormal systemic supply to the left lower lobe segments.

Clinical presentation

Many children are symptom-free and remain so through adult life.
• A common presentation is with dextroposition and abnormal right lung on a CXR requested because of a chest infection or recurrent chest infections (Figure 17.2).
• History of what is thought to be asthma.
• Troublesome recurrent chest infections.
• Initial diagnosis may be primary pulmonary hypertension.
• Particularly in those with extreme right lung hypoplasia and a large systemic-to-pulmonary collateral, tachypnea and heart failure may be the presenting feature in infancy and occasionally an infant cannot be weaned from a ventilator.

Investigations

The diagnosis can usually be made from the CXR appearances and cross-sectional echocardiogram.

Although one option is to do nothing in patients who are symptom-free, the ideal method of investigation is cardiac catheterization and angiography, which will then provide the opportunity for embolization of systemic-to-pulmonary collaterals and balloon dilatation of any pulmonary vein stenosis.

Management

Pulmonary hypertension might benefit from treatment with pulmonary vasodilators.

Some children benefit from surgical lobectomy, although this is not usually required. Some patients with significant partial anomalous pulmonary venous drainage will benefit from surgery, although connection of the anomalous vein to the left atrium without causing pulmonary vein stenosis may be difficult. Anomalous pulmonary venous connection is preferable to pulmonary vein stenosis! A large ASD should be closed.

Cerebral arteriovenous malformations

The vein of Galen aneurysm may present with cardiac manifestations during early infancy. The amount of

aneurysmal enlargement of the vein of Galen depends upon the size and number of arteriovenous connections; an additional cause of dilatation may be a rare angiomatous malformation draining through the Galenic system. Dural arteriovenous malformations are extremely rare.

Clinical presentation

The clinical presentation of the cerebral arteriovenous fistulae depends upon their size and severity.
• High output congestive heart failure in the neonatal period is the most common presentation often with a bruit over the occiput.
• Large volumes of oxygenated blood return under high pressure to the right atrium and pulmonary circulation.
• As well as intractable heart failure and myocardial ischemia, ischemic parenchymal brain damage may result.
• Cyanosis may be a striking feature because of persistent fetal circulation. Presentation during infancy can also be associated with obstructive hydrocephalus, seizures, subarachnoid hemorrhage and venous congestion of the scalp.
• In older children, hydrocephalus, persistent headache, or focal neurologic signs are sometimes encountered.

Investigations

• **EKG:** In infancy this shows right ventricular hypertrophy, myocardial ischemia or even infarction.
• **CXR:** Demonstrates cardiomegaly, right atrial enlargement, and increased pulmonary vascular markings.
• **Ultrasound:** Diagnosis can be made with ultrasound in the newborn.
• **CT and MRI:** Refine the details.
• **Echocardiography:** Features include ventricular enlargement, a hyperdynamic circulation, dilated superior caval vein, and ascending aorta.
• **Contrast echocardiography:** Can assist in the diagnosis.

Management

Cerebral vascular malformations can be treated by surgery, embolization or a combination of these. There is a high mortality and morbidity in symptomatic infants. Embolization of dural arteriovenous fistulae can sometimes be successful.

Congenital pulmonary arteriovenous malformations

Fistulous communications between the pulmonary arteries and veins are rare malformations resulting in a right-to-left shunt and varying degrees of cyanosis and finger clubbing. There may be a solitary or several connections or a multitude of microscopic shunts. Presentation sometimes occurs in adult life but more severe forms are encountered in infants and children. Acquired pulmonary arteriovenous malformations are well-recognized following surgical bidirectional cavopulmonary anastomosis where the pulmonary trunk is also ligated, effectively excluding hepatic blood flow to the lungs.

Major types of congenital pulmonary arteriovenous malformations

- Primary pulmonary telangiectasia
- Hereditary hemorrhagic telangiectasia
- Discrete fistulae
- Hepatogenic pulmonary angiodysplasia

Clinical presentation

- Cyanosis varies from mild to severe depending upon the extent of arteriovenous connections. May be present in the early neonatal period and tends to become more severe with increasing age.
- Large right-to-left shunt may result in tachypnea during infancy or even congestive cardiac failure.
- Exertional dyspnea or fatigue and recurrent chest infections in older patients.
- Brain abscess and systemic emboli caused by the right-to-left shunt.
- Hemoptysis and hemothorax have been described.

Investigations

- **CXR:**
  - Abnormal vascular patterns are often present
  - Pulmonary vascularity is often decreased and intrapulmonary opacities may be seen with a large fistulous communication
  - Alternatively a multitude of spider-like vessels may be identified when there are diffuse small fistulae.
- **Contrast echocardiography:** Used to demonstrate the right-to-left pulmonary shunting.
- **CT angiography and catheterization:**
  - May be useful for diagnosis
  - Coupled with contrast transesophageal echocardiography, this is a sensitive method of diagnosis.

- **MRI:** Limited applications. Association with hypoplasia of peripheral pulmonary arteries carries a poor prognosis.

Management

Treatment should be individualized for a particular patient; ligation or embolization of a segmental pulmonary artery or surgical resection of an affected lung segment or lobe is appropriate in some patients. A significant number of infants and children appear to have isolated arteriovenous connections and an encouraging outcome from initial transcatheter embolization techniques, but then go on to manifest additional shunts with recurrence of progressive central cyanosis. In many instances the natural history is of a progressive severe cyanosis with no effective treatment.

Peripheral arteriovenous malformations

There is a variety of rare congenital peripheral arteriovenous malformations in which shunting occurs from the arteries at high pressure to veins at low pressure. The most common arteriovenous malformations presenting to the pediatric cardiologist are those involving the intercostal, internal mammary, and subclavian vessels, resulting in dilated venous channels over the upper arm, neck, and chest.

With large communications, congestive cardiac failure can occur during infancy. More peripheral malformations may result in local growth disturbance giving rise to asymmetry. Localized pain is a frequent complaint but the cosmetic effects are often the most troublesome in older children.

Discrete arteriovenous malformations can sometimes be treated by embolization techniques. Great care should be exercised when treatment is purely for cosmetic reasons because of the risks of arterial occlusion and localized ischemia.

Further reading

Jacobs JP, Anderson RH, Weinberg P et al. The nomenclature, definition and classification of cardiac structures in the setting of heterotaxy. *Cardiol Young* 2007;00:1–28.

18 Pericardial disease and infectious endocarditis

Michael Y. Henein[1] and Koichiro Niwa[2]

[1]Umea University, Umea, Sweden
[2]St Luke's International Hospital, Tokyo, Japan

Pericardial disease

Anatomy and physiology

The pericardium consists of two layers, a visceral and a parietal layer lined by mesothelial cells. The mesothelial layer secretes a small amount of pericardial fluid that allows both surfaces to slide together during the cardiac cycle. Intrapericardial pressure falls during inspiration, resulting in a fall in right-sided cardiac pressures. This causes a modest increase in right heart filling velocities with inspiration.

Pleuropericardial defect

Congenital anomalies of the pericardium are rare. A pleuropericardial defect is the most common form. The left side is more commonly involved in the partial form, allowing the left atrial appendage or part of the left ventricle to herniate through the defects. In the majority of instances, pericardial defects are asymptomatic. Approximately one-third of cases are associated with congenital abnormalities of the heart and lungs.

Pericardial effusion
Etiology
Acute rapid collection (Figure 18.1) is usually caused by traumatic injury, iatrogenic ventricular puncture, intravenous central line extravasation, or aortic dissection with fluid collection inside the pericardium. Chronic effusion is more common.

Common causes of chronic effusion
- Idiopathic
- Viral infection
- Juvenile rheumatoid arthritis
- Leukemia/lymphoma
- Systemic lupus erythematosus
- Congestive cardiac failure
- Other infections, malignancy, hypothyroidism, renal failure, hepatic cirrhosis

Clinical features
- Rapidly accumulated effusion may result in raised pericardial pressure and development of symptoms.
- Slowly accumulating effusion may be asymptomatic even with large volumes.
- Symptoms and signs:
  - Often non-specific
  - Reduced exercise tolerance
  - Dull aching chest pain
  - Mediastinal syndrome (cough, dyspnea, hoarseness of voice)
  - Heart sounds distant and widespread dullness on percussion.

Investigations
- **CXR:** Does not always confirm the presence of pericardial effusion.

Pediatric Heart Disease: A Practical Guide, First Edition. Piers E. F. Daubeney, Michael L. Rigby, Koichiro Niwa, and Michael A. Gatzoulis.
© 2012 Blackwell Publishing Ltd. Published 2012 by Blackwell Publishing Ltd.

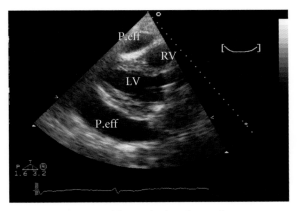

Figure 18.1 Parasternal long axis view shows a large pericardial effusion posterior to the left ventricle and anterior to the right ventricle. LV, left ventricle; P. eff, pericardial effusion; RV, right ventricle.

- **Echocardiography:**
  - ◦ Investigation of choice for confirming the presence of pericardial effusion and for assessing its volume
  - ◦ On 2D echocardiography, a 1-cm global collection around the heart in an adult suggests an approximate volume of 200 mL.

The hemodynamic effects of pericardial effusion depend on the speed of fluid collection and the volume of the effusion (Figure 18.1).

Pericardial tamponade

The most common cause of tamponade is an acute fluid collection after cardiac surgery or a malignant effusion. Right ventricular collapse is a sensitive (92%) and highly specific (100%) diagnostic sign for tamponade. It reflects transient negative transmural early diastolic pressure as pericardial pressure exceeds right ventricular pressure.

Pathophysiology

In adults, the pericardium is normally able to stretch to accommodate more than 2000 mL if slowly accumulated. Rapid accumulation of as little as 200 mL increases pericardial pressure. Inability of the pericardium to distend causes its pressure to rise above the right atrial pressure, then above the right ventricular pressure, and eventually results in right ventricular collapse. In tamponade during inspiration, the intrapericardial pressure does not fall as much as intrapleural pressures, resulting in a smaller pressure gradient between the intrathoracic pressure and pulmonary veins and left atrium and ventricle (Figure 18.2). On the right side of the heart, the increase

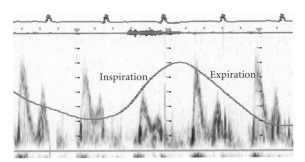

Figure 18.2 Transmitral Doppler flow in a patient with tamponade demonstrating compromised velocities during inspiration.

in right ventricular dimensions during inspiration enhances right-sided filling and ejection. These two mechanisms may eventually compromise cardiac output. Pericardial pressure greater than 10 mmHg results in right ventricular collapse and raised diastolic pressures of both ventricles. This leads to a fall in aortic pressure on inspiration and hence pulsus paradoxus and hypotension. Patients with such disturbed hemodynamics often present with raised jugular venous pressure (JVP), tachycardia, and tachypnea.

Clinical features and diagnosis
- Intrapericardial pressure greater than filling pressure of the ventricles.
- Common causes: acute fluid collection after cardiac surgery or malignant effusion.
- Tachycardia, tachypnea, raised JVP.
- Pulsus paradoxus.
- Hypotension.
- Right atrial and ventricular diastolic collapse on echocardiography.

Management
- Needle pericardiocentesis.
- Surgical pericardial drain insertion.

Pericardiocentesis is performed under ultrasound imaging. Substernal window drainage is usually recommended in patients with resistant, recurrent, or fast accumulating effusion. The procedure allows therapeutic symptomatic pressure relief, fluid drainage, diagnostic analysis of pericardial fluid for cytology and culture, and pericardial biopsy for cytology.

Constrictive pericarditis
Pericardial constriction is a pathologic condition characterized by pericardial thickening and fibrosis that results

in adhesion of its two layers and calcium deposition. The most common cause of constrictive pericarditis is viral infection, followed by tuberculosis, radiation, connective tissue disease, chronic renal failure, neoplastic disease, and previous cardiac surgery.

Pathophysiology

The stiff pericardium loses its ability to stretch to accommodate normal changes in intracardiac pressures. This is demonstrated by the equalization of end-diastolic pressures in the right and left ventricles: "dip and plateau pattern." Since this pathology is uniform, it manifests itself in the form of raised venous pressure.

A fibrosed and unstretchable pericardium adherent to the epicardial layer of the myocardium can limit its normal movement during the cardiac cycle. The chronic increase in venous pressure results in systemic congestion and dilatation of the hepatic veins.

Investigations and differential diagnosis

- **CXR:** Calcification of the pericardial border may be seen.
- **MRI/CT:** Thickened pericardium is a poorly sensitive marker.

A raised right atrial pressure during inspiration (Kussmaul's sign) and dilated inferior vena cava are non-specific signs for this condition.

The clinical similarity between constrictive pericarditis and restrictive cardiomyopathy makes the differential diagnosis difficult, i.e. both show raised venous pressure and fluid retention resistant to medical therapy. For more information about restrictive cardiomyopathy, see Chapter 19.

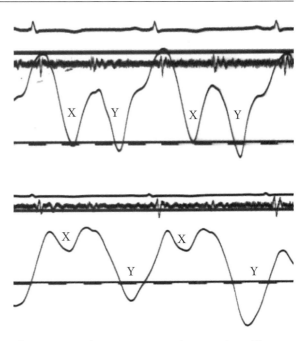

Figure 18.3 Jugular venous pressure from a patient with constrictive pericarditis before (top trace) and after (bottom trace) pericardiectomy. Note the diagnostic deep "X" descent and systolic right atrial filling before surgery which disappeared a few days after surgery.

Management

- Diuretics.
- Pericardiectomy (Figure 18.3):
  ○ Recommended in patients resistant to pharmacologic therapy
  ○ After surgical removal of the pericardium, the venous pressure drops within a few days or even weeks.

Pericardial complications after open heart surgery

Pericardial complications after open heart surgery are rare.
- **Pericardial clot:** Clot collection in the pericardial space is often associated with delayed postoperative recovery. With time, the clot results in increased intra-pericardial pressure and hence disturbed hemodynamics. This condition is managed with surgical removal of the clot.
- **"Tight" pericardium:** JVP is raised and right-sided physiology, filling and ejection, is predominantly inspiratory. On 2D echocardiographic images there is no evidence of right atrial or ventricular collapse. The condition tends to settle within days after surgery.
- **Restrictive pericarditis:** This presents with resistant fluid retention and raised venous pressure with a thickened pericardium. Patients who are resistant to medical

Differentiation between constrictive pericarditis and restrictive cardiomyopathy		
	Constrictive pericarditis	Restrictive cardiomyopathy
Pathophysiology	Extracardiac constraint	Intrinsic myocardial disease
Respiratory variation of ventricular filling and ejection velocities	Modestly present	Absent
Treatment	Pericardiectomy	Diuretics, transplantation

therapy may respond to surgical decortication of the pericardium.
• **Pericardial effusion:** See above.

Pericardial tumors

Pericardial tumors invade the pericardium either directly or via the lymphatics or hematogenous dissemination. Primary tumors are rare but usually include malignant mesothelioma and sarcomas. Lymphomas and leukemia present in the form of uniform pericardial infiltration and thickening, which may cause tumor incarceration of the heart and hence the clinical syndrome of "constrictive physiology." For a description of cardiac tumors, see Chapter 20.

Infective endocarditis

Despite the new generation of antibiotics and improved surgical techniques, infective endocarditis remains a potentially lethal disease. Although relatively rare in patients with congenital heart disease, its incidence is increasing due to dramatically increased survival. In addition, postoperative patients with or without residual artificial materials have a life-long risk for infective endocarditis. Infective endocarditis can occur despite appropriate preventive care.

Etiology

Endocarditis is more commonly found in right than left heart lesions in congenital heart disease. Often the source of infection remains unknown, with only about 40% of cases having an identifiable predisposing event such as dental or cardiac surgery.

The commonest lesions in which infective endocarditis occurs are:
• Unrepaired small ventricular septal defects;
• Tetralogy of Fallot including after a conduit repair;
• Complex congenital heart disease, either repaired or unrepaired;
• Prosthetic cardiac material (patches, valves, conduits), which is an additional risk factor for infection.

The most frequent causative organisms in children with congenital heart disease, especially beyond 1 year of age, are:
• Gram-positive cocci, including the viridans group;
• Alpha-hemolytic streptococci such as *Streptococcus sanguis*, *Streptococcus mitis*, *Streptococcus mutans*, etc.
• Staphylococci: *Staphylococcus aureus* endocarditis is virulent and aggressive, especially in the setting of prosthetic material.
• Enterococci – less frequent in children than adults.

Patients with cyanotic congenital heart disease may have a degree of immunocompromise, and therefore unusual organisms (e.g. fungal infections) may be more common. Fungal infective endocarditis is usually caused by a Candida species and may give rise to large vegetations, metastatic infection, and perivalvular invasion; the prognosis is poor.

The prevalence of **culture-negative infective endocarditis** may be 5–7%. The most common causes are current or recent antibiotic use, infection by fastidious organisms that grow poorly *in vitro*, and fungi (uncommon in children).

Prevention

Prevention needs to be regularly reinforced for patients with congenital heart disease. The patient should be educated to have:
• An understanding of the reason antibiotics are prescribed prophylactically in some types of congenital heart disease;
• An understanding that non-dental procedures may require prophylaxis;
• Simple instructions about the basic care of wounds to prevent bacteremia;
• Instructions about what to do in the event of febrile illness;
• In particular, patients should be encouraged to ask that blood cultures be taken before starting a course of blinded antibiotic therapy.

Diagnosis

• **Pathologic criteria:** Microbiologic and pathologic evidence from a vegetation, or intracardiac abscess
• **Clinical criteria:** Two major, or one major and three minor, or five minor:
  ○ Major criteria:
    Blood cultures: two separate positive blood cultures with a typical organism

    Persistently positive cultures with an organism consistent with infective endocarditis

    Endocardial involvement

    Positive echocardiograms with classic vegetation or abscess or new partial dehiscence of a prosthetic valve

    New valvular regurgitation
  ○ Minor criteria:
    Predisposition: heart condition or intravenous drug abuser

    Fever > 38 °C

    Vascular phenomena

    Immunologic phenomena

    Microbiologic evidence (not sufficient to be major)

    Echocardiography findings (suggestive but not sufficient to be major)

Prompt use of diagnostic microbiology laboratory tests and 2D echocardiography is critical in the diagnosis and management of children with infective endocarditis. A high index of suspicion should be maintained in high-risk patients, especially if they have had previous infective endocarditis.

While it should be remembered that the majority of patients with congenital heart disease with a temperature do not have infective endocarditis, the physician must be alert to its possibility.

Diagnostic approach to the patient with congenital heart disease and unexpected fever

- **History:**
  - History of predisposing event
  - Symptoms of hemodynamic decompensation
  - Systemic upset and symptoms of complications
- **Examination:**
  - Careful examination of skin: rashes, sites of possible infection, emboli (less common)
  - New murmurs (require previous description/documentation)
  - Exclusion of other causes of fever
  - Hemodynamic upset: heart failure
  - Reduced systemic oxygen saturation, e.g. in the context of a Blalock–Taussig shunt
  - Central nervous involvement: if new neurologic signs, reduction in level of consciousness or changes in behavior develop, consider mycotic aneurysm and cerebral abscess
- **Blood investigations:**
  - Blood cultures (three recommended)
  - Full blood count with differential white blood cell count
  - Renal function
  - Liver function and proteins
  - Immunoglobulin, autoantibodies (if diagnosis unclear)
  - C-reactive protein (serial)
  - PCR (useful tool for early detection of causative organism)
- **Specimens:**
  - Urine: urinalysis, culture and sensitivities (C&S)
  - Sputum for C&S
  - Other microbiology specimens as appropriate
- **EKG:** Arrhythmia, especially new conduction defect (less common)
- **CXR:** Change in cardiothoracic ratio
- **Echocardiography** (Figure 18.4):
  - Transthoracic generally suitable in children, but low threshold for transesophageal imaging
  - Particularly recommended for complex lesions requiring closer imaging in adolescents and adults
  - Remember failure to detect vegetations does not exclude infective endocarditis
  - Look for presence of vegetations or abscesses and new valvular insufficiency
- **CT/MRI:** For complications such as infective emboli and infarcts

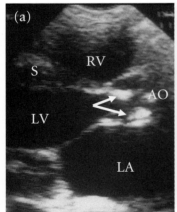 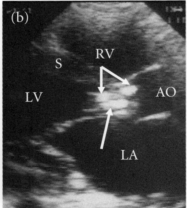 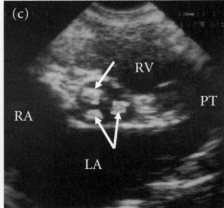

Figure 18.4 Endocarditis of the aortic valve. Echocardiographic appearance of several large vegetations of the aortic valve. The arrows demonstrate the vegetations. Parasternal long axis view in systole (a) and diastole (b), and short axis view (c). AO, aorta; LV, left ventricle; PT, pulmonary trunk; RV, right ventricle; S, septum.

Management

In general, the treatment of infective endocarditis in children is similar to that in adults.

Medical management

Bacteriocidal antibiotics should be chosen whenever possible to reduce the possibility of treatment failure.

Bacteremia generally resolves within several days after appropriate therapy has been initiated. Recommendations for antibiotic treatment of infective endocarditis in the adult population have been made by the American Heart Association and can be used in children with appropriate dose adjustment (Table 18.1). Good communication with the microbiologist or infectious disease specialist is key

Table 18.1 Suggested antibiotic treatment for infective endocarditis in children with congenital heart disease

Organism	Antimicrobial agent	Duration
Streptococci, e.g. viridans	1: PenG + Gent 2: Vanc + Gent*	PenG: 4–6 weeks** Vanc: 4–6 weeks** Gent: Stop after 2 weeks if organism fully/moderately sensitive to PenG
Staphylococci (methicillin sensitive)	1: Fluclox 2: Vanc + Rif*	Fluclox: 4–6 weeks** Vanc: 4–6 weeks** Rif: 4–6 weeks.** In prosthetic valve endocarditis add to Fluclox for 2 weeks
Staphylococci (methicillin resistant)	1: Vanc + Rif	Vanc: 4–6 weeks** Rif: 4–6 weeks**
Enterococci, e.g. *Enterococcus faecalis*	1: Amox or Amp + Gent 2: Vanc + Gent*	Amox/Amp: 4–6 weeks** Vanc: 4–6 weeks** Gent: 4–6 weeks**
"HACEK" organisms, e.g. haemophilus, actinobacillus, cardiobacterium, eikenella, kingella	1: Amox or Amp + Gent 2: Cefx + Gent	Amox/Amp: 4–6 weeks** Cefx: 4–6 weeks** Gent: Stop after 2 weeks
Culture negative (postoperative)	1: Vanc + Gent	Vanc: 4–6 weeks** Gent: 4–6 weeks**
Culture negative (non-operative)	1: Fluclox + Gent 2: Vanc + Rif + Gent* (or if cardiac prostheses)	Fluclox: 4–6 weeks** Gent: 4–6 weeks** Vanc: 4–6 weeks** Rif: 4–6 weeks**
Fungus	Amphotericin B	6 weeks

*Penicillin allergy
**Treat prosthetic valve endocarditis for at least 6 weeks

Doses (>1-month old; normal renal function: seek specialist advice if neonate or renal/liver impairment)

PenG (penicillin G; Benzylpenicillin): 25–50 mg/kg (max 2.4 g) q4h. Note: 600 mg = 1 000 000 U

Vanc (vancomycin): 15 mg/kg q8h (max 2 g/day). Adjusted to serum concentrations: trough 10–15 mg/L

Amox (amoxicillin): 50 mg/kg (max 2 g) q4–6h

Amp (ampicillin): 50 mg/kg (max 2 g) q4–6h

Amphotericin B: Dose depends on formulation (i.e. lipid, liposomal, conventional). Please seek specialist advice on dose

Gent (gentamicin): 2.5 mg/kg q8h (>12 years: 2 mg/kg q8h). Adjusted to serum concentrations: peak 3–5 mg/L, trough < 1 mg/L

Fluclox (flucloxacillin): 50 mg/kg (max 2 g) q6h

Rif (rifampicin): 10 mg/kg (max 600 mg) q12h

Cefx (ceftriaxone): 80 mg/kg (max 4 g) q24h

to effective treatment. Prolonged antibiotic therapy and intravenous access may be problematic in congenital heart disease patients who have multiple previous lines and procedures.

Surgical management

It is always wise to inform the congenital cardiac surgical team if patients with congenital heart disease develop infective endocarditis. Early discussion and planning for the eventuality of treatment failure or complications is essential should medical therapy fail. Perioperative mortality may be high but surgery may be better than not operating.

Possible indications for surgical intervention in infective endocarditis

- Pre-existing indication for surgery
- Enlarging vegetations despite appropriate antibiotic therapy
- Emboli despite antibiotic therapy
- Worsening valvular disease: increasing regurgitation
- Valve leaflet rupture/perforation
- Heart failure
- Perivalvular extension, e.g. aortic root abscess, new conduction defects
- *Staphylococcus aureus* infection, especially in the presence of prosthetic material

---

Key clinical points

- Maintain high index of suspicion in high-risk patients, especially if previous infectious endocarditis.
- *Staphylococcus aureus* endocarditis is virulent and aggressive, especially in the setting of prosthetic material.
- Aortic valve infective endocarditis may lead to severe aortic regurgitation or cardiac rhythm disturbances: heart block suggests root abscess. Communicate with surgeons, particularly if low diastolic pressures (coronary ischemia) and rapid onset of left ventricular and renal failure.
- Central nervous involvement: if new neurologic signs, reduction in level of consciousness, or changes in behavior develop, consider mycotic aneurysm and cerebral abscess.

Further reading

Pericardial disease

Appleton CP, Hatle LK, Popp RL. Cardiac tamponade and pericardial effusion: respiratory variation in transvalvular flow velocities studied by Doppler echocardiography. *J Am Coll Cardiol* 1988;11:1020–1030.

Cameron J, Oesterle SN, Baldwin JC, Hancock EW. The etiologic spectrum of constrictive pericarditis. *Am Heart J* 1987;113 (2 Pt 1):354–360.

Chandraratna PA. Echocardiography and Doppler ultrasound in the evaluation of pericardial disease. *Circulation* 1991;84 (3 Suppl):I303–I310.

Chuttani K, Pandian NG, Mohanty PK, *et al*. Left ventricular diastolic collapse. An echocardiographic sign of regional cardiac tamponade. *Circulation* 1991;83:1999–2006.

D'Cruz IA, Hoffman PK. A new cross sectional echocardiographic method for estimating the volume of large pericardial effusions. *Br Heart J* 1991;66:448–451.

Guberman BA, Fowler NO, Engel PJ, Gueron M, Allen JM. Cardiac tamponade in medical patients. *Circulation* 1981;64:633–640.

Henein MY, Rakhit RD, Sheppard MN, Gibson DG. Restrictive pericarditis. *Heart* 1999;82:389–392.

Isner JM, Carter BL, Roberts WC, Bankoff MS. Subepicardial adipose tissue producing echocardiographic appearance of pericardial effusion. Documentation by computed tomography and necropsy. *Am J Cardiol* 1983;51:565–569.

Kochar GS, Jacobs LE, Kotler MN. Right atrial compression in postoperative cardiac patients: detection by transesophageal echocardiography. *J Am Coll Cardiol* 1990;16:511–516.

Nishimura RA, Kazmier FJ, Smith HC, Danielson GK. Right ventricular outflow obstruction caused by constrictive pericardial disease. *Am J Cardiol* 1985;55:1447–1448.

Reddy PS, Curtiss EI, O'Toole JD, Shaver JA. Cardiac tamponade: hemodynamic observations in man. *Circulation* 1978;58:265–272.

Shabetai R, Fowler NO, Guntheroth WG. The hemodynamics of cardiac tamponade and constrictive pericarditis. *Am J Cardiol* 1970;26:480–489.

Singh S, Wann LS, Schuchard GH, *et al*. Right ventricular and right atrial collapse in patients with cardiac tamponade – a combined echocardiographic and hemodynamic study. *Circulation* 1984;70:966–971.

Infective endocarditis

Ferrieri P, Gewitz MH, Gerber MA, *et al*. Unique features of infective endocarditis in childhood. *Circulation* 2002;105: 2115–2127.

Kavey REW, Frank DM, Byrum CJ, *et al*. Two-dimensional echocardiographic assessment of infective endocarditis in children. *Am J Dis Child* 1983;137:851–856.

Li JS, Sexton DJ, Mick N, *et al.* Proposed modifications to the Duke criteria for the diagnosis of infective endocarditis. *Clin Infect Dis* 2000;30:633–638.

Li W, Somerville J. Infective endocarditis in the grown-up congenital heart (GUCH) population. *Eur Heart J* 1998;19: 166–173.

Niwa K, Nakazawa M, Tateno S, *et al.* Infective endocarditis in congenital heart disease: Japanese national collaboration study. *Heart* 2005;91:795–800.

Nomura F, Penny DJ, Menahem S. Surgical intervention for infective endocarditis in infancy and childhood. *Ann Thorac Surg* 1995; 60:90–95.

19 Cardiomyopathies and acute myocarditis

Steven A. Webber[1,2] and Brian Feingold[1,2]

[1]University of Pittsburgh School of Medicine, Pittsburgh, PA, USA
[2]Children's Hospital of Pittsburgh of UPMC, Pittsburgh, PA, USA

Definition and classification

The definition and classification of cardiomyopathies was revised in 2006 by an expert panel of the American Heart Association following their initial classification by the World Health Organization in 1995. Cardiomyopathies are considered "a heterogeneous group of diseases of the myocardium associated with mechanical and/or electrical dysfunction that usually (but not invariably) exhibit inappropriate ventricular hypertrophy or dilatation and are due to a variety of causes that frequently are genetic." Cardiomyopathies are generally considered as primary (disease solely or predominantly confined to heart muscle) or secondary, showing pathologic myocardial involvement secondary to a systemic or multiorgan disease process. Both forms are commonly seen in children, although primary forms predominate. The principle forms of cardiomyopathy in childhood are summarized in Table 19.1. Each type of cardiomyopathy likely comprises multiple distinct etiologies, many of which are genetic.

Dilated cardiomyopathy

Dilated cardiomyopathy (DCM) is characterized by dilatation of one or both ventricles (most commonly the left ventricle [LV]) often with thinning of the LV walls (Figures 19.1a and 19.2a). Varying degrees of hypertrophy may also be seen and LV mass tends to be increased, even when the ventricular walls are thin. The LV takes on a globular shape, and mitral regurgitation with annular dilation is frequently seen along with left atrial dilatation. LV systolic function is usually globally depressed, and there may be varying degrees of ventricular dyssynchronous contraction. In contrast, right ventricular (RV) systolic function is often well preserved. RV dilatation, when present, may be due to involvement from the primary disease process or secondary to pulmonary hypertension with or without tricuspid regurgitation.

Incidence and etiology

DCM is the commonest form of cardiomyopathy in childhood and occurred with an annual incidence of 0.57 cases per 100 000 children in the Pediatric Cardiomyopathy Registry (PCMR). It accounts for about 54% of pediatric cardiomyopathies. The incidence appears similar in different regions and countries.

The etiology of DCM is highly heterogeneous. The distribution of etiologies reported within the PCMR is as follows:
- Idiopathic (65%);
- Myocarditis (16%);
- Neuromuscular disorders (9%);
- Familial isolated DCM (5%);
- Inborn errors of metabolism (4%);
- Part of malformation syndromes (1%).

Autosomal dominant, recessive, X-linked, and mitochondrial inheritance have been reported. A detailed description of inborn errors of metabolism leading to DCM is outside the scope of this chapter and readers are referred to the excellent review by Cox (see Further reading). In Central and South America, **Chagas disease** due to the protozoan parasite *Trypanosoma cruzi* is an important cause of DCM. A secondary cause of great

Pediatric Heart Disease: A Practical Guide, First Edition. Piers E. F. Daubeney, Michael L. Rigby, Koichiro Niwa, and Michael A. Gatzoulis.
© 2012 Blackwell Publishing Ltd. Published 2012 by Blackwell Publishing Ltd.

Table 19.1 Principle forms of cardiomyopathy

Type	Proportion	Physiology	Predominant pathology
Dilated	55%	Systolic dysfunction	Dilated, poorly contractile LV (±RV)
Hypertrophic	40%	Diastolic dysfunction	Concentric and/or septal LV hypertrophy
Restrictive	3%	Diastolic dysfunction	Markedly dilated atria, preserved ventricular systolic function and dimensions
Non-compaction	<1%	Systolic and diastolic	Deep apical ventricular trabeculations and recesses
Arrhythmogenic RV dysplasia	<1%	Ventricular tachycardia	Fibro-fatty replacement of variable part of RV

LV, left ventricle; RV, right ventricle.

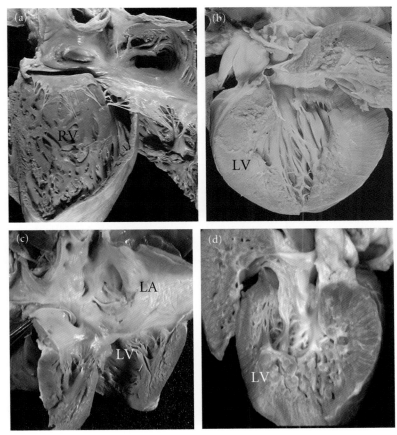

Figure 19.1 Spectrum of pediatric cardiomyopathies: pathologic specimens. (a) Dilated cardiomyopathy with marked ventricular dilatation and wall thinning (shown from RV side). (b) Severe hypertrophic cardiomyopathy with concentric hypertrophy, in this case secondary to Pompe disease (glycogen storage disease type II). (c) Restrictive cardiomyopathy with small left ventricular cavity size and marked dilatation of the left atrium. (d) Left ventricular non-compaction cardiomyopathy. LA, left atrium; LV, left ventricle; RV, right ventricle. (Courtesy of William Devine, Department of Pathology, Children's Hospital of Pittsburgh of UMPC, Pittsburgh, PA, USA.)

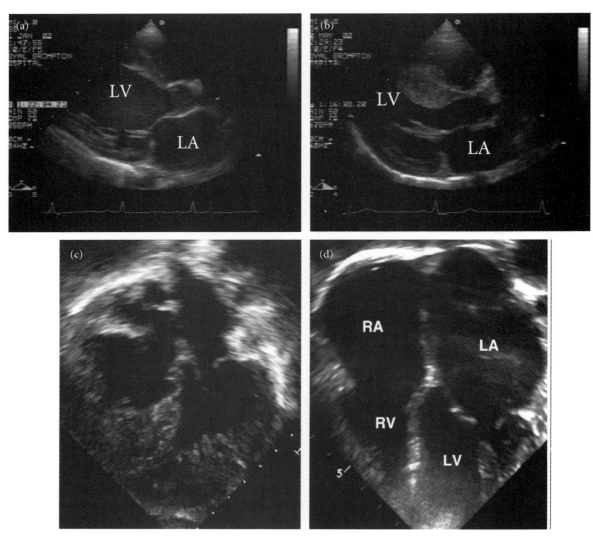

Figure 19.2 Spectrum of pediatric cardiomyopathies: echocardiographic views. (a) Dilated cardiomyopathy with marked ventricular dilatation and wall thinning. There is a dilated left atrium in addition. (b) Hypertrophic cardiomyopathy with asymmetrical septal hypertrophy. (c) Restrictive cardiomyopathy with dilated atria. (d) Biventricular non-compaction. Note the deep intertrabecular recesses. LA, left atrium; LV, left ventricle; RA, right atrium; RV, right ventricle.

importance in childhood in developed countries is **anthracycline-induced** cardiomyopathy.

Clinical features

Most cases of DCM present with congestive heart failure, often of acute onset. Presentations include:

• Heart failure: Exercise intolerance, shortness of breath on exertion, orthopnea, paroxysmal nocturnal dyspnea, abdominal pain (hepatic distension), edema (relatively rare in children);

• Cardiogenic shock;

• Acute arrhythmia with palpitations, pre-syncope, or syncope;

• Sudden death;

• Family screening (close relative diagnosed with DCM).

Key features of the physical examination of severe DCM

- Sinus tachycardia and hypotension
- Pallor, cool extremities, weak pulses
- Sweating (common in infants)
- Elevation of the jugular venous pulse and hepatomegaly
- Tachypnea and respiratory distress
- Displaced, diffuse apical impulse, muffled heart sounds, gallop rhythm (S3, or S3 and S4 summation gallop)
- Apical blowing pan-systolic murmur when mitral regurgitation is present
- Failure to thrive may be evident with chronic heart failure

Investigations

Investigations are focused on making the diagnosis and assessing the severity of the condition. The key initial investigations and characteristic findings are:

- **EKG:**
  - Sinus tachycardia, atrial enlargement, LV hypertrophy, non-specific ST-T changes
  - Some cases will show conduction delay
  - Holter monitor or continuous EKG monitoring (for hospitalized patients) to rule out atrial or ventricular arrhythmias, especially high-grade ventricular ectopy or tachycardia.
- **CXR:** Cardiomegaly ± pulmonary edema, left basal atelectasis, pleural effusions.
- **Echocardiography:** Left or biventricular dilatation, globally poor systolic function, mitral (and/or tricuspid) insufficiency, atrial dilation; exclude intracardiac thrombi and pericardial effusion; assess extent of pulmonary hypertension.

Additional studies may be warranted. It is critical to rule out anatomically correctable lesions, such as an anomalous left coronary artery from the pulmonary artery. This can usually be identified from non-invasive imaging, but cardiac catheterization may be required. Endomyocardial biopsy may be indicated when myocarditis is suspected (see below). When inborn errors of metabolism are suspected (including in all infants), additional metabolic work-up is required to assist in the diagnosis. Appropriate tests for metabolic causes of cardiomyopathy include:

- Full blood count with white cell differential, electrolytes, pH, glucose, liver function tests, ammonia, creatinine kinase, amino acids, carnitine and acylcarnitine profile, ketones, uric acid, free fatty acids, lactate, and pyruvate;
- Urine analysis for ketones, amino acids, organic acids;
- Muscle biopsy and skin biopsy for fibroblast culture in selected cases;
- Blood for DNA for potential genetic testing.

Management

Acute, new-onset cardiomyopathy may be due to acute myocarditis or sudden decompensation in a previously asymptomatic child with chronic DCM. This determination is vital, as most patients with fulminant myocarditis will recover, whereas those with severe heart failure from DCM may not without transplantation. Clearly, the utility and goals of mechanical support (extracorporeal membrane oxygenation [ECMO] or ventricular assist device [VAD]) and the consideration for listing for cardiac transplantation are directly impacted by the underlying diagnosis (DCM vs myocarditis).

The principles of management of acute and chronic heart failure are outlined in Chapter 32. The critically ill child (irrespective of etiology) requires aggressive therapy to augment tissue oxygen and substrate delivery, while minimizing oxygen consumption. Intubation with mechanical ventilation and sedation (±paralysis) is useful to eliminate the work of breathing while improving pulmonary edema. Intravenous diuretics are used to augment urine output and improve congestive symptoms. Continuous infusions of furosemide have been used with success in pediatric patients when intermittent dosing has failed. Nesiritide may be useful for inducing diuresis in acute pulmonary edema when there is poor response to intravenous diuretics. Although positive inotropes have minimal, if any, role in the chronic management of DCM in the clinic, inotropes are indicated in the setting of acute low cardiac output state. Milrinone ($0.1-1\,\mu g/kg/min$) is often used as the agent of choice since it both diminishes afterload through vasodilatation and also exhibits positive inotropy. Dobutamine or dopamine are added when further inotropy is required. Caution must be taken with regard to the arrhythmogenic potential of all inotropes, particularly with escalating doses. When there is evolving end-organ dysfunction, or refractory hypotension and oliguria, mechanical circulatory support is considered. If short-term support is anticipated, ECMO is generally preferred. When support is required as a bridge to transplant, VADs are the preferred method of support.

Outpatient therapy of DCM depends on the severity of disease and the presence of heart failure. When heart failure is present, digoxin, diuretics, and angiotensin converting enzyme (ACE) inhibitors are generally used in combination, though the value of digoxin in this setting is not well established. Aldosterone antagonists are widely used in adult heart failure, but their role in children is not well established. There is a risk of hyperkalemia when used with ACE inhibitors, so careful monitoring of electrolytes is required. Chronic therapy with beta-blockers (e.g. metoprolol or carvedilol) is of proven benefit in adults with chronic heart failure and they are widely used in children, though only one controlled trial has assessed their efficacy in this setting (with possible benefit in patients with systemic ventricle of LV morphology).

Other important aspects of chronic management of children with DCM (beyond control of heart failure) include:

• Screening, prevention, and treatment of arrhythmias;
• Prevention of sudden death;
• Prevention of thromboembolic complications;
• Screening of family members, including siblings and parents;
• Consideration of genetic testing, especially if positive family history.

Anticoagulation is generally recommended when there is severe LV dysfunction, evidence of intracardiac thrombus, or history of embolic event. Warfarin is used in older children. Aspirin and low molecular weight heparin have been used in infants.

Amiodarone is commonly used for treatment of ventricular tachycardia, as well as for refractory atrial tachycardias. The role of implanted cardioverter–defibrillators (ICDs) in the management of children and adolescents has not been as well defined as in adults. Evidence suggests children with DCM have a lower risk of sudden death as compared to adults with similar degrees of ventricular dysfunction. Furthermore, inappropriate shocks are common. Biventricular pacing has also been recommended to improve cardiac output and symptoms in DCM with evidence of electrical or mechanical dyssynchrony. Again, the indications for this therapy in children with DCM are not established.

Long-term outcomes

Traditionally, long-term outlook in children with DCM was said to follow the "rule of thirds," with one-third improving, one-third remaining the same, and one-third demonstrating progressive deterioration in cardiac function. Recent population data from several groups have improved our understanding of the natural history of DCM. The National Australian Childhood Cardiomyo-

pathy Study showed a 5-year freedom from death or transplantation of 63% for children with DCM. The PCMR showed a 5-year transplant-free survival of 54% for DCM in North America. Predictors of survival for DCM vary considerably between series. In a recent systematic review, it was noted that the most consistent findings associated with improved outcome were younger age at diagnosis, better fractional shortening and ejection fraction at diagnosis, and presence of myocarditis.

Hypertrophic cardiomyopathy

The most common morphology of hypertrophic cardiomyopathy (HCM) is that of asymmetric hypertrophy of the interventricular septum, with varying degrees of obstruction to the LV outflow due to the prominence of the subaortic septum and/or systolic anterior motion of the anterior leaflet of the mitral valve (Figures 19.1b and 19.2b). This typical morphology is seen most often in adults and adolescents. Less commonly, children with HCM demonstrate concentric LV hypertrophy. With infant presentation, involvement of both the LV and RV is common, and biventricular obstruction may be observed. In contrast to older patients, systolic dysfunction is more common in infant presentation. Histologically, there are varying degrees of myocyte hypertrophy, myofibrillar disarray, and interstitial fibrosis. In **Noonan syndrome**, mid-cavity LV hypertrophy and obstruction often predominate. Storage disease forms of HCM include **Pompe, Fabry, and Danon disease**.

Incidence and etiology

HCM is the second commonest form of cardiomyopathy in childhood and occurred with an annual incidence of 0.47 cases per 100 000 children in the PCMR, where it accounted for approximately 40% of pediatric cardiomyopathies. The distribution of etiologies of HCM as reported within the PCMR is as follows:

• Idiopathic (74%);
• Inborn errors of metabolism (9%);
• Part of malformation syndromes (9%);
• Neuromuscular disorders (8%).

HCM is most commonly an inherited disorder (usually autosomal dominant) with marked variability in clinical expression. Most mutations identified to date in older children (and adults) encode cardiac sarcomere proteins, including myosin heavy and light chains, myosin binding protein C, and the thin filaments, actin and cardiac troponin T and I. It is likely that many other disease-causing mutations will be identified. Other causes of pediatric HCM not due to sarcomeric protein mutations include **Noonan and Leopard syndrome**, and several metabolic conditions leading to cardiac storage disorders. The classic disease in this category is **glycogen storage disease type II** (**Pompe disease**) due to genetic deficiency of α-1,4 glucosidase, resulting in impaired breakdown of glycogen to glucose. A second, rare storage disorder, **Danon disease**, is an X-linked condition characterized by mutation in the lysosomal associated membrane protein 2 (LAMP2). This tends to present in teenage years with HCM and impaired systolic function. Various **mitochondrial myopathies** (with maternal inheritance) may also lead to a HCM phenotype.

Clinical features

Many cases of HCM in older patients are not associated with symptoms, and disease is often diagnosed during family screening or during evaluation of an asymptomatic murmur. Infants are much more likely to present with heart failure. Presentations of HCM thus include:

- Heart failure – mainly in infants;
- Family screening (close relative diagnosed with HCM);
- Evaluation of asymptomatic murmur or abnormal heart sound;
- Chest pain, exertional dyspnea or palpitations;
- Pre-syncope, syncope or sudden death (often during exercise).

Key features of the physical examination of HCM

- Failure to thrive and signs of heart failure in infants
- Dysmorphic features such as those of Noonan syndrome
- Poor muscle tone and delayed motor development (e.g. Pompe disease)
- Sustained, forceful systolic apical impulse on precordial palpation
- Ejection systolic murmur increased on standing (decreased LV volume, increased LV outflow gradient) and after exercise. Decreased murmur with squatting (due to increased LV volume)
- S4 gallop

Investigations

Investigations focus on making the correct diagnosis and assessing the pattern and severity of the hypertrophy, diastolic dysfunction, extent of mitral regurgitation, and severity of any outflow obstruction.

- **EKG:**
  - LV, or biventricular, hypertrophy, non-specific ST–T changes
  - Giant negative T waves in apical variant
  - Short PR interval and marked hypertrophy in Pompe disease
  - Superior axis in some cases of Noonan syndrome
  - Holter monitor: To rule out atrial or ventricular arrhythmias, especially high-grade ventricular ectopy or ventricular tachycardia
  - Exercise test: Document exercise performance and symptoms (e.g. dyspnea or chest pain) and evaluate for exercise-induced arrhythmias.
- **CXR:** Variable cardiomegaly (less severe than DCM) and only rarely pulmonary edema.
- **Echocardiography:** Assess severity and distribution of LV (±RV) hypertrophy, systolic anterior motion of mitral valve, mitral regurgitation, left atrial enlargement, LV (±RV) outflow gradient.

Additional genetic and metabolic studies may be warranted, especially in infants. The diagnostic work-up is similar to that for infantile cases of DCM, though it is guided by the clinical findings. For example, the classical presentation of Pompe disease requires biochemical confirmation of the enzyme deficiency.

Management

The goals of therapy for HCM are:

- To improve LV compliance and reduce symptoms of diastolic dysfunction;
- To reduce LV outflow obstruction;
- To reduce risk of serious arrhythmias;
- To reduce risk of sudden death.

Infants in severe heart failure may be best treated by heart transplantation. On occasion, infants with severe outflow obstruction without systemic disease have been treated surgically by relief of obstruction. Pompe disease is usually lethal within a few months of diagnosis, but a novel enzyme replacement therapy has been used in select infants and older children under research protocols, and more recently as clinical care, following approval of therapy by regulatory agencies in several developed countries. Older children with HCM are frequently asymptomatic and it is unclear if treatment will alter the natural history of the disease. When there are symptoms due to diastolic dysfunction (e.g. exertional dyspnea), non-dihydropyridine **calcium channel blockers** (e.g. verapamil) or **beta-blockers** (e.g. propranolol, atenolol), and occasionally disopyramide, are used with variable effect. Severe LV outflow obstruction has been treated with high-dose **beta-blockers, alcohol septal ablation** (mainly in adults) and surgical myectomy/myotomy. These procedures may relieve symptoms but have not been shown to prevent sudden death. Diuretics and other agents that decrease LV volume are generally contraindicated since they increase propensity for outflow obstruction.

Implantation of an ICD is generally considered indicated in children with HCM who experience syncope or aborted sudden death, or who have documented sustained ventricular tachycardia. Use of antiarrhythmic therapy (e.g. amiodarone) and ICDs for **primary prevention** of sudden death is not established, though some authorities have recommended that ICDs be used in high-risk asymptomatic patients, such as children with very severe LV hypertrophy, strong family history of sudden death, and "'high-risk mutations." In later life, systolic function may become impaired and heart failure may develop, leading to consideration of heart transplantation. This is rarely observed in childhood, and HCM remains a very rare indication for transplantation in children.

Long-term outcome

Survival for HCM is worse when presentation is in infancy, in those with inborn errors of metabolism, and in the presence of malformation syndromes and neuromuscular disease. However, for infants with **idiopathic disease** and who survive beyond 1 year of age, survival is independent of age at diagnosis with an annual mortality rate of about 1%, which is similar to that for patients who present at an older age. Overall, survival for idiopathic HCM is 90% at 5 years and 85% at 10 years. Patients who present at older than 1 year of age rarely die of progressive heart failure but may succumb to sudden death. Sudden death predominates in adolescents and young adults and is thought to be more likely in those with a family history of sudden death, with personal history of recurrent syncope or ventricular tachycardia, and with massive LV hypertrophy.

Restrictive cardiomyopathy

Restrictive cardiomyopathy (RCM) is a very rare form of cardiomyopathy characterized by normal or decreased volume of both ventricles associated with bi-atrial enlargement (often massive) and with normal LV wall thickness (Figures 19.1c and 19.2c). There is some phenotypic overlap with HCM, and mild LV hypertrophy is sometimes observed. Systolic function is generally normal.

Incidence and etiology

RCM accounts for only ~2–5% of pediatric cardiomyopathies with an annual incidence of approximately 0.03 per 100 000 children. The underlying cause(s) are generally unknown. This is in contrast to adult patients with RCM, in whom infiltrative diseases such as amyloidosis and sarcoidosis are sometimes identified. While some children may present with familial forms, most cases are sporadic. Cardiac troponin I and β-myosin heavy chain gene mutations have been reported as causes of restrictive (and hypertrophic) cardiomyopathy as have desmin mutations. The **desminopathies** are generally inherited in an autosomal dominant fashion and are associated with skeletal myopathy and conduction disease.

Clinical presentation

Many patients have relatively few symptoms at presentation. Overall, presentation of RCM is similar to HCM and includes:
• Family history (close relative diagnosed with RCM/HCM);
• Asymptomatic murmur or abnormal heart sound;
• Chest pain, exertional dyspnea or palpitations;
• Pre-syncope, syncope or sudden death (often during exercise).

Key features of the physical examination of RCM

• Relatively well appearing child without failure to thrive
• Absence of dysmorphic features
• Quiet precordium with normally positioned apex
• Prominent pulmonary component of second heart sound (when pulmonary hypertension present)
• S4 gallop
• Variable findings of right heart failure (elevated jugular venous pulse, hepatomegaly)

Investigations
• **EKG:**
  ○ Biatrial enlargement, variable LV hypertrophy, nonspecific ST–T changes
  ○ ST segment depression may be seen especially during tachycardia
  ○ Holter monitor to rule out arrhythmias (usually atrial).
• **CXR:** Mild cardiomegaly (mainly atrial enlargement) ± pulmonary venous congestion.

- **Echocardiography:**
  - Biatrial enlargement (often left greater than right), normal or small ventricular cavities, absent or mild ventricular hypertrophy, normal systolic function
  - Evidence of restrictive physiology and pulmonary hypertension.
- **Catheterization:**
  - Markedly elevated right and LV end-diastolic pressures, markedly elevated atrial pressures, elevated pulmonary artery pressure, and frequent elevation of pulmonary vascular resistance
  - Reduced cardiac output.

Cardiac catheterization should be performed during the evaluation process because of the high likelihood of increased pulmonary vascular resistance. Hemodynamic assessment may also help with the distinction from constrictive pericarditis (see Chapter 18). CT is indicated if pericardial disease is suspected. Since secondary causes of RCM, such as amyloidosis and sarcoidosis, are exceedingly rare in children, endomyocardial biopsy rarely contributes to the diagnosis.

Management

Therapeutic options for pediatric RCM are very limited. Gentle diuresis is indicated if there is pulmonary venous congestion or pulmonary edema, but excessive diuresis may lead to reduction in cardiac output. Vasodilators may lead to hypotension, since augmented cardiac output may not occur when stroke volume is relatively fixed. The role of beta-blockers is unclear. Slowing of the heart rate will prolong diastolic filling time, but since stroke volume is relatively fixed, increasing heart rate may be an important mechanism for augmenting cardiac output. Because short-term survival is poor after a diagnosis of RCM, many centers recommend early evaluation for cardiac transplantation. For patients managed out of hospital, implantation of an ICD in combination with antiarrhythmic agents may be considered, especially if prior near-syncope, syncope, or serious tachyarrhythmia has been documented.

Long-term outcomes

Children with RCM have a very poor prognosis in the absence of heart transplantation, with median survival of around 50%. Freedom from death or transplant at 5 and 10 years after diagnosis has been reported as 39% and 20%, respectively. The presence of symptoms at diagnosis did not correlate with survival in several series. Many patients have significant elevation in pulmonary vascular resistance and this should also lead to consideration of

early transplantation since excessive resistance is a risk factor for acute donor right heart failure at transplantation. Contemporary graft and patient survivals at 5 years after transplantation are approximately 50%, which far exceeds the natural history of the disease.

Non-compaction cardiomyopathy

LV non-compaction (LVNC) cardiomyopathy (also called "spongiform" or "fetal" myocardium) is an increasingly recognized form of cardiomyopathy. It is thought to reflect arrested development of the normal ventricular myocardium. The LV shows prominent trabeculations and deep intertrabecular recesses (Figures 19.1d and 19.2d). These findings are most commonly observed at the apex of the LV but can be seen to extend a variable distance superiorly towards the mid-cavity of the ventricle. Similar findings can be observed in the apex of the RV. There is phenotypic overlap with other forms of cardiomyopathy, including dilated, restrictive, and hypertrophic disease.

Etiology

As with other forms of cardiomyopathy, there are likely multiple etiologies giving rise to the LVNC phenotype. Both sporadic and familial forms have been described. When LVNC is inherited, X-linked inheritance appears to be most common, but autosomal dominant, recessive, and mitochondrial inheritance may also occur. Mutations in the *G4.5* gene at Xq28 (which encodes tafazzin) are responsible for X-linked LVNC, including **Barth syndrome**. The latter is characterized by cardiomyopathy (often with LVNC), intermittent neutropenia, peripheral myopathy, and growth delay.

Clinical features

Approximately half of children with LVNC have signs and symptoms of heart failure. Patients may also present with arrhythmias. Presentation in infancy with heart failure due to severe systolic ventricular dysfunction is not unusual and some of these cases show marked improvement over time, though this may be transient. A "waxing and waning" course is not uncommon.

Management

The principles of management are the same as those for other cardiomyopathies with comparable physiology and function. Transplant-free survival of infants presenting with LVNC and impaired ventricular function is approximately 50% at 5 years. Prognosis in later-onset presentation (including adults) is less well defined.

Arrhythmogenic right ventricular dysplasia

This is a rare inherited cardiomyopathy characterized by fibro-fatty replacement of normal myocardium, primarily of the free wall of the RV.

Etiology
Arrhythmogenic right ventricular dysplasia (ARVD) is most often inherited as an autosomal dominant condition with variable penetrance. Mutations in genes encoding desmosomal proteins appear to be the main etiology. It appears to be particularly common in Italy.

Clinical features
Affected patients may develop ventricular ectopy, ventricular tachycardia with left bundle branch block pattern, and ventricular fibrillation. It may present as sudden death, and accounts for about one-fifth of all causes of sudden death in the young.

Investigations
The extent of RV involvement may be very subtle, making the diagnosis very challenging with standard imaging techniques, though MRI can be very helpful. When myocardial replacement with fibro-fatty tissue is extensive, echocardiography may be sufficient to confirm the diagnosis. Recent data suggest that left ventricular disease may also be present in many cases. Genetic testing is now commercially available.

Management
Treatment may involve antiarrhythmic agents, catheter ablation of arrhythmogenic foci, and ICD implantation. RV failure may develop late in the course of the disease.

Myocarditis

Incidence and etiology
Myocarditis is an inflammatory disorder of the myocardium. Multiple etiologies exist, including infection with bacteria, fungi, protozoa, and viruses; drug toxicities; and systemic disorders, including Kawasaki disease, acute rheumatic fever, and various autoimmune disorders. Idiopathic giant cell myocarditis may also be seen in chil-

dren, though it is very rare. In practical terms, most cases in children are thought to be due to viral infection and this will be the focus of this section.

Viruses may cause cardiac dysfunction from direct viral invasion of myocytes leading to cell lysis and/or secondary to a delayed autoimmune process initiated by recent viral infection. In this setting, infiltration with T lymphocytes usually predominates. The presence of myocardial edema contributes to acute cardiac dysfunction with both systolic and diastolic dysfunction prominent in most cases. Rarely, myocarditis presents with new-onset arrhythmias with preserved function.

The incidence of myocarditis is unknown since most patients with acute viral infection are not screened for evidence of cardiac disease. It is likely that the incidence is markedly underestimated.

Clinical features
Myocarditis in childhood usually presents as an acute-onset cardiomyopathy and distinction from acute onset of chronic DCM is challenging (see above). Heart failure is often severe, with pulmonary edema and low-output state being evident at presentation. Frequently, the course is fulminant, with mechanical ventilation or mechanical circulatory support being required within 24 h of presentation. Presentation with new-onset atrial or ventricular arrhythmias, or atrioventricular block, but with preserved cardiac function has been observed.

Investigations
- **EKG:**
  - Sinus tachycardia with diffusely low QRS voltages
  - Pathologic Q waves may be present
  - Atrial or ventricular arrhythmias or atrioventricular block.
- **CXR:** Mild-to-moderate cardiomegaly with pulmonary venous congestion ± pulmonary edema.
- **Echocardiography:**
  - Mild-to-moderate left atrium and LV enlargement, depressed LV systolic function, variable RV dysfunction
  - Mitral regurgitation common
  - Myocardial hypertrophy due to myocardial edema.
- **Viral studies:** Stool, urine, and respiratory secretions for viral culture ± PCR; blood for viral PCR and viral serologies (IgM and IgG).

In many cases, clinical testing may help differentiate the diagnosis of acute myocarditis from the acute presentation of DCM. The presence of marked cardiomegaly on CXR and prominent left-sided precordial forces on

EKG suggest the underlying process occurred over some time, favoring a diagnosis of chronic DCM. In contrast, absence of (or mild) cardiomegaly and globally diminished voltages on EKG are more typical of acute myocarditis. Frank myocardial infarction may sometimes be observed on the 12-lead EKG of children with acute myocarditis. By echocardiogram, there is generally marked enlargement of the LV and left atrium in chronic DCM. In myocarditis, LV and left atrial dilatation tend to be less pronounced, and there may be myocardial hypertrophy with a "glistening" appearance secondary to myocardial edema.

Endomyocardial biopsy (EMB) appears safe in older children (>1 year) who are hemodynamically stable. Lymphocytic infiltrates with myocyte necrosis are consistent with a diagnosis of acute myocarditis (so-called "**Dallas criteria**"), whereas non-specific changes without inflammation, such as myocyte hypertrophy and interstitial fibrosis, favor a diagnosis of DCM. A fresh-frozen sample should also be obtained for PCR analysis of common viral causes of myocarditis.

Management

In acute myocarditis, therapy is primarily supportive. Only rarely is infection caused by a specific agent for which there is established antimicrobial therapy of proven efficacy. Intravenous immunoglobulin and corticosteroids have both been used, though no randomized clinical trials have been performed to prove their efficacy in children. Steroids are contraindicated when there is evidence of active viral infection. More potent immunosuppressive agents, including T-cell cytolytic agents (such as OKT3) and calcineurin inhibitors (e.g. cyclosporine [ciclosporin] or tacrolimus), have been used in some programs but without clinical trial data to support their use. When clinically indicated, mechanical circulatory support (usually ECMO) should be instituted since the prognosis is excellent if appropriate support can be provided in a timely fashion.

Late outcomes

In general, the outcomes of acute myocarditis in children are good. A number of studies have shown survival rates of between 75% and 100% for acute myocarditis in childhood, including fulminant cases that may require mechanical circulatory support. This emphasizes the benefit of knowing the diagnosis of myocarditis, since acute transplantation should be avoided even if mechanical support is required. This will provide the opportunity for cardiac recovery, as well as minimize the risks of transplantation during recent or active viral infection.

Further reading

Alvarez JA, Wilkinson JD, Lipshultz SE. Outcome predictors for pediatric dilated cardiomyopathy: A systematic review. *Prog Pediatr Cardiol* 2007;23:25–32.

Colan SD, Lipshultz SE, Lowe AM, *et al.* Epidemiology and cause-specific outcome of hypertrophic cardiomyopathy in children: Findings from the Pediatric Cardiomyopathy Registry. *Circulation* 2007;115:773–781.

Cox GF. Diagnostic approaches to pediatric cardiomyopathy of metabolic genetic etiologies and their relation to therapy. *Prog Pediatr Cardiol* 2007;24:15–25.

English RF, Janosky JE, Ettedgui JA, Webber SA. Outcomes for children with acute myocarditis. *Cardiol Young* 2004;14:488–493.

Hershberger RE, Lindenfeld J, Mestroni L, Seidman CE, Taylor MRG, Towbin JA. Genetic evaluation of cardiomyopathy – A Heart Failure Society of America Practice Guideline. *J Cardiac Failure* 2009;15:83–97.

Maron BJ, Towbin JA, Thiene G, *et al.* Contemporary definitions and classification of the cardiomyopathies: an American Heart Association Scientific Statement. *Circulation* 2006;113:1807–1816.

Shaddy RE, Boucek MM, Hsu DT, *et al.* Carvedilol for children and adolescents with heart failure: a randomized controlled trial. *JAMA* 2007;298:1171–1179.

Towbin JA, Lowe AM, Colan SD, *et al.* Incidence, causes, and outcomes of dilated cardiomyopathy in children. *JAMA* 2006;296:1867–1876.

Webber SA. Primary restrictive cardiomyopathy in childhood. *Prog Pediatr Cardiol* 2008;25:85–90.

Weintraub RG, Nugent AW, Daubeney PEF. Pediatric cardiomyopathy: The Australian experience. *Prog Pediatr Cardiol* 2007;23:17–24.

Wilkinson JD, Sleeper LA, Alvarez JA, Bublik N, Lipshultz SE. The Pediatric Cardiomyopathy Registry: 1995-2007. *Prog Pediatr Cardiol* 2008;25:31–36.

20 Cardiac tumors

Koichiro Niwa[1] and Shigeru Tateno[2]

[1]St Luke's International Hospital, Tokyo, Japan
[2]Chiba Cardiovascular Center, Chiba, Japan

The widespread use of non-invasive investigations has resulted in a marked increase in the detection of cardiac tumors. Their manifestations are non-specific and include systemic, embolic, and cardiac symptoms. Although cardiac tumors are usually benign in childhood, they may induce life-threatening arrhythmias or cardiac failure, and therefore surgical resection is indicated in symptomatic patients if feasible.

Incidence and etiology

The reported incidence varies from 0.027% among pediatric postmortem specimens to 0.49% among infants with congenital heart disease. The incidence of primary cardiac tumors is 0.2% among patients referred for assessment of potential cardiac defects. Cardiac tumors are benign in more than 90% of children. At least 80% of rhabdomyomas are associated with tuberous sclerosis and 40–86% of patients with this condition have cardiac rhabdomyomas. Familial atrial myxoma is occasionally encountered.

Clinical features

Although cardiac tumors are usually benign in childhood, they may induce life-threatening symptoms. The clinical features are best divided into systemic, embolic, and cardiac manifestations.

- **Systemic symptoms** include fever, general malaise, and digital clubbing; arthralgia is specific to myxomas.
- **Embolic manifestations** are caused by embolization of either fragments of the tumor itself or thrombus.
- **Cardiac manifestations** are dependent on the location and extent of the tumor within the heart:
  - Even small tumors may produce disturbance of atrioventricular conduction or arrhythmias
  - Infiltrative tumors of the myocardium can cause hemodynamic compromise
  - Pericardial effusion, eventually with cardiac tamponade, may be the first symptom of the epicardial location of the tumor
  - Primary cardiac tumors with an intracavitary extension may cause obstruction or interfere with valvular closure
  - Intermittent ventricular inflow or outflow obstruction may result in syncope as the primary symptom.

Physical examination reveals non-specific findings, including loud added heart sounds in mobile pedunculated tumors.

Investigations

- **EKG:** Non-specific, but arrhythmias and conduction disturbances or changes of voltage and ST–T wave abnormalities may be detected.
- **CX-R:** Cardiac tumors may alter the contour of the heart, but the changes are non-specific.

Pediatric Heart Disease: A Practical Guide, First Edition. Piers E. F. Daubeney, Michael L. Rigby, Koichiro Niwa, and Michael A. Gatzoulis.
© 2012 Blackwell Publishing Ltd. Published 2012 by Blackwell Publishing Ltd.

- **Echocardiography:** The gold standard for diagnosis, reliable for identification and useful for risk stratification.
- **MRI:** Provides not only information about the extension of the tumor and extracardiac structure, but also tissue characterization and differentiation of solid tissue, cystic, hemorrhagic, and fatty tumors.
- **Angiography:** Cardiac catheterization is rarely required but may be helpful in evaluating the blood supply in hemangiomas and malignant growths.

Management

Medical management

Treatment of cardiac tumors depends on the specific histologic type, location, and associated arrhythmias or embolic phenomena. Antiarrhythmic drugs are often effective in patients with ventricular tachycardia in whom surgical resection is not an option.

Surgical management

Surgical resection is indicated in symptomatic patients, usually those with significant obstruction of ventricular inlet or outlet, systemic or pulmonary embolization, or life-threatening arrhythmias. Single lesions, even large solitary intramural and extramural tumors, may be amenable to surgical resection if they are well circumscribed. Others with extensive myocardial invasion will be inoperable and conservative management or heart transplantation should be considered. In multiple lesions and in the absence of symptoms, surgery is better postponed or avoided.

Late complications and long-term outcome

Recurrence of tumors can be observed after surgical resection.

Long-term cardiologic follow-up is required for virtually all patients because of the ongoing risk of potentially fatal arrhythmias. The exception is patients with rhabdomyomas that have regressed spontaneously.

Reports on **pregnancy** are very limited. Care must be taken because of the continuing risk of arrhythmias and cardiac failure during pregnancy.

Following successful and complete resection of cardiac tumors, many patients have an excellent chance of symptom-free survival.

Types of cardiac tumors

Rhabdomyoma (Figure 20.1)

The most frequent tumors found in the fetus and infants are hamartomas, usually multiple and located in the ventricular myocardium. The natural history is spontaneous regression in the majority by the age of 2 years. Tuberous sclerosis is often present and the presence of multiple tumors may be the first indication of the condition.

Most infants with multiple rhabdomyomas are without cardiac symptoms, but the prognosis of the few with symptoms (cardiomegaly, cardiac failure, arrhythmias) is poor. Surgery is rarely required unless there is severe obstruction or refractory life-threatening arrhythmias.

Fibroma (Figure 20.1)

Fibromas are the second most frequent tumor in children and they have a distinct predilection for the ventricular septum and left ventricle. They are solid, firm, non-cystic lesions of variable size, and symptoms relate to arrhythmias or obstruction depending primarily on location. Conservative management is often the best approach because of extensive myocardial invasion, but surgery is employed in a few.

Myxoma (Figure 20.2)

Myxomas are the most common cardiac tumors in adult life and are diagnosed infrequently in infants and children (5–10%). Typically a single tumor is attached to the atrial septum in the region of the fossa ovalis and may protrude into the left or right atrioventricular junction during diastole, resulting in syncope in some patients. Sudden death and myocardial infarction have been described. Left atrial myxomas are more common (75%) and give rise to fever, anorexia, weight loss, malaise, and arthralgia. Raised ESR, C-reactive protein, leukocytosis, thrombocytopenia, hypergammaglobulinemia, and anemia may occur. All these features resolve following surgical removal but there is a risk of recurrence.

Cystic tumors

Teratomas are the most frequently encountered cystic tumors of the heart. They are usually located in the pericardium and are often associated with a pericardial effusion. Rarely, intracardiac teratomas have been described, usually located in the ventricular septum and bulging into the right ventricle. In most cases they are histologically benign, unless they have germ cell tumor

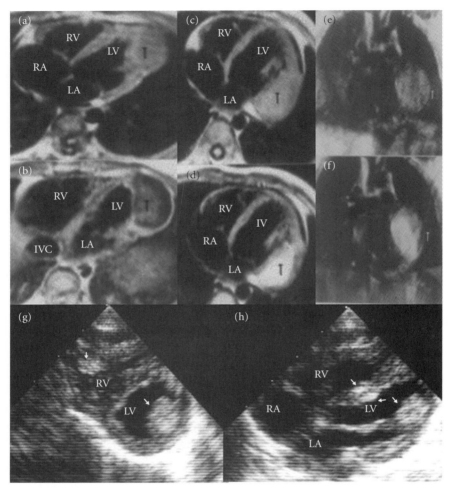

Figure 20.1 Various cardiac tumors. (a,b) MRI of fibroma. (c-f) MRI of unknown type of tumor (same patient): (c, d)axial view; (e,f) coronal view. (g,h) Echocardiogram of rhabdomyoma (arrowed). Note: a, c, and e are MRI spin-echo images; b, d, and f are of gadolinium-DTPA enhanced images; b shows edge enhancement d and f show tumor enhancement). IVC inferior vena cava; LA, left atrium; LV, left ventricle; RA, right atrium; RV, right ventricle. (Courtesy of Atsushi Mizuno, MD.)

elements, which are rare in the heart, and impossible to detect by observing the gross image obtained with echocardiography or MRI. There are reports of heart teratomas with metastases, but this is unusual. The malignant component of teratomas in young children in general is a **yolk sac tumor**, and is associated with a raised blood alpha-fetoprotein.

Surgical removal to prevent arrhythmias, complications of tumor growth, and risk of malignant change, and to establish the diagnosis is often advised but is not always feasible; unless a tumor causes significant ventricular inflow or outflow obstruction or is associated with intractable arrhythmias, conservative management may be a safer approach in the majority.

Other cystic tumors include bronchogenic, dermoid, and mesothelial cysts; they are also more likely to be found in the pericardium. An intracardiac bronchogenic cyst is considered to be ectopic tissue sequestered inside the heart during embryogenesis.

Other tumors

Benign tumors rarely encountered include lipoma, papillary fibroelastoma, and hemangioma. Malignant tumors are also rare and include rhabdomyosarcoma, angiosar-

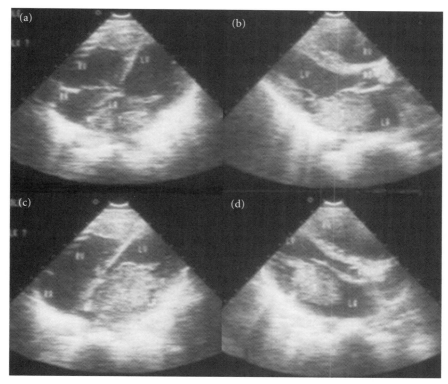

Figure 20.2 Myxoma in an 8-year old girl. Echocardiogram revealed left atrial myxoma. (a,b) Systole; (c,d) diastole. In diastole, myxoma occupies the inflow of the left ventricle. Ao, aorta; LA, left atrium; LV, left ventricle; RA, right atrium; RV, right ventricle. (Courtesy of Atsushi Mizuno, MD.)

coma, mesothelioma, fibrosarcoma, lymphoma, osteosarcoma, thymoma, neurogenic sarcoma, and the most common, malignant teratoma.

Summary

Clinical manifestations differ according to the type and extension of the tumor, and are divided into systemic, embolic, and cardiac manifestations. Surgical removal to prevent arrhythmias, complications of tumor growth, and risk of malignant change, and to establish the diagnosis is often advised but not always feasible. Unless a tumor causes significant ventricular inflow or outflow obstruction or is associated with intractable arrhythmias, conservative management may be a safer approach. While surgical resection can be performed successfully in some,

it is not always possible. Careful evaluation of cardiac MRI and echocardiography imaging is an essential prerequisite to correct patient treatment.

Further reading

Beghetti M, Gow RM, Haney I, Mawson J, Williams WG, Freedom RM. Pediatric primary benign cardiac tumors: a 15-year review. *Am Heart J.* 1997;134:1107–1114.

Bosi G, Lintermans JP, Pellegrino PA, Svaluto-Morelo G, Viers A. The natural history of cardiac rhabdomyoma with and without tuberous sclerosis. *Acta Pediatr* 1996;85:928–931.

Cho JM, Danielson GK, Puga FJ, *et al*. Surgical resection of ventricular cardiac fibromas: early and late results. *Ann Thorac Surg.* 2003;76:1929–1934.

Reynen K. Cardiac myxomas. *N Engl J Med* 1995;333:1610–1617.

21 Primary pulmonary arterial hypertension in children

Alan G. Magee

Royal Brompton Hospital, London, UK

In recent years there has been a revival of interest in idiopathic pulmonary arterial hypertension (IPAH; previously known as primary pulmonary hypertension) because of a better understanding of the underlying mechanism and the availability of new treatments. Without treatment, prognosis is poor, with a mean survival from diagnosis of only 10 months in children younger than 16 years and 2.8 years in adults.

Pulmonary hypertension in general is defined as a mean pulmonary artery pressure on direct catheter measurement of greater than 25 mmHg at rest or 30 mmHg with exercise. The diagnosis of IPAH is made when other causes of pulmonary hypertension, including left heart disease, congenital heart disease, collagen vascular disease, HIV infection, chronic thromboembolism, and portal hypertension are excluded: the last two being extremely rare causes in children.

Incidence and etiology

The reported incidence of IPAH is one to two cases per million per annum in the US, but the true incidence may be greater than this as incidence data have been obtained from large specialist centers and cases may well go unrecognized. IPAH is closely related to familial pulmonary arterial hypertension (FPAH), which has been found in approximately 100 families worldwide and is inherited in an autosomal dominant fashion with incomplete penetrance. It has a tendency to develop at earlier ages in subsequent generations (genetic anticipation). Mutations in the bone morphogenetic protein receptor II (BMPR2)

are found in approximately 50% of patients with FPAH and 25% of those with sporadic IPAH.

Pathophysiology

Much remains to be discovered regarding the pathophysiology of IPAH, which involves a triad of vasoconstriction, vascular remodeling, and thrombosis. Normal pulmonary arterial vascular tone is maintained by a balance between endogenous vasoconstrictors and vasodilators. When this balance is upset by a vascular insult, in presumably genetically susceptible individuals, then vasoconstriction leads to increased pulmonary vascular resistance. In addition many of these vasoactive substances have effects on both smooth muscle and endothelial cell proliferation and platelet activation (Figure 21.1). Cell proliferation and thrombosis in turn lead to further reduction in the total pulmonary vascular cross-sectional area and eventually to complete vascular occlusion with the appearance of plexiform lesions (Figure 21.2). These are areas of disorganized growth and abnormal angiogenesis. It is interesting that histologic findings are very similar in all forms of PAH whether idiopathic or secondary to other conditions.

Clinical features

The presentation of PAH is often insidious with progressive dyspnea on exertion, general fatigue, and later anginal chest pain and syncope. It may be confused with asthma in children and indeed presents with bronchospasm that does not respond to bronchodilators. Much later

Pediatric Heart Disease: A Practical Guide, First Edition. Piers E. F. Daubeney, Michael L. Rigby, Koichiro Niwa, and Michael A. Gatzoulis.
© 2012 Blackwell Publishing Ltd. Published 2012 by Blackwell Publishing Ltd.

anorexia, abdominal swelling, and peripheral edema develop as the right ventricle fails and tricuspid regurgitation worsens.

The principal clinical findings are an accentuated pulmonary component of the second heart sound together with a palpable left parasternal lift produced by the hypertrophied right ventricle. In more advanced disease the early diastolic murmur of pulmonary regurgitation and the pan-systolic murmur of tricuspid regurgitation may be heard. Eventually the signs of right heart failure are seen with evidence of a low cardiac output and a third heart sound gallop rhythm on auscultation.

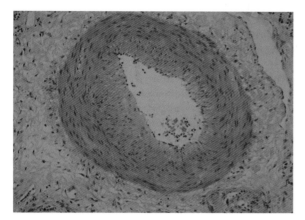

Figure 21.1 Cross-section of pulmonary arteriole showing hyperplasia of intimal and smooth muscle layers.

Key features of history and examination

- Progressive dyspnea on exertion
- Family history
- Syncope
- Left parasternal lift
- Prominent P2
- Raised jugular venous pressure, ascites, peripheral edema, hepatomegaly (late features)

Investigations

- **EKG:**
  - Right ventricular hypertrophy ± strain pattern, right atrial hypertrophy
  - Should be performed in any child suspected of having PAH, but lacks sufficient sensitivity to act as an effective screening tool
  - 6-minute walk test should be included for older children.
- **CXR:** May show enlargement of the central pulmonary arteries with peripherally oligemic lung fields (so-called "pruning"), but the absence of pruning does not exclude PAH.
- **Echocardiography with Doppler:**
  - Dilated hypertrophied right ventricle with elevated estimated systolic pressure
  - This is the best screening test

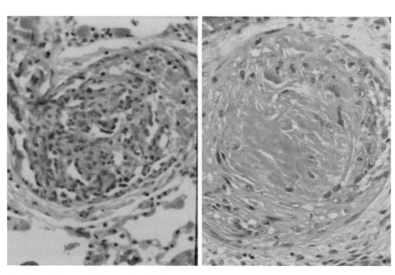

Figure 21.2 Plexiform lesions with complete vessel occlusion.

○ The right ventricular pressure is estimated by taking the right ventricular-to-right atrial pressure gradient from the jet of tricuspid regurgitation and adding the assumed right atrial pressure

○ Can also rule out left heart disease, including structural lesions such as mitral or less commonly pulmonary vein stenosis.

• **Right heart catheterization:**

○ Raised pulmonary vascular resistance ± response to vasodilator

○ This is the definitive investigation for PAH and, if possible, should be performed before treatment is started

○ In general, the pulmonary pressures and cardiac output are measured with calculation of the pulmonary vascular resistance in room air, in 100% oxygen, and with inhaled nitric oxide

○ Potentially hazardous investigation in pulmonary hypertension and must be performed in an experienced center with pediatric intensive care back-up and the facility to perform an urgent atrial septostomy in the event of an acute exacerbation. Patients with advanced disease who present with evidence of low cardiac output are at particularly high risk during catheterization, which should probably be deferred until some response to cautiously introduced treatment can be obtained. Chronic thromboembolism causing PAH is rare in children and in any case would be detected during cardiac catheterization.

It is also important to exclude secondary forms:
• Connective tissue disease;
• HIV infection;
• Chronic thromboembolism;
• Portal hypertension.

If there is a possibility of lung disease or upper airway obstruction, then a respiratory opinion should be sought. Lung biopsy is no longer routinely performed as the chance of altering the diagnosis based on histology is low and the risk is significant.

Management

An algorithm for current management was provided by the third World Symposium on Pulmonary Hypertension in Venice in 2003 (see Chapter 22).

Medical management (Table 21.1)

All patients should receive anticoagulation; those with desaturation should receive oxygen to maintain an oxygen saturation above 90%, and diuretics may be required if there is evidence of right heart failure. Following this, treatment depends on the results of acute vasodilator testing:

• Patients who respond to inhaled nitric oxide should receive oral calcium channel blockers. These are contraindicated in non-responders and response should be re-tested after around 1 year.

Table 21.1 Medical management of pulmonary arterial hypertension

Treatment	Indications	Comments
Warfarin	Prevention of thrombosis	Prolonged survival in IPAH, maintain INR around 2
Supportive therapy	Right heart failure	Diuretics best, digoxin may have some effect on cardiac output
Calcium antagonists	Positive vasodilator response during right heart catheter	Only around 40% children respond, fewer show sustained responseand use may be harmful in non-responders
Prostaglandins (epoprostenol, iloprost)	Treatment of IPAH (WHO Class III/IV)	Expensive, risk of rebound effect, first treatment to show prognostic benefit
Endothelin receptor antagonist (bosentan)	Treatment of IPAH (WHO Class III/IV)	Demonstrated to improve symptoms and survival, risk of hepatic toxicity
Phosphodiesterase inhibitors (sildenafil)	Patients who have failed, or are not candidates for, other treatments	Selective inhibition of cGMP-specific phosphodiesterase, further evidence required

IPAH, idiopathic pulmonary arterial hypertension.

• Non-responders are treated according to clinical severity with those in WHO class III or IV starting on an endothelin receptor antagonist (bosentan) or prostaglandin analog (intravenous epoprostenol or inhaled iloprost). The most severely ill would probably go directly to epoprostenol. If the response to treatment is inadequate or not sustained, treatment should be combined, possibly with the addition of sildenafil, or surgical treatment considered.

Surgical management

Surgical treatment consists of atrial septostomy and either lung or heart–lung transplantation. Atrial septostomy has been used in patients with advanced pulmonary hypertension to decompress the right ventricle, so increasing cardiac output at the expense of reduced systemic oxygen saturation. It carries a significant mortality and should only be performed electively by experienced operators in carefully selected cases. Patients with the most severe pulmonary hypertension and low cardiac output do particularly badly and the recommendation is that septostomy should only be performed if the right atrial pressure is between 10 and 20 mmHg.

The first heart–lung transplantation performed for primary pulmonary hypertension was in 1981 by Shumway and colleagues at Stamford University, but since then the use of transplantation has declined with the introduction of prostacyclin analogs such as epoprostenol. At present, patients with severe disease whose prognosis remains poor in spite of medical therapy should be considered for transplantation. This could either be a heart–lung transplant or bilateral lung transplant, the latter becoming more popular in children (see Chapter 35). Data from the International Society for Heart and Lung Transplantation would suggest a 5-year survival rate of 41%. Mortality is chiefly related to acute rejection, obliterative bronchiolitis, overwhelming infection, and coronary artery disease.

Prognosis

IPAH has a worse prognosis than pulmonary hypertension related to congenital heart disease; however, this is being modified by current treatment strategies. Six series have demonstrated improved survival with epoprostenol in adults and studies in children have shown similar improvement in longevity. Three series have shown a positive impact of anticoagulation on survival and of course calcium channel blockers improve survival in the small proportion of positive responders. A worse prognosis is associated with severe disease at the time of presentation, in particular evidence of low cardiac output, pericardial effusion, and poor exercise tolerance. In children, a younger age at diagnosis appears to be a poor prognostic feature.

Further reading

Barst RJ, Rubin LJ, Long WA, *et al.* A comparison of continuous intravenous epoprostenol (prostacyclin) with conventional therapy for primary pulmonary hypertension. The primary pulmonary hypertension study group. *N Engl J Med* 1996;334: 296–302.

Barst RJ, Ivy D, Dingemanse J, *et al.* Pharmacokinetics, safety and efficacy of bosentan in paediatric patients with pulmonary arterial hypertension. *Clin Pharmacol Ther* 2003;73:372–382.

D'Alonzo GE, Barst RJ, Ayers SM, *et al.* Survival in patients with primary pulmonary hypertension. Results from a national prospective registry. *Ann Intern Med* 1991;115:343–349.

Klepetko W, Mayer E, Sandoval J, *et al.* Interventional and surgical modalities of treatment for pulmonary arterial hypertension. *J Am Coll Cardiol* 2004;43 (Suppl S):73S–80S.

Moledina S, Hislop AA, Foster H, Schulze-Neick I, Haworth SG. Childhood idiopathic pulmonary hypertension: a national cohort Study. *Heart* 2010;96:1401–1406.

Rich S, Kaufmann E, Levy PS. The effect of high doses of calcium-channel blockers on survival in primary pulmonary hypertension. *N Engl J Med* 1992;327:76–81.

The Task Force for the Diagnosis and Treatment of Pulmonary Hypertension of the European Society of Cardiology (ESC) and the European Respiratory Society (ERS). Guidelines for the diagnosis and treatment of pulmonary hypertension. *European Heart Journal* 2009;30:2493–2537.

Thompson JR, Machado RD, Pauciulo MW, *et al.* Sporadic primary pulmonary hypertension is associated with germline mutations in BMPR2, a receptor member of the TGF-beta family. *J Med Genet* 2000;37:741–745.

22 Pulmonary arterial hypertension associated with congenital heart disease (including Eisenmenger syndrome)

Mark S. Spence[1,2] and Michael A. Gatzoulis[3,4]

[1]Royal Victoria Hospital, Belfast Trust, Belfast, UK
[2]Queen's University, Belfast, UK
[3]Royal Brompton Hospital, London, UK
[4]National Heart and Lung Institute, Imperial College, London, UK

Definition and clinical classification

Pulmonary hypertension is defined as an increase in mean pulmonary arterial pressure (PAP) $\geqslant 25$ mmHg at rest as assessed by right heart catheterization. This value has been used for selecting patients in all randomised controlled trials and registries of pulmonary arterial hypertension.

As a result of improved pathophysiologic understanding of the mechanisms involved in pulmonary hypertension, the earlier Evian classification was revised by the third World Symposium on Pulmonary Hypertension in Venice in 2003. The 2008 fourth World Symposium on Pulmonary Hypertension held in Dana Point, California, resulted in some further modifications while maintaining the philosophy and architecture of the previous clinical classifications. This classification divides pulmonary hypertension into five groups, one of which is pulmonary arterial hypertension (PAH), which in turn is divided into five subgroups.

Congenital heart disease is one of the conditions commonly associated with PAH and is further classified according to:

Clinical classification of pulmonary hypertension (adapted from the Dana Point classification)

- Pulmonary arterial hypertension:
  - Idiopathic PAH (IPAH)
  - Heritable
  - Drug and toxin induced
  - Associated with:
    Connective tissue diseases
    HIV infection
    Portal hypertension
    Congenital heart disease
    Schistosomiasis
    Chronic hemolytic anemia
  - Persistent pulmonary hypertension of the newborn
  - Pulmonary veno-occlusive disease (PVOD) and /or pulmonary capillary hemangiomatosis (PCH)
- Pulmonary hypertension owing to left heart disease
- Pulmonary hypertension owing to lung diseases and/or hypoxia
- Chronic thromboembolic pulmonary hypertension (CTEPH)
- Pulmonary hypertension with unclear multifactorial mechanisms

---

Pediatric Heart Disease: A Practical Guide, First Edition. Piers E. F. Daubeney, Michael L. Rigby, Koichiro Niwa, and Michael A. Gatzoulis.
© 2012 Blackwell Publishing Ltd. Published 2012 by Blackwell Publishing Ltd.

- Lesion type;
- Lesion size;
- Direction of shunt;
- Associated cardiac and extracardiac abnormalities
- Repair status.

Anatomic/pathophysiologic classification of congenital systemic-to-pulmonary shunts associated with pulmonary arterial hypertension

- Type of lesion:
  - Simple pre-tricuspid shunts:
    Atrial septal defect (ASD)
    Total or partial unobstructed anomalous pulmonary venous return
  - Simple post-tricuspid shunts:
    Ventricular septal defect (VSD)
    Patent ductus arteriosus (PDA)
  - Combined shunts (describe combination and define predominant defect)
  - Complex congenital heart disease:
    Atrioventricular septal defect (AVSD; see Chapter 9)
    Truncus arteriosus (see Chapter 16)
    Single ventricle physiology with unobstructed pulmonary blood flow (see Chapter 16)
    Transposition of the great arteries with VSD (without pulmonary stenosis) and/or PDA (see Chapter 14)
    Other
    Small to moderate (ASD < 2.0 cm and VSD < 1.0 cm)
    Large (ASD > 2.0 cm, and VSD > 1.0 cm)
- Dimensions (specify for each defect if >1 congenital heart defect)
  - Hemodynamic (specify Qp/Qs):
    Restrictive
    Unrestrictive
  - Anatomic:
- Direction of shunt
  - Predominantly systemic-to-pulmonary
  - Predominantly pulmonary-to-systemic
  - Bidirectional
- Associated cardiac and extracardiac abnormalities
- Repair status:
  - Unoperated
  - Palliated (specify type of operation(s), age at surgery)
  - Repaired (specify type of operation(s), age at surgery)

Classification of PAH in the setting of congenital heart disease is challenging due to the dynamic nature of the disease and the fact that patients with similar underlying cardiac lesions may develop PAH of variable severity. However, four quite distinct phenotypes can be recognized, providing a useful clinical classification:

A. **Eisenmenger syndrome** represents the extreme end of the spectrum of PAH associated with CHD. It is characterized by the presence of a large uncorrected central left-to-right shunt causing a progressive and eventually irreversible rise in pulmonary vascular resistance that leads to reversed or bidirectional shunt flow with resultant cyanosis, erythrocytosis and multiorgan involvement.

B. **PAH associated with systemic-to-pulmonary shunts.** Includes moderate to large defects; PVR is mildly to moderately increased, systemic-to-pulmonary shunt is still prevalent, and no cyanosis is present at rest.

C. **PAH with small defects.** Clinical picture is usually very similar to idiopathic PAH.

D. **PAH after corrective cardiac surgery.** Congenital heart disease has been corrected, but PAH is still present immediately after surgery or recurs several months or years after surgery in the absence of significant postoperative residual lesions.

Epidemiology

It has been reported that 5–10% of patients with congenital heart disease develop PAH, although this is only an estimate as pulmonary artery pressures are not available for many patients. The prevalence of Eisenmenger syndrome is more easily quantified and has declined from approximately 8% in the 1950s to approximately 4% of those followed up in tertiary adult congenital heart centers today. It is expected that the proportion of patients with simple lesions and PAH will decline further due to better and earlier correction. However, the numbers with complex congenital heart disease, such as those with single ventricle physiology who develop PAH after palliative procedures in childhood, will increase. Currently patients with VSD, AVSD, and PDA account for 70–80% of those with Eisenmenger syndrome. For individuals with Eisenmenger syndrome, a large variation in life expectancy exists. Reports that include pediatric patients have found an average age at death in the 25–35-year range. Alternatively, mean survival in the adult population is in the 50–55-year range.

Pathophysiology

The size and type of lesion are important determinants of the likelihood and rapidity of developing PAH. However, the fact that patients with similar underlying defects develop differing degrees of PAH is strongly suggestive of genetic factors being important in determining an individual's risk. In general terms, the penetrance of PAH is high, and the onset of Eisenmenger physiology is relatively early and inevitable in patients with large shunts at ventricular or arterial level. Since most patients with even large ASDs do not develop Eisenmenger physiology and those who do develop PAH usually do so much later on in life, it is doubted whether the severity of the PAH in patients with ASD can be directly attributed to the degree of shunting. It is generally accepted that the PAH in this situation is due to concomitant IPAH or other causes such as lung or thromboembolic disease. Support for this hypothesis comes from reported cases of severe pulmonary hypertension in children with small ASDs whose mothers had IPAH.

PAH is a dynamic and multifactorial process related to vasoconstriction and remodeling of the pulmonary vascular bed, which may be aggravated by thrombosis. Intrauterine pulmonary vascular disease is unusual in patients with congenital heart disease and the disease process starts at birth. There is a reduction in the size and number of respiratory units as normally about half of these form after birth. Several histopathologic abnormalities are associated with congenital heart disease and PAH. Extension of smooth muscle cells into peripheral pulmonary arteries, medial hypertrophy, formation of plexiform lesions, and rarification of the pulmonary arterial tree have been observed (see Figures 21.1 and 21.2). High flow and pressure initiate pulmonary vascular endothelial damage and are central to the pathogenesis of PAH in congenital heart disease. The role of mediators influencing pulmonary vascular tone such as endothelins, prostacyclin, and nitric oxide has attracted much research interest as they are potential targets for pharmacologic manipulation (see below).

Survival is substantially better for patients with PAH associated with congenital heart disease compared to those with IPAH. Two potential mechanisms are proposed to account for this:
• In PAH associated with congenital heart disease, the right ventricle is subjected to high pressures from birth or from infancy, and therefore may be better trained to support systemic pulmonary pressures, reducing the incidence of early right ventricular failure.

• In patients with IPAH, pulmonary hypertension *per se* limits pulmonary and thereby systemic blood flow during exercise. In contrast, patients with PAH and associated shunts maintain or increase their systemic cardiac output during exercise by shunting right to left, albeit at the expense of cyanosis.

Clinical presentation

Clinical signs and symptoms are variable and depend on the underlying heart defect, patient age, repair status, and degree and direction of shunting.

General symptoms suggestive of PAH are non-specific and may include breathlessness, fatigue, poor exercise capacity, syncope, and chest pain.

The dramatic changes in pulmonary vascular resistance in early life must be borne in mind when assessing children with congenital heart disease and suspected PAH. Before birth the pulmonary vascular resistance is greater than the systemic resistance and pulmonary blood bypasses the lungs via the ductus arteriosus (see Chapter 30). Immediately after birth, pulmonary vascular resistance falls by half with the first breath and continues to fall over the next 3 months. The pulmonary artery pressure should therefore also normally fall as it is dependent on the product of the pulmonary vascular resistance and blood flow. The signs and symptoms of the CHD patient are therefore modified accordingly.

For example, at birth a neonate with a large VSD will have equal pressures in the left and right ventricle and thus immediate signs such as a murmur may not be detectable. Only when the pulmonary vascular resistance begins to fall will significant left-to-right shunting develop, resulting in the typically detectable signs and symptoms of heart failure (often around 2–6 weeks after birth). Eventually the increased pulmonary blood flow will cause progressive pulmonary vascular disease and PAH will develop. If left untreated, shunt reversal and cyanosis is likely to occur and the patient will have been transformed into one with **Eisenmenger physiology** that is not reversible by corrective surgery:
• **Central cyanosis and clubbing:** Most visible clinical consequences. The chronic cyanosis has multisystem effects.
• **Exercise intolerance:** Most adult patients with Eisenmenger physiology are very symptomatic, with over 90% of patients in NYHA class II or higher. They are the most limited subgroup of adult congenital patients with a mean peak oxygen uptake well within the transplant range (below 14 mL/kg/min).
• **Transcutaneous oxygen saturations:** At rest are typically in the low-to-mid 80s. Importantly, not all Eisenmenger

patients are cyanotic at rest and some may exhibit differential cyanosis (e.g. a patient with a PDA and Eisenmenger physiology will have no clubbing of the right hand but cyanosis and clubbing of the left hand and both feet).

• **Secondary erythrocytosis:** Physiologic adaptation to chronic cyanosis and essential in maintaining adequate tissue oxygenation and preventing hypoxic end-organ damage.

• **Iron deficiency:** Important cause of symptoms and morbidity and must be regularly tested for.

• **Hyperviscosity symptoms,** such as headaches, dizziness, visual disturbances, paresthesia, and myalgia, have been linked with raised hematocrit levels; however, **iron deficiency** causes very similar symptoms and must be sought and treated first.

• **Neutropenia, thrombocytopenia, platelet dysfunction, and clotting abnormalities:** Commonly present, contributing to the infection, bleeding, and clotting risk in these patients.

• **Intrapulmonary thrombosis:** Detected in up to a third of adult patients with Eisenmenger physiology and is associated with hemoptysis and pulmonary infarction. Hemoptysis is common in patients with Eisenmenger physiology (incidence between 11% and 100%, increasing with age). It is usually mild and self-limiting, and, although troublesome, is rarely fatal.

• **Infections:** There is a high risk of developing bacterial endocarditis and attention to oral hygiene and maintaining healthy dentition is therefore vital for patients with PAH and congenital heart disease. Intracerebral abscess is a particular risk and requires diagnostic vigilance and a low threshold for investigation, particularly as subtle signs may easily be misinterpreted as iron deficiency or hyperviscosity symptoms.

• **Arrhythmias and sudden cardiac death:** In one series 42% of Eisenmenger patients were found to have supraventricular arrhythmias on routine EKG or 24-h Holter monitoring during long-term follow-up. Their presence is a marker for increased mortality associated with congestive heart failure and sudden cardiac death, modes of death in 30% and 25% respectively of adult patients with Eisenmenger syndrome.

Multiorgan involvement in patients with chronic cyanotic congenital heart disease and pulmonary arterial hypertension

• **Ischemic and embolic complications:**
  ○ Cerebrovascular accidents (stroke or transient ischemic attack)

• **Bleeding and thrombotic diathesis:**
  ○ Hemoptysis
  ○ Intrapulmonary thrombosis
  ○ Pulmonary hemorrhage
  ○ Cerebral bleeding
  ○ Menorrhagia
  ○ Epistaxis
• **Hematologic involvement:**
  ○ Secondary erythrocytosis
  ○ Thrombocytopenia
• **Infections:**
  ○ Bacterial endocarditis
  ○ Cerebral abscess
  ○ Pneumonia
• **Progressive right ventricular failure**
• **Cardiac arrhythmias and sudden cardiac death**
• **Renal dysfunction:**
  ○ Glomerular abnormalities
  ○ Hyperuricemia and gout
• **Hepatic dysfunction:**
  ○ Cholelithiasis (calcium bilirubinate) and cholecystitis
• **Acne**
• **Skeletal disease:**
  ○ Scoliosis
  ○ Hypertrophic osteoarthropathy

Clinical assessment

Typical physical findings in PAH include:

• Central cyanosis with clubbing (which may be differential);

• Right ventricular heave, palpable pulmonary component of the second heart sound, right-sided S4, and sometimes a pulmonary ejection click;

• Murmurs associated with tricuspid or pulmonary valvular regurgitation may be present;

• As Eisenmenger physiology develops, the defects responsible for the PAH no longer generate murmurs due to equalization of the pressure difference between the pulmonary and systemic circulations;

• Signs of right heart failure, such as elevated jugular venous pressure, peripheral edema, abdominal tenderness, and heptomegaly.

Investigations

- **Routine laboratory testing:** In patients with Eisenmenger physiology abnormalities are to be expected and comparison should always be made with previous results if available. Some of the typical findings are:
  - **Full blood count:** Hematocrit is typically elevated due to secondary erythrocytosis. Low platelet count. White cell count slightly low or at the lower limit of normal
  - **Iron status:** It is important to measure transferrin saturation and serum ferritin as microcytosis and hypochromia may be found in only 16% of cyanotic patients with iron deficiency. The hemoglobin is often in excess of 18 g/dL, even when iron deficiency is present
  - **Coagulation:** Mild increases in INR and activated partial thromboplatin time (aPTT) are present due to decreased levels of Factors V, VII, VIII, and X, thrombocytopenia, platelet dysfunction, and increased fibrinolytic activity
  - **Renal function:** Proteinuria typically less than 1 g/24 h in patients with Eisenmenger physiology due to hypoxic glomerulopathy. Serum creatinine may be mildly elevated; hematuria can also be found; uric acid and bilirubin are typically elevated.

Practical points

- As secondary erythrocytosis increases the hematocrit and decreases the plasma volume; this needs to be corrected for when measuring coagulation parameters. The laboratory should be asked to provide sample bottles containing a volume of liquid anticoagulant adjusted according to the hematocrit. Simple formulae exist for this purpose; otherwise inaccurate results will be obtained.
- Hypoglycemia is not uncommon and is usually spuriously low due to increased *in vitro* glycolysis due to the increased red cell mass. This can be avoided by adding sodium fluoride to the tube.
- **EKG:**
  - Useful in assessing underlying heart rhythm and may indicate atrial dilatation or right ventricular strain (in addition to showing abnormalities related to the underlying cardiac defect)
  - Right ventricular hypertrophy defined by voltage criteria may provide prognostic information in patients with Eisenmenger physiology.
- **Formal exercise testing:**
  - Exercise capacity in patients with PAH may reflect disease severity and assist prognostic evaluation

  - For patients with Eisenmenger physiology, also provides information on change in arterial oxygen saturations during exercise
  - Exercise capacity is assessed either by measurement of the 6-minute walk test (SMWT) distance or cardiopulmonary exercise testing with measurement of peak oxygen consumption. Both measurements have been successfully employed to evaluate objective exercise limitation in patients with PAH of various etiologies, including congenital heart disease. Currently the SMWT represents the preferred method to assess exercise capacity and appraise therapeutic effects in patients with PAH.
- **CXR:** Radiographic findings are variable and the CXR may be remarkably normal. If present, typical abnormalities in patients with PAH associated with congenital heart disease include:
  - Dilatation, aneurysm or calcification of the central pulmonary arteries. In contrast to IPAH, attenuation of peripheral vascular markings (pruning) is not a common feature in these patients
  - Signs of right atrial and right ventricular enlargement (the cardiothoracic ratio should be recorded)
  - Consolidations suggestive of pulmonary infiltrates or pulmonary hemorrhage.
- **Cardiac MRI:**
  - Can be employed to determine the exact intracardiac anatomy and confirm the location and size of intra- or extra-cardiac communications, especially in patients with inadequate echocardiographic windows
  - Provides additional information on right ventricular function and the pulmonary vascular bed.
- **High-resolution CT:**
  - Useful in the assessment for pulmonary arterial thrombi and to exclude intrapulmonary hemorrhage or infarction in patients with PAH
  - Imaging modality of choice for assessing the lung parenchyma.
- **Cardiac catheterization:**
  - Diagnostic gold standard
  - Allows accurate measurement of pulmonary artery pressure and pulmonary vascular resistance
  - Depending on the individual case and available non-invasive imaging, it provides complimentary invasive hemodynamic data and determines the potential vasoreactivity of the pulmonary vascular bed (using 100% oxygen via a rebreathing mask, inhaled nitric oxide, intravenous adenosine or prostacyclin)
  - Assessment of operability in patients with PAH entails accurate determination of pulmonary vascular resistance and its response to pulmonary vasodilators

○ Pulmonary vasoreactivity was recently shown to have prognostic value for adult patients with Eisenmenger physiology. However, there is also evidence to suggest that pulmonary hemodynamics and clinical status may improve irrespective of the response to acute vasodilator testing

○ Therefore, whilst cardiac catheterization provides diagnostic and prognostic information, an absent pulmonary vasoreactivity study should not preclude initiation of the newer disease targeting therapy.

• **Additional tests:**

○ Pulmonary function testing, overnight oximetry for sleep apnea (particularly common in patients with Down syndrome), ventilation–perfusion lung scintigraphy, and blood screening for connective tissue disease may be particularly useful in patients where there is apparent discrepancy between the underlying congenital heart disease and severity of PAH, in order to exclude additional causes of PAH

○ Lung biopsy is occasionally performed to help clarify the severity of pulmonary vascular disease and help determine the risk of surgical repair, but this should only be performed after careful consideration in centers experienced in the technique.

Management

General strategies

The most important advance in the prevention of morbidity and mortality of patients with congenital heart disease and high pulmonary blood flow is early operation to prevent the development of pulmonary vascular disease and progressive PAH.

Most children with lesions repaired before the age of 9 months will have a normal pulmonary resistance at 1 year and therefore should not go on to develop PAH. If the repair is performed after 2 years of age, the resistance may fall, but not to normal levels.

It is essential not to miss the opportunity to identify individuals who have sufficient reversibility of their pulmonary vascular disease that may enable a surgical repair of the defect and prevent progression of PAH. It is however cautionary to remember that at any age, repairing congenital cardiac lesions in the presence of established PAH accelerates the progression of PAH and worsens outcome.

The mainstay of management for patients with established PAH associated with congenital heart disease has generally been not to destabilize the balanced equilibrium between the systemic and pulmonary circulation.

The recent emergence of new drug treatments that have been shown to be effective in PAH and that show early promise in congenital heart disease, however, has challenged this convention.

The comprehensive evaluation of patients with PAH associated with congenital heart disease should therefore occur in a specialist center by cardiologists experienced in managing these patients. They should also undergo periodic reassessment, ideally 6–12 monthly, in such a center.

Specific management strategies in Eisenmenger syndrome

• Preservation of **fluid balance** and avoidance of **dehydration**.

• **Iron deficiency** limits exercise tolerance and increases the risk of stroke. It should be routinely tested for and promptly treated with iron supplementation (intravenously if oral therapy fails).

• Relief of **hyperviscosity symptoms**: Routine phlebotomy in cyanotic patients with congenital heart disease and PAH is contraindicated and should be discouraged as it may impair oxygen transport capacity, reduce exercise tolerance, induce iron deficiency, and increase the risk of stroke. On the rare occasion phlebotomy is deemed necessary, it should be performed by withdrawing 250–500 mL of blood, with appropriate intravenous volume replacement and the incorporation of air filters.

• **Contraception and avoidance of pregnancy counseling:** Should begin in adolescence to avoid unplanned pregnancies. Pregnancy is associated with high maternal and fetal mortality and should be strongly discouraged. Maternal mortality has been reported to be as high as 50% and spontaneous abortion to occur in 40% of pregnancies. Maternal deaths usually occur 1–2 weeks postpartum. Laparoscopic sterilization or the use of an intrauterine coil impregnated with progestogen (e.g. the Mirena coil) is recommended in women of child-bearing age. If pregnancy occurs and abortion is declined, a multidisciplinary approach including experienced cardiologists, obstetricians, and anesthesiologists is essential.

• **Antiarrhythmic therapy:** Arrhythmias are common and generally poorly tolerated in patients with Eisenmenger physiology and prompt restoration and maintenance of sinus rhythm is an important objective.

• **Pacing:** May be required for bradyarrhythmias. The risks and benefits of transvenous versus epicardial pacing need careful consideration. The presence of a transvenous lead has been reported to be an independent predictor of risk for thromboembolism in patients with intracardiac shunts. However, epicardial leads were associated with higher atrial and ventricular thresholds and shorter generator longevity. The implantation of an epicardial system may be associated with greater risks, particularly of bleeding. This study suggests that an epicardial approach should generally be favored over a transvenous approach in the presence of intracardiac shunts.

• The role of **implantable cardiac defibrillators** in this patient group needs to be investigated, as sudden cardiac death is the most common mode of death.

• **Anticoagulation:** Large intrapulmonary thrombi occur in up to a third of adult patients with Eisenmenger physiology. Whether routine prophylactic anticoagulation with warfarin (a common practice for other forms of PAH) or antiplatelet therapy is warranted in patients with congenital heart disease and PAH remains unknown due to a paucity of data; therapy decisions are usually empirical. When used, warfarin needs to be slowly and carefully titrated and requires special blood tubes (see above).

• **Oxygen therapy and air travel:** Available data suggest that long-term nocturnal oxygen therapy does not improve symptoms, exercise capacity or outcome in adult patients with Eisenmenger syndrome. Although some patients report subjective improvement, routine use of long-term oxygen therapy is not recommended as it is cumbersome and has a drying effect that predisposes some to epistaxis. Cabin pressures in commercial airplanes are maintained at levels corresponding to approximately 2000 m of altitude throughout the flight. This is generally well tolerated by congenital heart disease patients with PAH and air travel is therefore not contraindicated. Sensible precautions are to avoid rushing, stress, dehydration, and prolonged immobility.

• **Transplantation:** Heart–lung transplantation or lung transplantation in combination with repair of the underlying cardiac defect represents a therapeutic option for selected patients, although the timing of this decision is very difficult. In practice, transplantation is currently restricted to highly symptomatic patients and those in whom life expectancy is considered to be very short.

• **Other considerations:** Patients can perform light exercise as tolerated but should avoid strenuous exercise and have annual immunization against influenza and pneumococcal infections. Essential surgery should be carefully planned and performed in a center familiar with the significant mortality risks in this population.

• **Therapeutic interventions:** There is increasing data on the use of various drugs, which have been demonstrated to be beneficial in patients with IPAH (see Chapter 21), and in both children and adults with PAH and congenital heart disease:

○ **Prostacyclin analogs** improve functional capacity, oxygen saturations, and pulmonary hemodynamics in patients with congenital heart disease and PAH. However, prostacyclin administration is invasive and prolonged intravenous therapy is associated with frequent complications such as sepsis and line dislocation. Only preliminary data on the efficacy of oral (beraprost) and subcutaneous (treprostinil) prostacyclin analogs are available.

○ Inhalation of **nitric oxide** reduced total pulmonary resistance in 30% of patients with Eisenmenger syndrome and responsiveness was associated with a mid-term survival benefit in patients with PAH and congenital heart disease. Although delivery systems are improving, the administration of nitric oxide remains challenging.

○ **Sildenafil**, an oral phospodiasterase-5-inhibitor, is effective in reducing pulmonary vascular resistance and improving functional class and SMWT in patients with IPAH. Reports of the use of sildenafil in both children and adults with PAH, including those with congenital heart disease have described improved SMWT distance and hemodynamics.

○ In several intention-to-treat open label pilot studies and now randomized placebo controlled trials, **bosentan**, an oral dual-receptor endothelin antagonist, has shown efficacy in improving SMWT distance and pulmonary hemodynamics in adults with Eisenmenger physiology. It has an acceptable safety profile and is a promising treatment option for symptomatic patients with PAH and congenital heart disease. Longer-term studies are required before these drugs can be recommended in all patients with PAH and CHD. Favorable reports using Ambrisentan, an orally active selective endothelin receptor antagonist in this patient group have been published. Combination therapies are another area of interest and further clinical trial results are awaited with interest.

Conclusions

The success of early reparative surgery for "simpler" congenital heart defects means that in coming years patients with PAH associated with congenital heart disease will increasingly be those with complex lesions surgically palliated in childhood (such as those with single ventricle physiology).

Improved understanding of the underlying pathophysiologic mechanisms, earlier diagnosis, careful medical management, and the introduction of novel disease targeting therapies are now benefiting patients with PAH and congenital heart disease. Commitment to ongoing education of both patients and healthcare professionals is vital to translate our improving knowledge into better clinical outcomes.

Further reading

Avila WS, Grinberg M, Snitcowsky R, *et al*. Maternal and fetal outcome in pregnant women with Eisenmenger's syndrome. *Eur Heart J* 1995;16:460–464.

Galiè N, Hoeper MM, Humbert M, *et al*. ESC Committee for Practice Guidelines (CPG). Guidelines for the diagnosis and treatment of pulmonary hypertension: the Task Force for the Diagnosis and Treatment of Pulmonary Hypertension of the European Society of Cardiology (ESC) and the European Respiratory Society (ERS), endorsed by the International Society of Heart and Lung Transplantation (ISHLT). *Eur Heart J* 2009;30(20):2493–2537. Erratum in: *Eur Heart J* 2011;32(8):926.

Galie N, Beghetti M, Gatzoulis MA, *et al*; Bosentan Randomized Trial of Endothelin Antagonist Therapy-5 (BREATHE-5) Investigators. Bosentan therapy in patients with Eisenmenger syndrome: a multicenter, double-blind, randomized, placebo-controlled study. *Circulation* 2006;114:48–54.

Heath D, Edwards JE. The pathology of hypertensive pulmonary vascular disease: a description of six grades of structural changes in the pulmonary arteries with special reference to congenital cardiac septal defects. *Circulation* 1958;18:533–547.

Oechslin E. Eisenmenger syndrome. In: Gatzoulis MA, Webb GD, Daubeney PEF, eds. *Diagnosis and Management of Adult Congenital Heart Disease*. Philadelphia: Elsevier Saunders, 2011, p. 358–370.

Rabinovitch M, Haworth SG, Castaneda AR, Nadas AS, Reid LM. Lung biopsy in congenital heart disease: a morphometric approach to pulmonary vascular disease. *Circulation* 1978;58: 1107–1122.

Rosenzweig EB, Kerstein D, Barst RJ. Long-term prostacyclin for pulmonary hypertension with associated congenital heart defects. *Circulation* 1999;99:1858–1865.

Simonneau G, Robbins IM, Beghetti M, *et al*. Updated clinical classification of pulmonary hypertension. *J Am Coll Cardiol* 2009;54(1 Suppl):S43–54.

23 Bradyarrhythmias

Jan Till

Royal Brompton Hospital, London, UK

For bradyarrhythmia resuscitation guidelines, see Appendix A.

Presentation

A bradyarrhythmia can present with:
- Tiredness;
- Inability to keep up with peers;
- Poor exercise tolerance;
- Dizziness;
- Syncope (see Chapter 37).

Diagnosis

The diagnosis can be difficult as symptoms are often mistaken for other conditions. General tiredness is extremely common in adolescents and is usually unrelated to their hearts.

Syncope is also fairly common and more often due to vasovagal episodes and epilepsy than cardiac in aetiology (see Chapter 37). When investigating a child with syncope it is important to take a detailed history. Cardiac syncope is more often sudden with little warning and patients may well injure themselves during their abrupt fall to the floor. Vasovagal syncope often occurs shortly after a minor injury, at the sight or thought of blood, or in a hot room. It may also happen shortly after exercise; as he/she walks to the changing rooms. Syncope during exercise, however, should always lead to urgent investigation for a cardiac cause. Epilepsy is far more common than cardiac syncope and since there is no test that can exclude epilepsy, children may well be mistakenly treated with antiepileptic drugs before the cardiac origin of their problem is recognized.

Investigations

- **EKG:**
  - A resting EKG may reveal the diagnosis, such as heart block or long QT syndrome, or suggest a problem with a junctional escape rhythm
  - Further helpful tests include 24-h tapes, exercise testing, event monitoring or implantation of a loop recorder.
- **Tilt testing:** Of some value in providing additional evidence if vasovagal syncope is suspected, but it is not a perfect test and the physician needs to keep an open mind.

Vasovagal syncope (see also Chapter 37)

Vasovagal syncope is common in older children and it is important to distinguish this from potentially more dangerous causes of collapse. Although generally considered benign, in some cases the practical problems associated with frequent attacks and the anxiety this evokes in schools and parents, make it a very difficult condition to live with. Vagal episodes may cause a pronounced slowing of heart rhythm. This is generally sinus bradycardia or arrest, but a degree of atrioventricular nodal block can occur. Alternatively, the heart rate is little affected but there is a precipitous fall in blood pressure.

Management
- Initial advice should be to increase fluid intake and supplement the diet with salt.
- Avoidance of situations such as standing in line on hot days is recommended.
- Initially the patient is unaware of warning symptoms, but if episodes continue to occur, he/she can usually

Pediatric Heart Disease: A Practical Guide, First Edition. Piers E. F. Daubeney, Michael L. Rigby, Koichiro Niwa, and Michael A. Gatzoulis.
© 2012 Blackwell Publishing Ltd. Published 2012 by Blackwell Publishing Ltd.

recognize subtle signs and may avoid complete loss of consciousness by lying down or performing isometric maneuvers as soon as he/she is aware of the symptoms.
• Fludrocortisone or midodrine may prove useful in symptom control but rarely prevent all attacks.
• Very rarely a dual chamber pacemaker is needed.
• The patient should be encouraged that he/she will usually grow out of the attacks.

Sick sinus syndrome

This is unusual in a child with a structurally "normal" heart. An EKG and 24-h tape may show slow sinus rhythm with little rate response to exercise. With a slower sinus node there may be a junctional escape rhythm or escape capture bigeminy. Further confirmation is usually available on a 24-h tape and an exercise test.

Management
Sick sinus syndrome is not as life-threatening as heart block, but if the symptoms are frequent or disabling, treatment with **pacing** is usually the best option. Attempts to increase heart rate with theophylline derivatives can be made but these are difficult to administer, requiring frequent administration with little selective effect. When pacing, attempts should be made to avoid pacing the ventricle if possible unless there is more extensive conduction disease.

Following cardiac surgery, such as the Mustard or Senning operation (see Chapter 14), Fontan or total cavopulmonary connection (TCPC) procedure (see Chapter 34), **loss of sinus node function** is common. In the immediate post-surgical setting, "bruising," atrial distension or atrial collapse can result in an inadequate sinus rate and cardiac output may be increased with temporary pacing. Long-term loss of sinus node function was the first arrhythmic complication of the Mustard procedure noted by the surgeons pioneering this surgery and many revisions of surgical technique were made in an attempt to prevent this. In this situation the majority of patients exhibit a good junctional rhythm and loss of sinus node function rarely appears to cause symptoms in itself. Sinus node dysfunction is not thought to be a cause of sudden death; however, it would appear to be a factor in the development of re-entry atrial tachycardias (see Chapter 24). The latter are not benign and frequently cause collapse and the need for acute hospital management and even sudden death.

• **Atrial pacing in the Mustard circulation** is usually possible with current active fix leads. A position in the baffle has to be chosen. If the left atrial appendage is selected, phrenic nerve stimulation should be carefully avoided. An antitachycardia pacemaker should be considered.
• **Atrial pacing in the Fontan or TCPC patient** can be challenging. Access to the heart chambers may be limited. Scarring may limit sensing and cause high thresholds. Again an antitachycardia pacemaker should be considered as re-entry atrial arrhythmias are common in these patients.

Heart block

First degree
First-degree heart block (prolongation of the PR interval beyond 200 ms; Figure 23.1), can represent the initial stages in a progressive genetically-determined conduction disease or may be acquired following infection by such organisms as *Borrelia burgdorferi* in Lyme disease. Alternatively, it may simply represent the delay in atrial excitation as a result of atrial distension or hypertrophy. In itself it does not require treatment.

Causes of first degree atrioventricular block

• Enhanced vagal tone
• Athlete's heart
• Myocarditis
• Hypokalemia
• Lyme disease

Second degree
There are two types of second-degree heart block. The first is often present in a well child found to have a variable heart rate. However, the most common cause is normal sinus arrhythmia.

• **Wenckebach block (Möbitz type 1):** Progressive prolongation of PR interval until the P wave is no longer followed by a QRS complex (Figure 23.2a). Often seen in well children during the night and should be considered normal.
• **Möbitz type II:** Two P waves for every QRS complex (Figure 23.2b). This type is not normal and may be a prelude to chronic third-degree heart block.

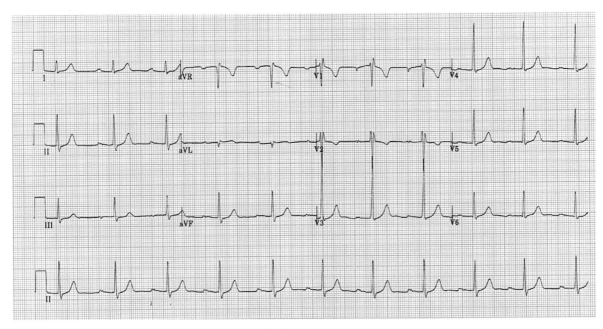

Figure 23.1 First-degree heart block. Note the PR interval of 240 ms.

Third degree (complete)

Complete heart block (Figure 23.3) may be congenital or acquired.

Acquired heart block

Although there has been enormous progress in the understanding of the conduction tissue in structurally abnormal hearts, sadly surgical damage to the conduction system is sometimes inevitable or unavoidable. In such cases temporary pacing is usually necessary in the immediate postsurgical period to support cardiac output (Figure 23.3). Recovery may occur, generally within the first week. Thereafter the chances of recovery diminish, but many cardiologists wait for 2 weeks before placing a permanent pacing system.

The long-term outcome of children left unpaced with surgically-created atrioventricular nodal block is poor.

Congenital heart block

Congenital heart block for many years was thought of as a benign phenomenon in children and was treated as such. Many children born with atrioventricular nodal block are well and able to cope with normal life at school. They are at small risk throughout their lives of sudden Stokes Adams attacks when their rhythm will suddenly become inadequate.

During the first few weeks of life a slow heart rate that initially appears to be adequate may slowly result in heart failure. Parents and staff should be alert to increasing tachypnea, poor perfusion, and/or feeding difficulties. Heart failure can result not only because of inadequate ventricular rate but also lack of atrioventricular synchrony. Congenital heart block has a strong association with antibodies usually detectable in both the mother and child, e.g. anti-Ro and -La. Although the mother may be asymptomatic, the presence of these antibodies is associated with the development of connective tissue disease. These antibodies can be demonstrated in the neonatal heart on the conduction system and myocardium. In addition to the rhythm problem, there may be an element of myocardial dysfunction.

Although many children remain very well with congenital complete atrioventricular block, the incidence of collapse, sudden death, and heart failure increases once they become adults unless they are paced. It is therefore generally accepted practice to implant a permanent pacemaker in adults with congenital heart block (Figure 23.3).

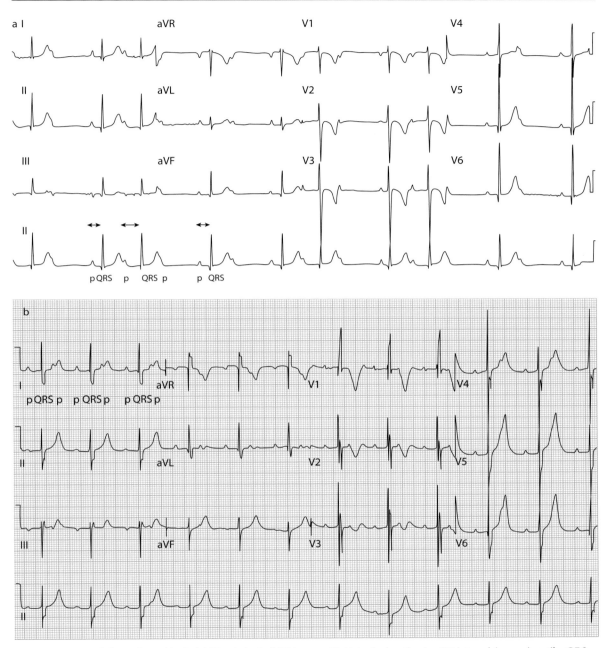

Figure 23.2 Second-degree heart block. (a) Wenckebach (Möbitz type 1). Note the lengthening PR interval (arrows) until a QRS complex is dropped. At this point there are two P waves (one buried in the T wave) for one QRS complex. (b) Möbitz type 2. Note the two P waves for every QRS.

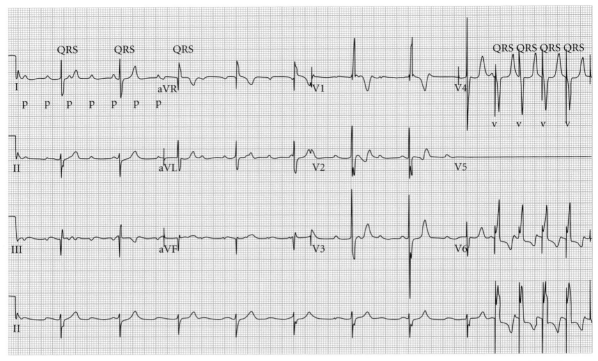

Figure 23.3 Third-degree (complete) heart block. Note how the P waves "walk through" the QRS complexes (see lead I). In lead V4, ventricular pacing has been initiated with each pacing spike (v) leading to a resultant QRS.

24 Tachyarrhythmias

Jan Till

Royal Brompton Hospital, London, UK

For tachyarrhythmia resuscitation guidelines, see Appendix A.

Presentation

The infant or small child is very dependent on rate for cardiac output and so a tachyarrhythmia can rapidly result in a reduced cardiac output. The diagnosis can be difficult as signs may be subtle and not specific.

> **Early signs of tachyarrhythmia**
> - Irritability
> - Reluctance to feed
> - Cold peripheries
> - Pallor
> - Increasing tachypnea

If early signs are missed, cardiogenic shock may follow. Older children may be able to recognize that their heart is beating rapidly or describe a discomfort, particularly in their throat, and therefore the diagnosis is made earlier. As older children are far less rate dependent, they are usually able to tolerate a tachycardia for longer. However, a minority of older children will experience an initial fall in blood pressure, which can result in syncope with the sudden increase in rate associated with a tachyarrhythmia.

Diagnosis

- There is no absolute heart rate that can be used to distinguish an abnormal from a normal rhythm.
- Heart rates above 220 bpm in childhood are suspicious of a tachyarrhythmia, but there are many abnormal rhythms that can exist at a rate less than this and equally there are children who can mount a sinus tachycardia greater than this.
- An EKG, preferably with 12 leads, is required to confirm the diagnosis and establish the mechanism wherever possible.
- If attacks are daily, a 24-h tape may be able to document the events or high rates in question, and then the behavior of the tachycardia may be helpful in distinguishing appropriate from inappropriate.
- Attempts should be made to examine the start and finish of the tachycardia.
- Event recorders that can be worn for a longer period or an implantable loop recorder may be useful if attacks are less frequent.
- Unfortunately, formal exercise testing may not always precipitate a tachyarrhythmia even if there is a correlation with exercise in the clinical setting.

Atrial arrhythmias

Supraventricular tachycardia

Supraventricular tachycardia (SVT) is the commonest fast heart rhythm seen in children. The different types of SVT are outlined in Figure 24.1. Unfortunately there is no worldwide agreement on nomenclature or classification.

Atrioventricular re-entry tachycardia

Atrioventricular re-entry tachycardia (AVRT) is thought to account for 90% of SVT in small children. The tachycardia arises from a re-entry circuit employing the atrioventricular (AV) node and His–Purkinje system as one

Pediatric Heart Disease: A Practical Guide, First Edition. Piers E. F. Daubeney, Michael L. Rigby, Koichiro Niwa, and Michael A. Gatzoulis.
© 2012 Blackwell Publishing Ltd. Published 2012 by Blackwell Publishing Ltd.

limb and an accessory pathway of conduction connecting ventricle to atrium as the other.

EKG

The EKG is characteristic (Figure 24.1a). The ventricular rate in a neonate is usually about 280 bpm, and slower in infants and older children. The tachycardia is typified by a regular narrow QRS complex. A P wave with superior axis can be seen at least 80 ms following the onset of the QRS complex. This appearance results from the usual circuit with the AV node involved from atrium to ventricle and the accessory pathway from ventricle to atrium (orthodromic AVRT). The retrograde limb of this circuit involves conduction through the ventricular myocardium and along the accessory pathway, which takes on average longer than 80 ms.

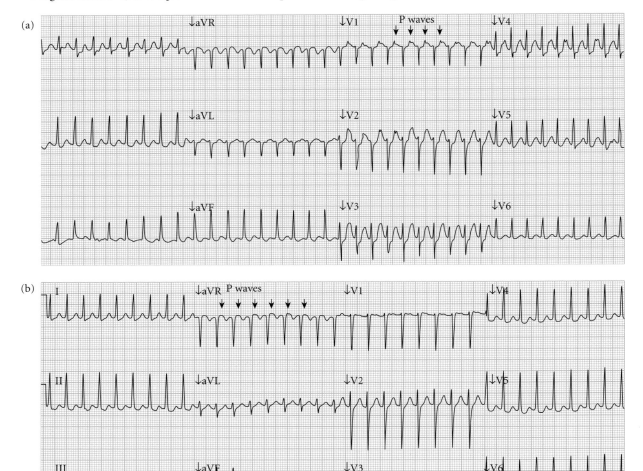

Figure 24.1 Types of supraventricular tachycardia. (a) Atrioventricular re-entrant tachycardia (AVRT). The ventricular rate is 214 bpm. There is a retrograde P wave seen embedded in each T wave, giving it a notched appearance (arrows). This is approximately 120 ms after the onset of the preceding QRS complex. (b) Atrioventricular nodal re-entrant tachycardia (AVNRT). The ventricular rate is 214 bpm. There is a retrograde P wave seen at the end of each QRS (arrows). This is approximately 75 ms after the onset of the preceding QRS complex. (c) Permanent junctional reciprocating tachycardia (PJRT). The ventricular rate is 190 bpm. There is a retrograde P wave seen after each T wave (arrows). This is approximately 190 ms after the onset of the preceding QRS complex.

(c)

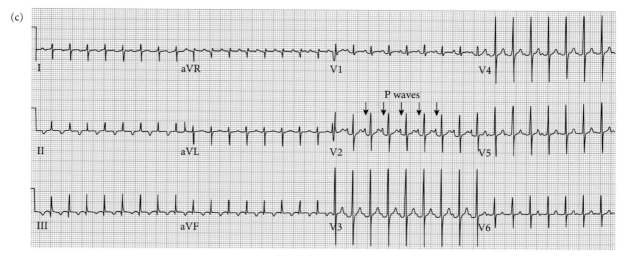

Figure 24.1 (*Continued*)

If there is existing bundle branch block on the same side as the accessory pathway or the bundle branch becomes refractory because of the sudden increase in rate (rate-related bundle branch block), the time to the retrograde P on the EKG will be delayed, and the cycle length slowed.

In some cases the accessory pathway between atria and ventricles only conducts from ventricle to atrium and the EKG in sinus rhythm appears normal. In other cases the accessory connection can conduct both from ventricle to atrium (retrograde) and from atrium to ventricle (antegrade). In the latter situation, a short PR interval and delta wave (pre-excitation) may be apparent during sinus rhythm; when associated with AVRT this is **Wolff–Parkinson–White syndrome** (Figure 24.2).

Rarely a tachycardia circuit occurs which involves the accessory pathway antegradely and the AV node retrogradely (antidromic AVRT). This tachycardia is typified by a regular wide QRS complex, the morphology of which resembles the pattern of pre-excitation in sinus rhythm.

Acute treatment

Most infants and small children require immediate treatment. Older children may tolerate SVT and so treatment can be delayed in the hope that the tachycardia might terminate on its own.

If treatment is given, the first option should be vagal maneuvers. There are a number of ways in which the vagal nerve can be stimulated. The method should be appropriate to the child's age and understanding:

- Vagal activation by cold stimulation of nerve endings across the cheek bones;
- Ice applied to the face;
- Patient encouraged to submerge his or her face in cold water;
- Neonates plunged face first into cold water;
- Older children may cooperate in increasing their intrathoracic pressure by blowing against a fixed pressure or standing on their head;
- Carotid pressure is difficult to apply in small children.
  If simple vagal maneuvers fail:
- Intravenous adenosine;
- DC cardioversion;
- Overdrive pacing.

All are equally acceptable as therapy if they are readily available.

Transesophageal pacing is rarely available outside a cardiac center and DC cardioversion may not always be practical. Adenosine needs to be given rapidly, followed by a flush as it is quickly deaminated to the inactive inosine. Doses of 200–500 µg/kg can be used and it is helpful if the EKG is recorded at the time, since it can be extremely useful in confirming the diagnosis by showing transient pre-excitation and echo beats, and in distinguishing atrial tachycardia.

If adenosine fails to work, the question needs to be asked if this is because the tachycardia stops and re-initiates or because the tachycardia is unaffected by adenosine. If the former and maximum doses have been given, another drug needs to be given to prevent re-initiation. If the latter, the diagnosis may be in question.

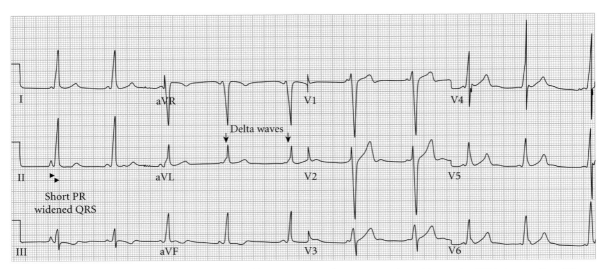

Figure 24.2 Wolff–Parkinson–White. Pre-excitation with an anteroseptal accessory pathway. The resting EKG shows a short PR interval of 60 ms and prolonged QRS of 140 ms (arrowheads). There is a prominent delta wave seen as a notched upstroke to the QRS complex (arrows).

Administration of drugs other than adenosine to potentially sick and deteriorating infants can be dangerous because of their negative inotropic properties and long-lasting effects. Advice and/or transfer to a cardiac unit should be strongly considered. A cardiac echocardiogram should be performed. Whilst an echocardiogram is informative as to the anatomy of the heart, it can be difficult to perform during tachycardia to assess function.

Amiodarone can be used and may represent one of the safest drugs. It appears to be less negatively inotropic than the class 1C or 1A drugs. It can however take some time to load and should be given in a central or large cannula. Rapid intravenous therapy has been reported to occasionally cause ventricular fibrillation and some operators advise oral loading if at all possible.

Flecainide can be very effective in the structurally normal heart, where function is not badly compromised, and in this situation has the advantages that it can be given through a peripheral vein and an effect is seen in 10–15 min. However, in a ventricle that is struggling to compensate, flecainide can cause deterioration in cardiac output, which may need prompt supportive therapy. Administration needs to be performed with an EKG running so that it can be stopped immediately if QRS widening beyond 25% is witnessed.

Chronic management

Prevention of further attacks should be considered. In an infant or neonate who can rapidly decline into advanced heart failure, the risk-to-benefit ratio is positive and chronic treatment is advisable. This decision is made more appealing in the knowledge that the great majority of infants will not have attacks of AVRT after 1 year of age, and therefore medication can be safely stopped at 1 year.

The natural history of AVRT has been verified by a number of researchers and is thought to occur as a result of:

• A change in the electrical properties of the cardiac tissue, i.e. both the AV node and accessory pathway exhibit a change in conduction and refractory period (recovery) such that the circuit involved in AVRT is less able to happen.

• There may also be a change in the events that trigger the tachycardia, i.e. AVRT in the young infant is initiated by sinus tachycardia whilst ectopic beats usually trigger the circuit in older children.

Families should be warned however, that AVRT can recur in later life and be advised on a plan of action in this event. They can be reassured that recurrence is rarely as difficult a situation as the first episodes of neonatal AVRT.

Prevention should also be considered in older children where attacks are frequent or intrusive, particularly if attacks cannot be terminated by vagal maneuvers and therefore require hospital treatment.

Many drugs can be considered for prevention. If there is a history suggestive of a relationship with excitement or exercise or in an infant, a beta-blocker can be effective. If partial prevention is achieved, digoxin and a beta-blocker is often a very effective combination. Flecainide is a good choice in an infant or child with a structurally and functionally normal heart. Amiodarone is useful in neonates who are refractory and may only require treatment until they are 1 year of age. It has few side effects if given in this limited fashion to this age group.

It is possible to ablate most cases of AVRT safely. Pathways that lie in close proximity to the AV node are an exception. Parents are increasingly more reluctant to give long-term drugs to their children. Ablation techniques are improving. It is therefore possible to offer radiofrequency ablation to many older children with good curative rates and limited risk.

Atrioventricular nodal re-entry tachycardia

Atrioventricular nodal re-entry tachycardia (AVNRT) is more typically seen in adults and older children. It involves fast and slow atrial pathways within the atrium.

EKG

AVNRT typically manifests on the EKG as a regular narrow QRS tachycardia (Figure 24.1b). The retrograde P wave is less easily seen than in AVRT as it appears within 80 ms of the onset of the QRS complex. The typical 12-lead EKG has a small positive deflection at the end of the QRS complex in V1.

Acute treatment

The approach and initial treatment is similar to AVRT: vagal maneuvers, DC cardioversion, and overdrive pacing are all effective.

Chronic management

A patient suffering from this tachycardia can be offered several options as it is not life-threatening.
• **Observation only:** This option is acceptable if the tachycardia is infrequent or easily controlled with vagal maneuvers.
• **Drug therapy:** If the patient has frequent episodes and/or is syncopal with them, drug therapy is recommended; or
• **Radiofrequency ablation.**

AVNRT may well respond to digoxin or a beta-blocking agent. Verapamil can be used in older children. Flecainide is also a very effective drug in prevention.

Radiofrequency ablation involves identifying and modifying or ablating the slow pathway, but because of the proximity to the AV node, it carries a risk of AV nodal

block. In a fully-grown adult this risk is 1%. The risk is likely increased in smaller patients and therefore elective ablation should be delayed dependent on the size of the child and the clinical need for the procedure.

Permanent junctional reciprocating tachycardia (PJRT)

Permanent junctional reciprocating tachycardia (PJRT) is an unusual tachycardia and is usually slightly less rapid than the other junctional re-entry arrhythmias. It is also one of the long R–P tachycardias. There is a regular narrow QRS complex and the retrograde P wave can be seen just before the QRS complex. This appearance results from the long conduction time of the accessory connection. When there is a long R–P time the differential diagnosis is PJRT or atrial tachycardia. The arrhythmia is often persistent in nature, stopping and starting continually throughout the day. It may not give rise to symptoms until after many years when the high rate causes ventricular dysfunction.

EKG

The EKG is characteristic with a regular narrow QRS complex and retrograde P wave that precedes the QRS complex (Figure 24.1c). The P wave is inverted in the inferior leads.

Treatment

This tachycardia is fairly drug resistant. Digoxin and beta-blockers rarely work. Class 1C drugs have better success. When the child is big enough, radiofrequency ablation is a good option as the accessory connection can usually be located just at the mouth of the coronary sinus and can be effectively abolished.

Atrial tachycardias
Atrial flutter

Atrial flutter is a relatively common rhythm problem in the fetus and is not unusual in the newborn. These babies usually have a structurally normal heart. In fetal life, flutter can result in hydrops fetalis but with treatment *in utero* outcome is usually good. Likewise the newborn is rarely severely compromised and can be effectively treated.

EKG

The rhythm is best recognized in the inferior limb leads where atrial flutter waves are usually most clearly seen (Figure 24.3). The ventricular response depends on the

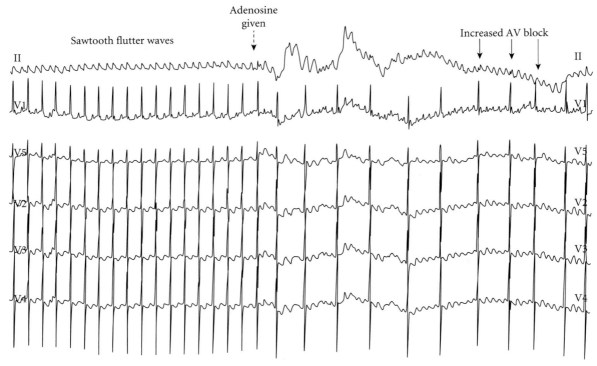

Figure 24.3 Atrial flutter. There is initially 2:1 block with a resultant ventricular rate of 212 bpm. On administration of adenosine (dotted arrow), the level of atrioventricular (AV) block is increased to about 5:1 (black arrows denote QRS complexes). Sawtooth flutter waves are then clearly seen. This can be used as a diagnostic test.

degree of AV nodal block. It can be regular with 1:1 or 2:1 atrioventricular conduction or irregular. Adenosine can be used as a diagnostic tool as it increases the degree of AV block, thereby revealing the underlying flutter waves (Figure 24.3).

Acute treatment
In the neonate prompt cardioversion is recommended. Chemical cardioversion with drugs is associated with potential problems as it is slow or may fail, during which time the newborn remains in a low output. There are also a small number of newborns who present in flutter but who have underlying pre-excitation, so use of drugs such as digoxin can precipitate ventricular flutter.

Atrial flutter is sometimes seen in an older child and then is almost always associated with structural heart disease and generally follows surgery. In this setting it can be managed initially as atrial re-entry tachycardia. However, if radiofrequency ablation is contemplated, isthmus-dependent atrial flutter has a higher success rate

as the cavotricuspid isthmus is a target with familiar electrical and anatomic landmarks.

Re-entry atrial tachycardia
These tachycardias are predominantly seen in children with structurally abnormal hearts who have undergone surgery. The substrate is a re-entry circuit within the atrium circulating around scar tissue or using an anatomic obstacle that has arisen either from surgical intervention or as part of the disease process.

EKG
This tachycardia can be recognized by rapid atrial activity in the presence of AV nodal block.

Treatment
This type of atrial tachycardia can be overdriven by pacing; alternatively cardioversion is a good option. Chemical cardioversion is slower and not as effective. The

agent of choice depends upon the state of ventricular function. Amiodarone is usually selected as the least negatively inotropic drug if chemical cardioversion is contemplated.

Prevention can be obtained with amiodarone, but also class 1 agents and beta-blockers can be effective in certain circumstances with careful delivery and monitoring. Bisoprolol can be used with good effect, administered alone or in combination. Drugs such as flecainide or disopyramide should only be given in combination with an AV nodal blocking agent in case they slow the atrial cycle length and therefore allow 1:1 conduction to the ventricle.

Radiofrequency ablation may be possible in these tachycardias, depending on the anatomy. The re-entry circuit will use a critical isthmus of tissue, functional or structural, around which it circulates. Identification and ablation of these is achieved by traditional electrophysiologic techniques alongside the use of newer advanced mapping systems.

Atrial fibrillation

Atrial fibrillation in young children is incredibly rare. It is occasionally seen in a very sick heart. It also rarely occurs in the teenager with Wolff–Parkinson–White syndrome.

Junctional arrhythmias

Junctional ectopic tachycardia

This tachycardia appears to arise from the His bundle region of the conducting system and therefore is peculiar in that it has a narrow QRS complex similar to that seen in sinus rhythm. It is usually a rapid and regular rhythm but as it does arise from below the AV node tissue, it can be associated with AV dissociation. Alternatively, in small infants and children, the AV node is fully functional. The impulse may be conducted back up the AV node from the ventricle and there may be ventricular–atrial association.

Junctional ectopic tachycardia (JET) can be seen in children with normal hearts but this is rare. Much more commonly JET is seen in the child returning from open heart surgery. In both situations it can be an extremely difficult arrhythmia to suppress. It is unresponsive to adenosine and cardioversion. It may respond to flecainide but in a postoperative setting, this drug is rarely used because of its negative inotropic effect on the ventricle. The most effective treatments are cooling the child to

reduce the tachycardia rate, whereupon atrial overdrive pacing to restore AV synchrony may be effective or amiodarone infusion. Usually the rhythm settles 4–10 days after surgery.

Ventricular arrhythmias

Idiopathic ventricular tachycardia of infancy

This is characterized on the surface EKG by a rapid, regular, broad complex tachycardia. If the rate is not too rapid, independent atrial activity can be seen with P waves marching through at a slower rate and dissociated from the QRS complexes.

• If the atria do happen to depolarize at the correct timing within the cycle, it may be able to conduct through the AV node and capture the ventricle, giving rise to a normal narrow QRS complex termed a **capture beat**. This will appear slightly early in the cycle in between the wide, broad QRS complex rhythm.

• If the atria depolarize slightly later in the cycle, yet still conduct through the AV node, there may be a **fusion beat**.

It is more common in children than in adults that the AV node conducts retrogradely from the ventricle and there is ventricular–atrial transmission after every QRS complex, giving rise to a retrograde P wave with a 1:1 association with the QRS complexes. It is important to realize that the QRS complex in a child or infant does not have to be very broad when it is coming from the ventricle; in fact, a very wide QRS complex is more likely to be bundle branch block in the setting of SVT than VT. Therefore VT is commonly mistaken for SVT. Vagal maneuvers and intravenous adenosine will not work in VT, although they may change the relationship between the ventricle and the atrium if there is conduction retrogradely through the AV node.

Management
• Cardioversion is usually effective
• Intravenous flecainide
• Intravenous lignocaine
• Intravenous amiodarone

Fascicular ventricular tachycardia

This ventricular tachycardia characteristically occurs in the "normal" heart. It presents in the older child and young adult. It is often mistaken for supraventricular tachycardia, not only because SVT is far more common but because symptoms are similar and the EKG is difficult to differentiate. It is thought to represent re-entry around the posterior fascicle from the left ventricle.

EKG

The EKG appearance is of a regular QRS with right bundle branch block. Because of its fascicular origin, the QRS is usually not very wide and because it occurs in young people with a good AV node there is often retrograde conduction to the atria. Therefore AV dissociation may not be present. The QRS axis is superior in the commonest form.

A distinct electrical signal identifying the posterior fascicle can be found two-thirds of the way down the septum on the left ventricular side.

Management

It responds both acutely and chronically to a class 1C drug, but in the long term radiofrequency ablation should be considered. Radiofrequency ablation is successful in 90% of cases.

Arrhythmogenic right ventricular cardiomyopathy

It is now known that the term arrhythmogenic right ventricular cardiomyopathy (ARVC) encompasses a number of genetic conditions that seem to present in late childhood and early adult life. Ventricular tachycardia arising from the right ventricle on exercise should always raise alarm bells.

The condition may be difficult to diagnose because the myocardium may appear "normal" on echocardiography. There is a wide spectrum of disease. MRI may show fibrous or fatty replacement of myocardium. The familial incidence is 40%. There are several phases to the disease:
• Concealed phase: subtle right ventricular structural changes ± ventricular arrhythmias. **Sudden death** may occur.
• Overt electrical, functional, and structural abnormality.
• Right ventricular failure.
• Biventricular cardiomyopathy.

EKG

The ventricular tachycardia is usually of left bundle branch block morphology and regular (Figure 24.4). It may occur in salvos or be sustained. Often the outflow tract is the initial electrically active area and so the QRS axis is inferior and resembles the so-called benign condition of right ventricular outflow tract tachycardia. It is

still not clear what distinguishes the two conditions and if they are truly separate entities, but many young individuals who appear to fulfill the criteria for ARVC have a very benign course.

Management
• Beta-blockers (sotalol)
• Radiofrequency ablation
• Implantable defibrillator

Catecholaminergic polymorphic ventricular tachycardia

This is one of the polymorphic ventricular tachycardias and was first described by Coumel. It characteristically occurs in what is believed to be a normal heart. It is rare but important to recognize because it is a well-described cause of sudden death in childhood or adolescence.

It presents between the ages of 5 and 10 years, although it has been reported in infants. Symptoms usually appear on emotion or exercise. Characteristically the child gives a history of dizziness or syncope on exercise. It is caused by a mutation in the gene coding for the ryanodine receptor in 30% of cases.

EKG

The resting EKG is normal, but the exercise test is positive in more than 90%.

Coumel described couplets, short salvos, and finally bidirectional ventricular tachycardia, which can then degenerate to ventricular fibrillation or revert to sinus rhythm (Figure 24.5).

Treatment
• Beta-blockers; as long as compliance is achieved there is an excellent prognosis with treatment. Nadolol is the drug of choice.
• Flecainide can be considered if beta-blockers fail.
• Left stellate ganglionectomy should be considered for resistant patients.
• A defibrillator may be used in unresponsive patients.

Long QT

The long QT syndromes typically produce a different type of polymorphic ventricular tachycardia. Torsades de pointes (Figure 24.6) has a characteristic sinusoidal amplitude (see below).

There have now been multiple genetic types described. The most common three, accounting for 90% of cases, are the best recognized.

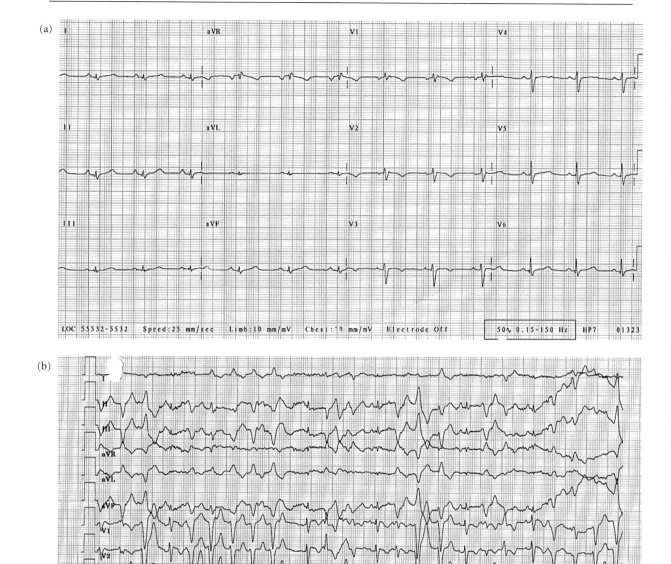

Figure 24.4 Arrhythmogenic right ventricular dysplasia in a 14-year old with a syncopal episode on the rugby pitch. (a) Resting EKG – shows a subtle delay in QRS in V1 and V2. (b) Exercise EKG – polymorphic ventricular tachycardia.

- **Long QT1:**
  - Patients are more susceptible to attacks on exercise and swimming
  - Broad-based T wave
  - Frequent attacks
  - Presents in childhood
- **Long QT2:**
  - Patients adversely respond to sudden noise such as an alarm call
  - T waves of low amplitude, notched
  - Frequent attacks
- **Long QT3:**
  - Patients are more likely to have attacks during rest/sleep
  - T wave is late appearing with prolonged isoelectric portion
  - Less frequent attacks but more lethal

The child presents with syncopal episodes often with a clear trigger.

EKG

The diagnosis can be extremely difficult from the resting EKG alone, which is why screening with EKGs is fraught with difficulty. Twenty percent of children with genetically proven long QT have a "normal" QTc interval on EKG. Multiple EKGs are helpful over a period of time and additional information can be gained from a 24-h tape or exercise testing. However, in some individuals the QTc is obviously long and once drugs and metabolic derangements (such as hypocalcemia) have been excluded, a safe diagnosis can be made. Recording Torsade de pointes is rewarding but should not delay treatment. The EKG patterns for the differing types of long QT syndrome are shown in Figure 24.6.

Treatment

- Beta-blockers such as nadalol remain the treatment mainstay; 81% of long QT1 will respond (81%), compared with 50% of long QT2, and 40% of long QT3.

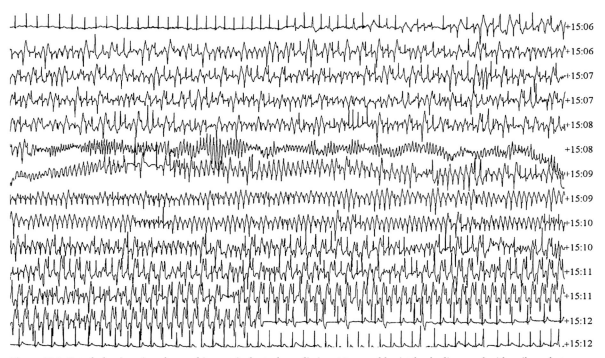

Figure 24.5 Catecholaminergic polymorphic ventricular tachycardia in a 13-year old mistakenly diagnosed with epilepsy but resistant to antiepileptics. EKG recorded during a syncopal episode shows characteristic polymorphic ventricular tachycardia. This reorganizes to bidirectional ventricular tachycardia before spontaneously recovering to sinus rhythm.

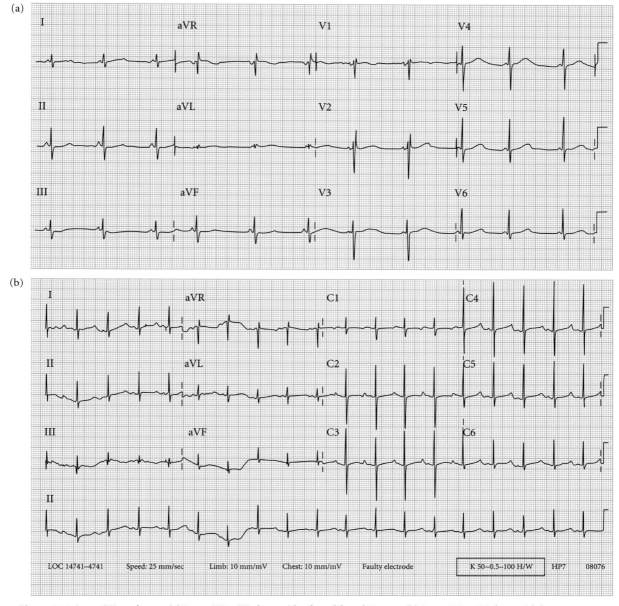

Figure 24.6 Long QT syndrome. (a) Long QT1: QTc long with a broad-based T wave. (b) Long QT2: QTc long with low-amplitude, notched T waves. (c) Long QT3: QTc long with late appearance of T wave due to prolonged isoelectric portion. (d) Torsades de pointes. Note the sinusoidal amplitude with changing QRS axis.

(c)

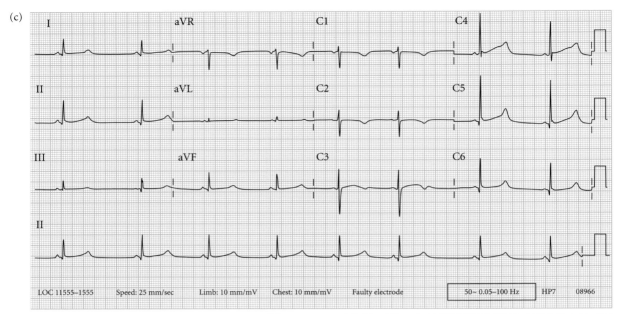

(d)

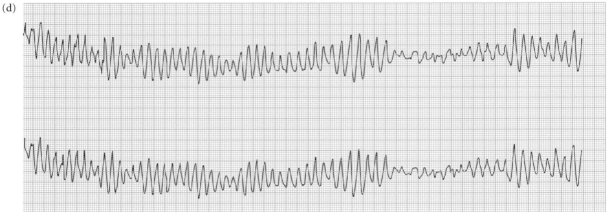

Figure 24.6 (*Continued*)

• Other drugs may be considered in the event of non-response, such as mexiletine in long QT3.

• An implantable defibrillator has proven efficacy in saving lives.

Ventricular tachycardia in the child with structural congenital heart disease

Ventricular tachycardia can occur following surgery either early or late in childhood, but more often in adult life. It is usually not well tolerated and may present with sudden collapse. The most common conditions in which it is seen are truncus arteriosus (see Chapter 16), tetralogy of Fallot (see Chapter 15), and transposition of the great arteries late after atrial switch procedures (see Chapter 14) and VSD closure.

EKG

The EKG will reflect the structural heart condition and from where the ventricular tachycardia is coming, but often shows a wide regular QRS complex with AV dissociation.

(a)

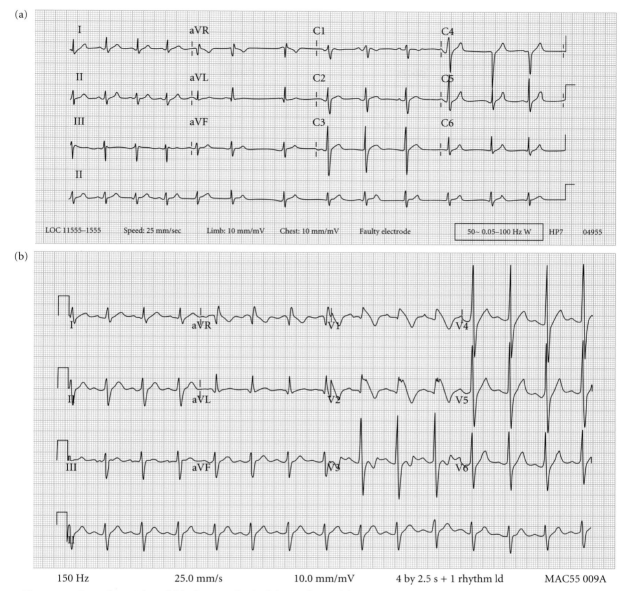

(b)

Figure 24.7 Brugada EKG in a child whose mother had the syndrome. (a) Resting EKG – normal. (b) Same child on provocation with ajmaline. EKG shows typical Brugada pattern with right bundle branch block, ST segment elevation by >2 mm, and deeply inverted T wave.

Acute treatment
- DC cardioversion
- Amiodarone
- Lignocaine if ventricular function is good

Brugada syndrome

This is another condition which predisposes to sudden death. Sudden death may result from ventricular fibrillation and, although described, is rare in childhood. The syndrome may result from a mutation of the *SCN5A* gene in 15–20%. This mutation results in decreased function of the sodium channel. Children are particularly at risk, with fever precipitating a storm of ventricular fibrillation.

EKG

The typical EKG characteristics are highly dynamic and therefore only appear at certain times, e.g. after an attack, with a fever, etc. In some patients the typical EKG pattern may only be revealed by giving ajmaline (Figure 24.7).

Management
- Avoid drugs that challenge the sodium channel
- Manage fever aggressively (with paracetamol ± ibuprofen ± hospital admission)
- Implantable defibrillator
- Ventricular fibrillation storm may require quinidine

Sudden death

Sudden unexpected death is unusual in childhood. Immediately following such a death a comprehensive autopsy by a specialist cardiac pathologist is essential. The heart needs to be examined both macroscopically and microscopically with multiple sections examined for evidence of arrhythmogenic cardiomyopathy and hypertrophic cardiomyopathy with myocardial disarray. Ideally splenic tissue or DNA should be carefully stored for future genetic studies if the family consent.

Depending on the autopsy findings, family screening should be offered and family members evaluated in an Inherited Cardiac Disease clinic. Ongoing screening may be required.

Etiology of sudden death in childhood includes:
- Cardiomyopathy:
  - Hypertrophic cardiomyopathy
  - Arrhythmogenic cardiomyopathy
  - Dilated cardiomyopathy
- Channelopathies:
  - Brugada syndrome
  - Catecholaminergic polymorphic ventricular tachycardia Long QT
  - Short QT
- Anomalous coronary artery

Standard tests used to screen individuals at risk of sudden death comprise:
- EKG
- Signal averaged EKG
- 24-h Holter monitor
- Exercise test
- Echocardiogram
- MRI (possibly).

In some cases a genetic diagnosis can be established from analysis of the DNA. In these cases genetic screening of other family members can be very valuable.

Further reading

Raju H. Inherited cardiomyopathies. *BMJ* 2011;343:1106–1110.

25 Rheumatic fever

Maria Virginia Tavares Santana and
Cleusa Cavalcanti Lapa Santos

Instituto Dante Pazzanese, São Paulo, Brazil

Rheumatic fever (RF) is a delayed non-suppurative sequela of Group A streptococcal pharyngitis. In developing countries it remains a serious health problem, responsible for approximately 40% of all hospital admissions for cardiovascular diseases in children over 5 years old and young adults. Valve involvement is a frequent reason for surgical intervention and a continuing socioeconomic burden throughout life.

Epidemiology

A significant reduction in the incidence has occurred in developed countries, although a resurgence of RF was recently reported in certain areas of the United States. The disease remains common in many developing countries.

Pathogenesis

In genetically predisposed individuals untreated Group A streptococcal throat infections (sore throat) trigger an exaggerated humoral and cellular immunologic response against streptococcal antigens. Why specific organs and particularly the heart should respond in this way is not certain; the concept of molecular mimicry has been introduced to explain the response of specific organs to the streptococcal antigen.

Clinical features

Acute pharyngotonsillitis caused by Group A β-hemolytic streptococci is characterized by:

- Most common in age group 5–15 years;
- Acute onset of sore throat and malaise;
- Headache;
- High fever;
- Pharyngeal erythema with exudates;
- Tender and enlarged cervical nodes;
- General malaise.

From the development of pharyngitis and sore throat to the appearance of the full-blown clinical picture, there is a latent period of 1–4 weeks during which pallor, myalgia, abdominal pain, tiredness, and epistaxis may be observed.

Major clinical manifestations

- **Carditis:**
  - Often described as "pan-carditis" (pericarditis, myocarditis, and endocarditis), this is without doubt the most important manifestation; it may even result in death during the acute phase and will certainly determine late sequelae
  - The mitral valve is the most frequently involved, followed by the aortic valve; the tricuspid and pulmonary valves are rarely affected
  - Persistent tachycardia, gallop rhythm, new murmurs or changes in pre-existing ones and a pericardial friction rub are all characteristic
  - Heart failure can be a predominant feature; it may vary from mild to severe, and sometimes is refractory to clinical treatment, demanding urgent surgical valve replacement during the acute phase
  - A systolic murmur is most frequently indicative of mitral regurgitation, whereas aortic valve involvement gives rise to an early diastolic murmur of aortic insufficiency

Pediatric Heart Disease: A Practical Guide, First Edition. Piers E. F. Daubeney, Michael L. Rigby, Koichiro Niwa, and Michael A. Gatzoulis.
© 2012 Blackwell Publishing Ltd. Published 2012 by Blackwell Publishing Ltd.

○ In patients with the clinical manifestations of acute RF, color flow Doppler echocardiography can detect silent mitral or aortic regurgitation, which has been called "subclinical carditis"; this should not be confused with the milder physiologic regurgitation often encountered in normal individuals and the established echocardiographic criteria should be followed (see below). Whether subclinical carditis has a different prognosis to clinical carditis is as yet unknown.

• **Arthritis:**
  ○ Occurs in the first attack in about 75% of cases
  ○ More common in older children and adults
  ○ Characterized by asymmetric, migratory, and self-limiting involvement of large joints that respond well to large doses of salicylates.

• **Sydenham's chorea:**
  ○ The most delayed manifestation, having a latency period from 1 to 6 months, and is sometimes the only manifestation
  ○ More frequent in females
  ○ Characterized by emotional lability, uncoordinated, abrupt, erratic movements and muscular weakness
  ○ Providing other causes have been excluded, the presence of chorea alone allows the diagnosis of RF to be made.

• **Subcutaneous nodules:** Painless, small, firm, mobile structures, often occurring in clusters and situated on the extensor surface of the joints, and observed predominantly on knees, elbows, knuckles, and over the spinal column (Figure 25.1).

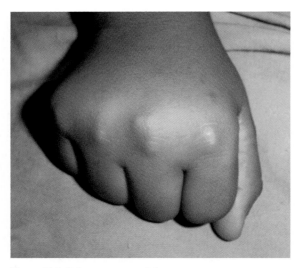

Figure 25.1 Subcutaneous nodules.

• **Erythema marginatum:**
  ○ Uncommon manifestation
  ○ Macular rash with circular form, copper pink at the border and lighter in the center
  ○ Located mainly on the trunk and inner surface of the proximal limbs, but does not involve the face
  ○ Usually transient but can appear intermittently and become accentuated by heat.

Echocardiographic criteria for the evaluation of subclinical carditis

• Jet persists through systole (mitral valve) and diastole (aortic valve)
• Regurgitant jet >1 cm in length
• Regurgitant jet in at least two planes
• Mosaic color jet with a peak velocity of >2.5 m/s

Diagnosis

It was Jones who first established the criteria for diagnosis. It has been subsequently modified and the most recent revision is recommended for diagnosis. Two major or one major and two minor criteria, plus evidence of an infection by streptococcus, is sufficient for there to be a high probability of acute RF.

Major criteria

• Carditis
• Polyarthritis
• Subcutaneous nodules
• Erythema marginatum
• Chorea

Minor criteria

• Clinical:
  ○ Fever
  ○ Polyarthralgia
  ○ Prolonged PR interval
• Laboratory:
  ○ Elevated acute phase reactants
  ○ Erythrocyte sedimentation rate
  ○ C-reactive protein

Supporting evidence of Group A streptococcal infection

• Positive throat culture, rapid streptococcal antigen test, elevated or rising antistreptolysin-O or other streptococcal antibody

Management

• A period of rest until the most severe symptoms have subsided is advisable.
• Benzathine penicillin 0.6–1.2 mU by intramuscular injection or oral phenoxymethylpenicillin 250 mg (under 27 kg) or 500 mg (over 27 kg) two or three times daily for 10 days to eradicate streptococci. In the event of penicillin allergy, erythromycin 40 mg/kg/day orally, bid or qid for 10 days is used.
• Anti-inflammatory treatment should be started when the diagnosis is confirmed. Aspirin 100 mg/kg/day, divided into four daily doses, leads to rapid resolution of fever and arthritis. The use of steroids is indicated when there is clear evidence of moderate or severe carditis; this often results in significant clinical improvement. Prednisone 1–2 mg/kg/day can be given once or divided into two or three doses.
• Valve insufficiency and heart failure are treated with digoxin, diuretics, and ACE inhibitors.
• The treatment of chorea is rest in a quiet place. Haloperidol, diazepam, or valproic acid is used for control of excessive movements. There is no evidence for the value of steroids.

Secondary prophylaxis

• Benzathine penicillin intramuscularly every 3 or 4 weeks is the best drug, although oral phenoxymethyl-penicillin is acceptable. Allergic patients should be prescribed sulfadiazine; a third choice is erythromycin (Table 25.1).
• Duration of secondary prophylaxis must be adapted to each patient:

  ◦ Patients without carditis: for 5 years after the last attack or until 18 years of age (whichever is longer)
  ◦ Patients with carditis (mild mitral regurgitation or healed carditis): for 10 years after the last attack or at least until 25 years of age (whichever is longer)
  ◦ More severe valvular disease or after valve surgery: lifelong.

Long-term outcome

The most important sequelae of RF are permanent and progressive damage to cardiac valves. The mitral valve is most commonly affected, followed by a combination of mitral and aortic, and then isolated aortic valve disease. Early or later involvement of the tricuspid valve is rare, while the pulmonary valve is hardly ever affected.

The optimal time for surgery in these patients often remains uncertain; many factors are taken into consideration, including symptoms, ventricular function, end-systolic and -diastolic left ventricular dimensions, changes in ventricular size, as well as estimates of pulmonary artery pressure. The social circumstances of some patients in developing countries can also require careful consideration.

Further reading

Folger GM Jr, Hajar R, Robida A, Hajar HA. Occurrence of valvar heart disease in acute rheumatic fever without evident carditis: colour-flow Doppler identification. *Br Heart J* 1992; 67:434–438.

Guilherme L, Kalil J. Rheumatic fever and rheumatic heart disease: cellular mechanisms leading autoimmune reactivity and disease. *J Clin Imunol* 2010;30:17–23.

Table 25.1 Secondary prophylaxis

Drug	Dose	Route of administration
Benzathine penicillin	600 000 U < 25 kg 1 200 000 U > 25 kg 3–4 weekly	Intramuscular
Phenoxymethylpenicillin	250 mg twice daily	Oral
Sulfadiazine	0.5 g < 25 kg once daily 1.0 g > 25 kg once daily	Oral
Erythromycin	250 mg twice daily	Oral

Marijon E, Mirabel M, Celermajer DS, Jouven X. Rheumatic heart disease. *Lancet* 2012;379:953–964.

Minich LL, Tani LY, Pagotto LT, Shaddy RE, Veasy LG. Doppler echocardiography distinguishes between physiologic and pathologic "silent" mitral regurgitation in patients with rheumatic fever. *Clin Cardiol* 1997;20:924–927.

Narula J, Virmani R, Reddy KS, Tandon R, eds. *Rheumatic Fever.* Washington: American Registry of Pathology, 1999, pp. 103–194.

Reményi B, Wilson N, Andrew S, *et al.* World Heart Federetion criteria for echocardiographic diagnosis of rheumatic heart disease – an evidence-based guideline. *Nat Rev Cardiol* advance online publication 28 February 2012.

Veasy LG, Wiedmeier SE, Orsmond GS, *et al.* Resurgence of acute rheumatic fever in the intermountain area of the United States. *N Engl J Med* 1987;316:421–427.

World Health Organization. *Rheumatic Fever and Rheumatic Heart Disease.* Report of a WHO Expert Committee (Technical Report Series n° 923). Geneva: WHO, 2001.

26 Marfan syndrome and connective tissue disorders

Koichiro Niwa[1] and Shigeru Tateno[2]

[1]St Luke's International Hospital, Tokyo, Japan
[2]Chiba Cardiovascular Center, Chiba, Japan

Marfan syndrome

There is marked variation in clinical expression in Marfan syndrome, and the diagnosis can be made from the newborn period through adulthood. Marfan syndrome affects the following systems:
- Skeletal;
- Ocular;
- Cardiovascular;
- Skin;
- Pulmonary;
- Central nervous.

The diagnosis is made primarily on clinical manifestations. Cardiovascular abnormalities, particularly those affecting the mitral valve and aorta, are common. Mortality is primarily related to aortic root dissection or rupture, usually preceded by progressive root dilatation. Severe mitral regurgitation (MR) or a dilated aortic arch warrants surgical replacement. Beta-blockers slow the progression of aortic dilatation and reduce the risk of dissection. The combination of beta-blocker therapy and elective surgical treatment has improved the survival. Recent studies have suggested a role for angiotensin receptor blockers such as losartan.

Incidence and etiology

Marfan syndrome is classified as a heritable connective tissue disorder caused by a defect in fibrillin protein encoded by the *fibrillin-1* gene on chromosome 15. Fibrillin is an element of elastic tissue and is abundant in tissues affecting patients with this disease. Cystic medial necrosis with the destruction of medial elastic fibers is found in the aortic media (Figure 26.1).

The incidence is approximately 1 in 10 000 individuals and equal between males and females. Approximately 55% of cases are sporadic and there is a 50% risk of recurrence in offspring.

Presentation and course in childhood

The diagnosis can be made even in fetal life. Patients with the severe neonatal form have mitral valve prolapse and MR, as well as significant pulmonary and tricuspid regurgitation. The skeletal and ocular complications present at birth and these children may die within the first year of life due to heart failure.

MR occurs more frequently and earlier in life than aortic regurgitation (AR). Presentation with significant MR or AR is more common in childhood than with aortic dissection or rupture.

Examination

Physical examination reveals skeletal, ocular, and cardiovascular manifestations.
- **Skeletal manifestations:** Tall stature, long arms, legs, fingers, and toes, hyperextensibility, scoliosis, and high-arched palate.
- **Cardiovascular manifestations:**
  ○ AR, MR, or pulmonary/tricuspid regurgitation
  ○ Dilatation of the aorta may occur gradually before any change in physical examination or appearance of symptoms
  ○ Cardiac failure is usually due to MR and/or AR.

Progressive enlargement of the aorta is usually asymptomatic; therefore regular assessment is necessary.

Pediatric Heart Disease: A Practical Guide, First Edition. Piers E. F. Daubeney, Michael L. Rigby, Koichiro Niwa, and Michael A. Gatzoulis.
© 2012 Blackwell Publishing Ltd. Published 2012 by Blackwell Publishing Ltd.

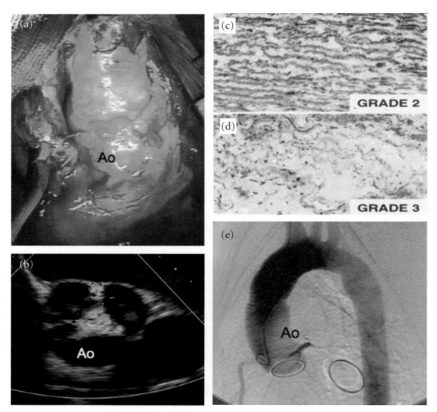

Figure 26.1 (a) Operative findings, dilated ascending aorta (Ao). (b) Echocardiogram. Aortic root dilatation with aortic regurgitation. Ao, aorta. (c,d) Light microscopy of the aortic wall with polychromatic stain. Moderate (c) and marked degeneration of the elastic fibers (d). (e) Digital angiogram of the aorta after the Bentall procedure and mitral valve replacement (note the annular rings of the artificial valves). Ao, aorta. (Courtesy of Atsushi Mizuno, MD.)

Investigations
- **EKG:** Left ventricular dilatation (Figure 26.2b).
- **CXR:** Left atrial, ventricular, and aortic dilatation (Figure 26.2a).
- **Echocardiogram:** MR, AR, aortic root dilatation, and left heart dilatation. Interval change is important (Figures 26.1b and 26.2d–f).
- **CT or MRI:** Accurate assessment of aortic root dilatation, dissection or rupture (Figure 26.2c).
- **Cardiac catheterization:** Not usually necessary.

The size of the aortic root correlates with body surface area and is usually normalized to this in children using Z scores. A dilated aortic root is generally defined as having a diameter exceeding 37 mm.

Diagnosis
Although molecular diagnosis is now available, diagnosis is currently made primarily on clinical manifestations using the Ghent diagnostic criteria (see Further reading).

Management
Medical management
Beta-blockers slow the progression of aortic dilatation and reduce the risk of dissection. They should be used in all patients at any age when the aortic root diameter is 40 mm or more and considered in those with a diameter under 40 mm. There is some evidence that angiotensin receptor blockers such as losartan play a role in reducing/preventing

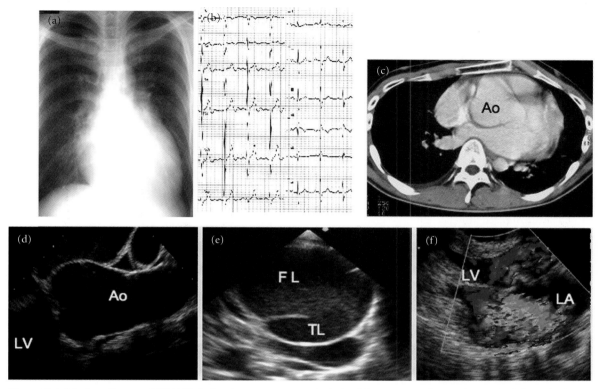

Figure 26.2 (a) Chest X-ray and (b) EKG. Left atrium, ventricle, and ascending aorta are dilated. (c) CT showing aortic root dilatation, aorta (Ao), aortic valve, and sinuses of Valsalva. (d) Echocardiogram showing aortic root dilatation, particularly of the sinuses of Valsalva. Ao, aorta, LV, left ventricle. (e) Echocardiogram showing dissection of the aorta. An intimal flap separates the true lumen (TL) from the false lumen (FL). (f) Echocardiogram. Mitral valve prolapse with regurgitation into the left atrium is shown by color flow mapping. LA, left atrium, LV, left ventricle. (Courtesy of Dr Tomohiko Toyoda, MD, Chiba University, and Atsushi Mizuno, MD.)

dilatation. In those unable to tolerate beta-blockers, ACE inhibitors or calcium antagonists are alternatives.

Catheter and surgical management

A mildly dilated aortic root only very infrequently dissects but the risk increases with progressive aortic dilatation. Elective replacement of the aorta should be considered when:

- Maximal diameter of the root exceeds 55 mm;
- Diameter exceeds 50 mm in a patient with a family history of aortic dissection or rupture or where there is a rapid annual change in size (>2 mm/year);
- Diameter exceeds 45 mm and pregnancy is desired or surgery is indicated for another reason such as severe AR or MR.

Urgent surgery is indicated for ascending aortic dissection and contained rupture. The operative mortality for elective replacement is <2%, while it is 12% for emergency operations.

Late complications and long-term outcome

The combination of beta-blocker therapy (and perhaps losartan) with elective surgical treatment has significantly improved survival, with average life expectancy now about 60 years. Survival after elective replacement of the aortic root at 10 years is 75%. The prognosis of infantile Marfan patients is still poor irrespective of management strategy.

Follow-up recommendations

Marfan patients should be under the care of experienced pediatricians and pediatric cardiologists, preferably in a multidisciplinary clinic. Yearly follow-up with assessment of aortic root size and MR is recommended, with more frequent assessment as the diameter approaches 50 mm. After surgical replacement of the aorta, patients are still at risk for dissection or dilatation of the arch and descending thoracic aorta and therefore need ongoing monitoring.

Exercise
Contact sports and strenuous exercise should be avoided to reduce excessive stress on the aorta.

Pregnancy
- 50% recurrence rate.
- Increased risk of aortic dissection during pregnancy, peripartum, and after delivery.
- Patients with an aortic root diameter above 44 mm should be discouraged from becoming pregnant. Surgical root replacement should be considered beforehand if pregnancy is contemplated. An aortic diameter below 40 mm is rarely a problem.

> **Key clinical points**
> - Mortality is primarily related to aortic root dissection or rupture
> - This is usually preceded by progressive aortic root dilatation, which is rare during childhood
> - In infantile Marfan, mortality is high
> - MR occurs more frequently and earlier in life than AR, and both are more common than aortic dissection or rupture in childhood
> - Progressive enlargement of the aorta is usually asymptomatic; therefore, regular assessment is necessary
> - Beta-blocker therapy (and perhaps losartan) combined with elective surgery has improved survival

Ehlers–Danlos syndrome

There are at least 11 different forms of Ehlers–Danlos syndrome. The diseases are inherited as an autosomal dominant disorder and are uncommon but with unknown incidence. The presumed defect involves synthesis of normal collagen.

The features of the diseases include:
- Hypermobility of the joints;
- Hyperextensibility of the skin;
- Cardiac features:
  - Mitral valve prolapse
  - Aortic root dilatation

- Dissecting aortic aneurysm in type IV Ehlers–Danlos.

The prognosis depends on the severity of the cardiovascular features.

Ehlers–Danlos syndrome type IV (vascular)
Complications from severe aortic root dilatation are rare in childhood, but 25% have a first complication by the age of 20 years. Survival has been estimated at 48 years and most deaths result from arterial rupture. Two-thirds of patients experience arterial complications, half involving thoracic or abdominal arteries. Forty-one percent of those undergoing surgery in one series died. Eleven percent died in the peripartum period. There is a 50% risk of having an affected child.

Management
This is similar to the management of Marfan syndrome with close observation of the mitral valve and ascending aortic size. Aortic root dilatation is treated with beta-blockade and surgical intervention if sufficiently enlarged.

Further reading

Marfan syndrome

De Paepe A, Devereux RB, Dietz HC, Hennekam RC, Pyeritz RE. Revised diagnostic criteria for the Marfan syndrome. *Am J Med Genet* 1996;62:417–426.

Finkbohner R, Johnson D, Crawford ES, Coselli J, Milewicz DM. Marfan syndrome. Long-term survival and complications after aortic aneurysm repair. *Circulation* 1995;91:728–733.

Geva T, Sanders SP, Diogenes MS, Rockenmacher S, Van Praagh R. Two-dimensional and Doppler echocardiographic and pathologic characteristics of the infantile Marfan syndrome. *Am J Cardiol* 1990;65:1230–1237.

Geva T, Hegesh J, Frand M. The clinical course and echocardiographic features of Marfan's syndrome in childhood. *Am J Dis Child* 1987;141:1179–1182.

Gillinov AM, Zehr KJ, Redmond JM, et al. Cardiac operations in children with Marfan's syndrome: indications and results. *Ann Thorac Surg* 1997;64:1140–1144.

Milewicz DM, Dietz HC, Miller C. Treatment of aortic disease in patients with Marfan syndrome. *Circulation* 2005;111: e150–e157.

Niwa K, Perloff JK, Bhuta SM, et al. Structural abnormalities of great arterial walls in congenital heart disease. Light and electron microscopic analyses. *Circulation* 2001;103:393–400.

Shores J, Berger KR, Murphy EA, Pyeritz RE. Progression of aortic dilatation and the benefit of long-term beta-adrenergic blockade in Marfan's syndrome. *N Engl J Med* 1994;330: 1335–1341.

Silverman DI, Burton KJ, Gray J et al. Life expectancy in the Marfan syndrome. *Am J Cardiol* 1995;75:157–160.

van Karnebeek CD, Naeff MS, Mulder BJ, Hennekam RC, Offringa M. Natural history of cardiovascular manifestations in Marfan syndrome. *Arch Dis Child* 2001;84:129–137.

Ehlers–Danlos syndromes

Pepin M, Schwarze U, Superti-Furga A, Byers PH. Clinical and genetic features of Ehlers-Danlos syndrome type IV, the vascular type. *N Engl J Med* 2000;342:673–680.

27 Kawasaki disease and Takayasu arteritis

Koichiro Niwa[1] and Shigeru Tateno[2]

[1]St Luke's International Hospital, Tokyo, Japan
[2]Chiba Cardiovascular Center, Chiba, Japan

Kawasaki disease

Kawasaki disease is an acute febrile multisystem vasculitic syndrome of unknown etiology occurring predominantly in infants and young children. The vasculitis involves medium- and small-sized arteries, especially the coronary arteries. It is characterized by the risk of developing coronary artery lesions accompanied by aneurysms, stenoses, and myocardial infarction.

Incidence and etiology

More than 180 000 cases have been recognized and there are around 10 000 new patients each year in Japan and 2000–4000 in the United States. The male-to-female ratio is 1.5:1. The etiology remains unknown, but may be the result of an immune response to an infectious agent.

Presentation and course in childhood

Diagnosis is entirely on clinical grounds.

> • Prolonged high fever (>5 days)
>   Plus four of the following five features:
> • Stomatits
> • Truncal rash
> • Erythema or swelling of the hands and feet
> • Conjunctival injection
> • Lymphadenopathy (>1.5 cm)

In atypical cases, particularly in infants, fewer features may be present and the fever shorter. There is characteristically late peeling of the hands and feet.

The cardiac examination may demonstrate a tachycardic hyperdynamic heart due to the fever and illness.

There may be a flow murmur or mitral regurgitant murmur.

The acute systematic vasculitis subsides within several weeks or months. Coronary artery aneurysms (CAAs) may appear as early as 7 days and as late as 4 weeks. Persistent large or giant CAAs are at risk of developing coronary artery stenoses with resultant myocardial ischemia. Regression may occur within 2 years of onset and there may be no progression to stenosis.

Investigations

The following may be found in the acute phase.
- **Blood tests:**
  - Thrombocytosis
  - Normocytic anemia
  - Raised acute-phase reactants (ESR and CRP)
  - Raised liver function tests
  - Low albumin.
- **Urinalysis:** Proteinuria and sterile pyuria.
- **Ultrasound:** Hydrops of the gall bladder.
- **EKG:**
  - Raised ST segments
  - Prolonged QRS
  - Prolonged QT interval
  - Features of pericarditis.
- **Echocardiogram:**
  - Should be performed when diagnosis is suspected
  - Left ventricular dysfunction (myocarditis)
  - Mitral regurgitation
  - Coronary artery dilatation and aneurysm formation
  - Serial studies required at presentation, 2 weeks, 6 weeks, and 6 months as a minimum, as aneurysm formation can occur up to 4 weeks after the onset of the disease
  - Normal echocardiography does not exclude diagnosis.

Pediatric Heart Disease: A Practical Guide, First Edition. Piers E. F. Daubeney, Michael L. Rigby, Koichiro Niwa, and Michael A. Gatzoulis.
© 2012 Blackwell Publishing Ltd. Published 2012 by Blackwell Publishing Ltd.

- **CT angiogram or MRI coronary arteries:** Useful where large aneurysms detected on echocardiography.
- **Coronary angiography:**
  ○ Generally performed once out of the acute phase if large coronary artery aneurysms detected
  ○ Detects coronary artery stenoses.

Management
Treatment should not be withheld while awaiting an echocardiogram.

Medical management
- Intravenous immunoglobulin. Risk of CAA is 15–25% when immunoglobulin is given in the first 10 days of illness.
- High-dose aspirin until the inflammatory markers and temperature subside.
- Corticosteroid occasionally added for resistant pyrexia.
- Low-dose aspirin (3–5 mg/kg/day):
  ○ Given until absence of coronary dilatation or CAA is confirmed 4–8 weeks after the onset of illness.
  ○ In persistent coronary dilatation/aneurysm formation, low-dose aspirin is continued.
- More aggressive therapy with addition of warfarin or dipyridamole if giant (>8 mm) CAAs.

Catheter and surgical management
Patients with obstructive coronary lesions or signs of ischemia should be evaluated for surgical and catheter intervention. Stent implantation, rotablator angioplasty, coronary artery bypass grafting (CABG), and cardiac transplantation have all been employed for patients with serious coronary artery pathology. Mitral regurgitation due to coronary ischemia may need mitral valve replacement.

Late complications and long-term outcome
Major late complications are:
- Ischemic heart disease;
- Acute myocardial infarction (AMI);
- Sudden cardiac death;
- Arrhythmia;
- Heart failure;
- Systemic artery aneurysm;
- Valvulopathy (mitral regurgitation);
- Early-onset atherosclerosis.

Large and medium aneurysms may progress to coronary artery stenosis with risk of myocardial ischemia, AMI, and sudden death. The mortality rate is approxi-

mately 0.1%. AMI is the most common cause of death and is most common in the first year after onset of illness. The first MI is fatal in 22% and asymptomatic in 37%. Fatal infarctions tend to involve the left main trunk and left anterior descending artery.

The results over the first decade after CABG are encouraging. Rotablator therapy with/without stenting is promising, especially for severe calcified lesions, but requires further assessment (Figures 27.1 and 27.2).

Follow-up
The level of follow-up depends on the degree of coronary artery involvement.
- **Patients with no evidence of coronary artery abnormalities:**
  ○ No need for antiplatelet medication beyond 6–12 weeks after onset or for restriction of physical activities
  ○ Cardiac evaluation every 5 years may be prudent (not universal advice)
  ○ Childhood Kawasaki disease may lead to long-term endothelial dysfunction, but whether this increases the risk for coronary atherosclerosis remains unknown.
- **Patients with transient CAA (resolving by 8 weeks):**
  ○ Treatment with aspirin 3–5 mg/kg/day until resolution of abnormalities
  ○ Cardiac evaluation every 3–5 years
  ○ Regression of small aneurysms appears to be common.
- **Patients with small-to-medium CAA (3–6 mm):**
  ○ Treatment with aspirin 3–5 mg/kg/day until resolution of abnormalities
  ○ Cardiac evaluation every year
  ○ Exercise stress test every 2 years in the second decade
  ○ Angiography if abnormal stress test.
- **Patients with large (>6 mm) and giant (>8 mm) CAA:**
  ○ Cardiac evaluation 6 monthly (or more frequently)
  ○ Treatment with aspirin and either warfarin or dipyridamole indefinitely for giant aneurysms
  ○ Exercise stress test every year in the second decade may reveal ischemia or infarction
  ○ Coronary angiography 6–12 months after initial illness and then if abnormal stress test
  ○ CT coronary angiography will show aneurysms, proximal and distal
  ○ MRI may show evidence of AMI, wall motion abnormalities and thinning after AMI.
- **Patients with coronary artery obstruction on angiography:**
  ○ As above
  ○ Beta-blockade to reduce myocardial work

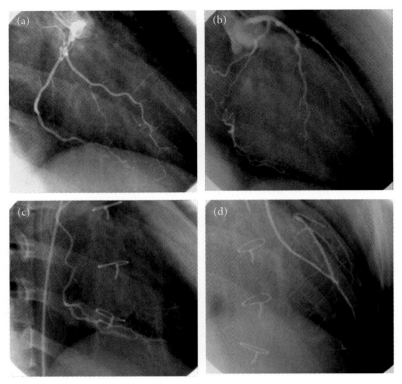

Figure 27.1 Coronary arteriography in a 17-year-old female with prior Kawasaki disease. (a) Right coronary artery (RCA) occlusion with recanalization and collateral arteries. (b) Left descending artery (LAD) aneurysm and severe LAD stenosis. Coronary artery bypass grafting was performed. (c) Right intrathoracic artery to RCA. (d) Left intrathoracic artery to LAD.

○ Coronary angiography is important to evaluate patients for thrombolytic therapy, catheter intervention, and possible CABG.
Endocarditis prophylaxis is not required.

Exercise
• No need to restrict physical activities in patients without ischemic lesion.
• Contact sports should be avoided by those on warfarin.
• Those with ischemic lesions should be allowed to self-limit their activity.

Pregnancy
• Successful pregnancy and delivery in patients with CAA can be achieved with careful care and management.
• Low-dose aspirin during pregnancy is thought to be useful.

Key clinical points
• Diagnosis is clinical
• Echocardiography should be performed when diagnosis is suspected and may show coronary artery dilatation and aneurysms
• Treatment should not be withheld whilst awaiting an echocardigram
• Normal echocardiography does not exclude the diagnosis
• Aneurysm formation can occur up to 4 weeks after the onset of the disease: echocardiography needs repeating at 2 and 6 weeks
• Beware atypical cases!
• Large and medium aneurysms may progress to coronary artery stenoses with risk of myocardial ischemia, AMI, and sudden death
• Patients with obstructive coronary lesions or signs of ischemia should be evaluated for surgical and catheter intervention

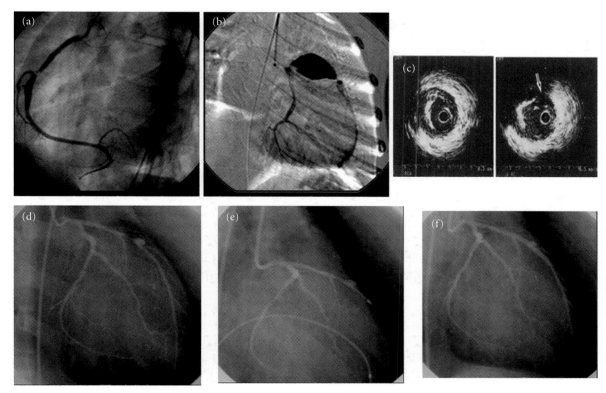

Figure 27.2 Coronary arteriography in a different patient with Kawasaki disease. (a) Moderate stenosis (90%) in the right coronary artery (RCA). (b) Severe stenosis (99%) in the left descending artery (LAD). (c) Pre-intervention, severe LAD stenosis. (d) During rotablator procedure. (e, f) Post-intervention, LAD was dilated with stent after intervention. (Courtesy of Dr Koji Higashi, Department of Pediatrics, Chiba University, Chiba, Japan).

Takayasu arteritis

Takayasu arteritis is a chronic inflammatory vasculitic arteriopathy of the aorta and the proximal portions of its major branches. It predominantly affects young women in Asian populations. Varying degrees of narrowing or dilatation develop in the involved segments, leading to clinical features related to limb or organ ischemia.

Incidence and etiology
The incidence is 20.7 cases per million in Japan and 2.6 cases per million in the United States. There is inflammation in the media and adventitia in the aorta and its branches. The etiology is unknown.

Presentation and course in childhood and adulthood
Systemic complications such as fever, arthralgia, and myalgia are observed during the inflammatory phase (20–65% in childhood series). The arterial lesions can lead to secondary hypertension, retinopathy, cardiac involvement, and cerebrovascular events. Although symptoms can appear after 10 years of age, they usually do so in the third decade of life.

Criteria for diagnosis

Three or more of the following:

- Onset at age ≤40 years
- Claudication of an extremity
- Decreased brachial arterial pulse
- Blood pressure difference between the arms of >10 mmHg
- Bruit in the subclavian arteries or aorta
- Angiography: narrowing or occlusion of the entire aorta, its primary branches, or large arteries in the proximal upper or lower extremities

Investigations
• **Erythrocyte sedimentation rate:** Elevated, indicator of disease activity.
• **CXR:** Contour irregularity of the descending aorta, aortic calcification.
• **MRI (or CT):** Mural thickening and aneurysm of the aorta.
• **Aortography:** Narrowed or obstructed subclavian arteries.
• **Echocardiography:** Aortic dilatation/regurgitation, arterial stenosis.

Management
Medical management
• Corticosteroid during active inflammatory phase (remission rate: 60%).
• Medication for hypertension and cardiac failure.

Catheter and surgical management
• Severe arterial stenosis or aneurysm may require surgical treatment.
• Catheter intervention is useful for renovascular stenosis.

Late complications and long-term outcome
Rarely causes death, but may be more lethal in children. Causes of premature deaths are major cardiovascular complications. In the long term, there is a significant incidence of morbidity.

Follow-up
Meticulous care is required in the case of progressive vascular lesions.

Pregnancy
Successful pregnancy is possible, but care must be taken in the presence of hypertension and aneurysm formation.

Further reading

Kawasaki disease
Dajani AS, Taubert KA, Takahashi M, et al. Guidelines for long-term management of patients with Kawasaki disease. Circulation 1994;89:916–922.

Kato H, Ichinose E, Kawasaki T. Myocardial infarction in Kawasaki disease. J Pediatr 1986;108:923–928.

Kato H, Sugimura T, Akagi T, et al. Long-term consequences of Kawasaki disease. A 10–21 year follow-up study of 594 patients. Circulation 1996;94:1379–1385.

Kitamura S, Kameda Y, Seki T, et al. Long-term outcome of myocardial revascularization in patients with Kawasaki coronary artery disease. A multicenter cooperative study. J Thorac Cardiovasc Surg 1994;107:663–673.

Newburger JW, Takahashi M, Burns JC, et al. The treatment of Kawasaki syndrome with intravenous gammaglobulin. N Engl J Med 1986;315:341–347.

Sugimura T, Yokoi H, Sato N, et al. Interventional treatment for children with severe coronary artery stenosis with calcification after long-term Kawasaki disease. Circulation 1997;96:3928–3933.

Takayasu arteritis
Arend WP, Michel BA, Block DA, et al. The American College of Rheumatology 1990 criteria for the classification of Takayasu arteritis. Arthritis Rheum 1990;33:1129–1134.

Ishikawa K. Diagnostic approach and proposed criteria for the clinical diagnosis of Takauyasu's arteriopathy. J Am Coll Cardiol 1988;964:964–972.

Kerr GS, Hallahan CW, Giordano J, et al. Takayasu arteritis. Ann Intern Med 1994;120:919–929.

Miyata T, Sato O, Koyama H, Shigematu H, Tada Y. Long-term survival after surgical treatment of patients with Takayasu's arteritis. Circulation 2003;108:1474–1480.

28 Hyperlipidemia

Eric Quivers

Dean Health System, Middleton, WI, USA

Atherosclerosis in the form of coronary artery disease and stroke remains a major cause of death worldwide, trailing only HIV/AIDS, tuberculosis, and traffic accidents. Coronary artery disease is becoming more prevalent in developing countries, while decreasing in the United States and many western European countries as treatment and prevention have proved effective. Though genetic factors play a role, 80–90% of affected individuals have modifiable risk factors for atherosclerosis which include hyperlipidemia, hypertension, obesity, diabetes, tobacco use, and sedentary lifestyles. The prevalence of some of these risk factors, such as obesity and type 2 diabetes, is increasing in children and adolescents.

Atherosclerosis appears to have its origins in early adolescence and rapidly progresses in early adulthood. The Korean Conflict Casualty Study demonstrated the presence of atherosclerotic lesions in the coronary arteries in asymptomatic young men, whose average age was 22 years. The Bogalusa study demonstrated a correlation between systolic blood pressure, elevated total and low density lipoprotein (LDL)-cholesterol, but lower high density lipoprotein (HDL)-cholesterol concentrations, and the degree of coronary and aortic atherosclerosis in children and adolescents. In the Pathobiological Determinants of Atherosclerosis in Youth Study, which analyzed the aortas and right coronary arteries at autopsy of African-American and white men and women between the ages of 15 and 34 years, over half the youngest age group had intimal lesions in the right coronary artery. These increased rapidly in prevalence and extent with an increase in age.

Clinical features

Most of the hyperlipidemia in children is secondary to exogenous factors or clinical illness. Newer medications such as HIV protease inhibitors and immunosuppressants can elevate various cholesterol fractions.

Addressing the primary condition or removal of the offending medication is the initial approach in the management of a child with secondary hyperlipidemia. If the hyperlipidemia persists, then consideration should be given to the possibility that the patient has a primary hyperlipidemia.

Causes of secondary hypercholesterolemia

- **Exogenous:**
  - Drugs: corticosteroids, isotretinoin (Accutane®), thiazides, anticonvulsants, beta-blockers, anabolic steroids, certain oral contraceptives
  - Alcohol
  - Obesity
- **Endocrine and metabolic:**
  - Hypothyroidism
  - Diabetes mellitus
  - Lipodystrophy
  - Pregnancy
  - Idiopathic hypercalcemia
- **Storage diseases:**
  - Glycogen storage diseases
  - Sphingolipidoses
- **Obstructive liver diseases:**
  - Biliary atresia
  - Biliary cirrhosis
- **Chronic renal diseases:**
  - Nephrotic syndrome
- **Others:**
  - Anorexia
  - Progeria
  - Collagen disease
  - Klinefelter syndrome

Pediatric Heart Disease: A Practical Guide, First Edition. Piers E. F. Daubeney, Michael L. Rigby, Koichiro Niwa, and Michael A. Gatzoulis.
© 2012 Blackwell Publishing Ltd. Published 2012 by Blackwell Publishing Ltd.

Genetic conditions resulting in primary hypertriglyceridemia are rare. Of men and women who have their first myocardial infarction before 50 and 60 years, respectively, one-third has hyperlipidemia. About half of these individuals have an inherited lipoprotein metabolism disorder. The two most common disorders are familial hypercholesterolemia (autosomal dominant; heterozygous and homozygous) and familial combined hyperlipidemia.

Heterozygous familial hypercholesterolemia

- Occurs in approximately 1 in 500 individuals worldwide; one of the most common single-gene disorders.
- Characterized by elevated total and LDL cholesterol levels with normal triglycerides and a family history of hypercholesterolemia or premature cardiovascular disease.
- Affected individuals have about 50% of LDL receptor activity of the normal population.
- Total cholesterol levels are usually above 240 mg/dL (6.2 mmol/L) and average 300 mg/dL (7.8 mmol/L), with LDL cholesterol above 160 mg/dL (4.1 mmol/L) and average 240 mg/dL (6.2 mmol/L).
- Physical finding of tendon xanthomas, more easily appreciated on the Achilles tendon, is virtually diagnostic.
- Diagnosis is made on clinical grounds.

Homozygous familial hypercholesterolemia

- Occurs in approximately 1 in 1 million persons worldwide.
- Caused by the inheritance of two mutant LDL receptor alleles, resulting in the absence or near absence of these receptors. "Receptor negative" patients have about 2% of normal receptor activity.
- Clinical course is much worse than in the heterozygote form.
- Patients can present in childhood with cutaneous xanthomas on the hands, wrists, elbows, buttocks, knees, and heels.
- Total cholesterol levels range from 500 mg/dL to 1200 mg/dL (12.9–31.0 mmol/L).
- Untreated individuals usually experience coronary artery disease before age 30 years.
- Family history and clinical findings are important in making the diagnosis.

Familial combined hyperlipidemia

- More common than familial hypercholosterolemia and may be present in as many as 1 in 300 people.

- Primary defect is the overproduction of apolipoprotein B containing very low density lipoprotein (VLDL) particles by the liver with subsequent conversion to LDL particles. The accumulation of VLDL and LDL particles depends on their removal.
- Most affected individuals lack tendon xanthomas.
- Visceral abdominal adiposity, glucose intolerance, hyperinsulinemia, and hypertension are common findings.
- Diagnosis is suggested by the presence of mixed hyperlipidemia with both fasting triglyceride and cholesterol levels greater than the 90th percentile and low HDL levels.
- Severely elevated cholesterol levels are not seen in childhood. Affected children may have total cholesterol levels between 190 and 220 mg/dL (4.9 and 5.7 mmol/L), mildly elevated LDL cholesterol, and moderately elevated triglycerides [120 mg/dL (3.1 mmol/L) or greater].
- Formal diagnosis requires the presence of dyslipidemia in at least two first-degree relatives.

Management

The National Cholesterol Education Program Expert Panel on Cholesterol in Children and Adolescents (NCEP) recommendations for the screening and treatment of children, published in 1991, advocate a dual approach and include a population approach and selective screening.

The NCEP's classification of total cholesterol and LDL cholesterol levels is given in Table 28.1. Fasting triglyceride levels should be <150 mg/dL (<3.9 mmol/L) and HDL-cholesterol >35 mg/dL (>0.9 mmol/L).

Screening

- Children older than 2 years of age should be screened for hypercholesterolemia if there is a parental history of elevated cholesterol levels >240 mg/dL (>6.2 mmol/L) or a family history of premature coronary artery disease, before 55 years of age, in a parent or grandparent.

Table 28.1 Classification of total and LDL-cholesterol levels in children and adolescents

Category	Total cholesterol (mg/dL) [mmol/L]	LDL-cholesterol (mg/dL) [mmol/L]
Acceptable	<170 [4.4]	<110 [2.8]
Borderline	170–199 [4.4–5.1]	110–129 [2.8–3.3]
High	≥200 [5.2]	≥130 [3.4]

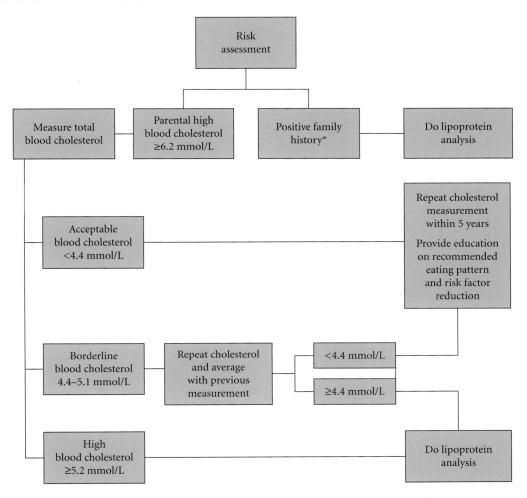

*Family history of premature (before 55 years) cardiovascular disease in a parent or grandparent

Figure 28.1 Risk assessment in children and adolescents with a positive family history.

Guidelines for risk assessment are shown in Figure 28.1. Subsequent follow-up, determined by the level of LDL cholesterol, is shown in Figure 28.2.
• Children with incomplete or unknown family histories or with other recognized risk factors for atherosclerosis, such as obesity, inactive lifestyles, diabetes, and hypertension, should be screened at the discretion of the investigating physician.

Lifestyle and diet
• Healthy lifestyle with regular activity and a diet with 30% or less of calories from fat.

• Dietary intervention is the primary approach in the hypercholesterolemic child who is 2 years of age or older.
• The American Heart Association's (AHA) Step-One diet is recommended for initial therapy and focuses on the reduction of total and saturated dietary fat (Table 28.2).
• If unsuccessful after 3–6 months, the AHA Step-Two diet, which recommends further reduction of total and saturated dietary fat, can be tried (Table 28.2).
• A child should be encouraged to eat a wide variety of foods, particularly those rich in soluble fiber.

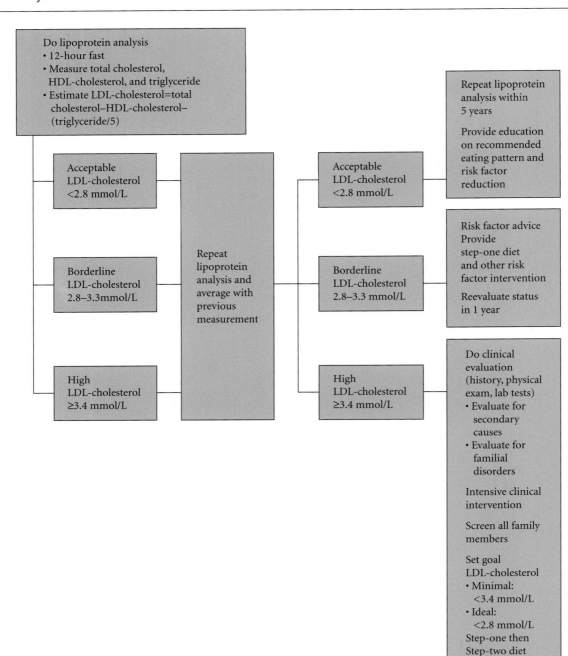

Figure 28.2 Follow-up based on LDL-cholesterol.

Table 28.2 Characteristics of Step-One and Step-Two Diets for lowering blood cholesterol

Nutrient	Recommended intake	
	Step-One Diet	Step-Two Diet
Total fat	Average of no more than 30% of total calories	Same
Saturated fatty acids	<10% of total calories	<7% of total calories
Polyunsaturated fatty acids	Up to 10% of total calories	Same
Monounsaturated fatty acids	Remaining total fat calories	Same
Cholesterol	<300 mg/day	<200 mg/day
Carbohydrates	About 55% of total calories	Same
Protein	About 15–20% of total calories	Same
Calories	To promote normal growth and development, and to reach or maintain desirable body weight	Same

• Goal is to reduce LDL-cholesterol to 110 mg/dL (2.8 mmol/L) or less and in the case of a high LDL-cholesterol, 130 mg/dL (3.4 mmol/L) is the minimal goal.

Drug therapy
• Should be considered for children 10 years of age or older who do not respond to a 6–12-month trial of adequate diet therapy and have:

  ◦ LDL-cholesterol levels ≥190 mg/dL (4.9 mmol/L), or
  ◦ LDL-cholesterol remains >160 mg/dL (4.1 mmol/L) and a positive family history of premature coronary artery disease or two or more risk factors such as obesity, diabetes, smoking or hypertension.
• Recommended first-line medications include the bile acid-binding sequestrants, cholestyramine, and colestipol, or statins. The sequestrants increase the secretion of bile acids in the stool and increase LDL receptor activity. Ezetimibe is a new medication that has been approved for use in children aged 10 years or older. It inhibits the uptake of cholesterol from the intestine. Niacin, fibric acids, and salmon fish oil medications are useful in the patient with elevated triglycerides.
• Goal of medical therapy is the same as for diet (see above).

Further reading

Enos WH, Holmes RH, Beyer J. Coronary disease among United States Soldiers killed in action in Korea. *JAMA* 1986;256:2859–2862.

Kavey REW, Daniels SR, Lauer RM, *et al.* American Heart Association Guidelines for Primary Prevention of Atherosclerotic Cardiovascular Disease Beginning in Childhood. *Circulation* 2003;107:1562–1566.

National Cholesterol Education Program, Lipid Metabolism Branch, Division of Heart, Lung, and Blood Institute. *The Report of the Expert Panel on Blood Cholesterol Levels in Children and Adolescents (Draft)*. Bethesda, MD: National Institutes of Health, 1991.

Newman WP, Wattigney W, Berenson GS. Autopsy studies in U. S. children and adolescents. Relationship of risk factors to atherosclerotic lesions. *Ann NY Acad Sci* 1991;623:16–25.

Strong JP, Malcom GT, McMahan CA, *et al.* Prevalence and extent of atherosclerosis in adolescents and young adults. Implications for prevention from the pathological determinants of atherosclerosis in youth study. *JAMA* 1999;281:727–735.

World Health Organization. Cardiovascular disease and control. http://www.who.int/dietphysicalactivity/publications/facts/cvd/en/, 2005.

29 Systemic hypertension

Eric Quivers

Dean Health System, Middleton, WI, USA

Significance and prevalence

Systemic hypertension is recognized as a major risk factor for the development of cardiovascular diseases, stroke, and renal failure if left untreated. In fact, the prevalence of hypertension increases with age with 25–35% of adults affected in the United States. The estimated prevalence of hypertension in children has been between 1% and 2%, but a recent study showed that 4.5% of school-age children were hypertensive. If hypertension is found in infants and younger children, it usually is indicative of the presence of an underlying disease. Primary or essential hypertension is on the rise in adolescence and it is usually multifactorial in origin with obesity and lifestyle playing major roles.

Natural history

In children, blood pressure (BP) increases gradually during the first week of life. Systolic BP stabilizes during the first year of life and then rises gradually during the remainder of childhood and adolescence. Diastolic BP demonstrates a gradual decline over the first 6–8 weeks of life and then it is stable for the next 4–5 years. Thereafter, it rises gradually throughout the remainder of childhood and adolescence. Height and weight play a role in a child's BP as a heavier and/or taller child generally has a higher BP than a smaller child of the same age and gender.

Definition

All children over the age of 3 years should have their BP measured during medical encounters. Children under the age of 3 years should have their BP measured under the following circumstances:

- History of premature birth;
- Low birth weight;
- NICU care;
- Congenital heart disease;
- Family history of congenital renal disease;
- Recurrent urinary tract infections.
- **Normal BP in children** – average systolic and diastolic BPs <90th percentile for age and gender
- **High normal or prehypertension BP** – between the 90th and 95th percentiles
- **Stage 1 hypertension** – between the 95th and 99th percentiles plus 5 mmHg
- **Stage 2 hypertension** – >99th percentile plus 5 mmHg

All children suspected of having hypertension are rechecked over a period of weeks to months, sooner and more frequently if Stage 2 hypertension is found. The term labile hypertension is reserved for the individual whose BP is inconsistently elevated above the 95th percentile for age and gender. As with adults, children and adolescents with BP readings of 120/80 mmHg or above should be considered prehypertensive, even if the readings are below the 95th percentile. BP percentiles for age and gender, as provided by the Fourth Report on the Diagnosis, Evaluation and Treatment of High Blood Pressure in Children and Adolescents, are given in Tables 29.1 and 29.2.

Measuring blood pressure

Technique is extremely important in obtaining the BP accurately. The process includes the selection of the appropriate size cuff as well as a properly calibrated BP recording device. Every pediatric office should have a selection of cuffs for the various age groups from infant to adult. However, these cuffs may not be appropriate for

Pediatric Heart Disease: A Practical Guide, First Edition. Piers E. F. Daubeney, Michael L. Rigby, Koichiro Niwa, and Michael A. Gatzoulis.
© 2012 Blackwell Publishing Ltd. Published 2012 by Blackwell Publishing Ltd.

Table 29.1 Blood pressure levels for bosy by age and height percentile. (Courtesy of the US National Heart Lung and Blood Institute, http://www.nhlbi.nih.gov/guidelines/hypertension/child_tbl.htm)

Age (year)	BP Percentile ↓	Systolic BP (mmHg) ← Percentile of Height →							Distolic BP (mmHg) ← Percentile of Height →						
		5th	10th	25th	50th	75th	90th	95th	5th	10th	25th	50th	75th	90th	95th
1	50th	80	81	83	85	87	88	89	34	35	36	37	38	39	39
	90th	94	95	97	99	100	102	103	49	50	51	52	53	63	54
	95th	98	99	101	103	104	106	106	54	54	55	56	57	58	58
	99th	105	106	108	110	112	113	114	61	62	63	64	65	66	66
2	50th	84	86	87	88	90	92	92	39	40	41	42	43	44	44
	90th	97	99	100	102	104	105	106	54	55	56	57	58	58	59
	95th	101	102	104	106	108	109	110	59	59	60	61	62	63	63
	99th	109	110	111	113	115	117	117	66	67	68	69	70	71	71
3	50th	86	87	89	91	93	94	95	44	44	45	46	47	48	48
	90th	100	101	103	105	107	108	106	59	59	60	61	62	63	63
	95th	104	105	107	109	110	112	113	63	63	64	65	66	67	67
	99th	111	112	114	116	118	119	120	71	71	72	73	74	75	75
4	50th	88	89	91	93	95	96	97	47	48	49	50	51	51	52
	90th	102	103	105	107	109	110	111	62	63	64	65	66	66	67
	95th	106	107	109	111	112	114	115	66	67	58	69	70	71	71
	99th	113	114	116	118	120	121	122	74	75	76	77	78	78	79
5	50th	90	91	93	95	96	98	98	53	51	52	53	54	55	55
	90th	104	105	106	108	110	111	112	65	66	67	68	69	69	70
	95th	108	109	110	112	114	115	116	69	70	71	72	73	74	74
	99th	115	116	118	120	121	123	123	77	78	79	80	81	81	82
6	50th	91	92	94	96	98	99	100	53	53	54	55	56	57	57
	90th	105	106	108	110	111	113	113	68	68	69	70	71	72	72
	95th	109	110	112	114	115	117	117	72	72	73	74	75	76	76
	99th	116	117	119	121	123	124	125	90	80	81	82	83	84	84
7	50th	92	94	95	97	99	100	101	55	55	56	57	58	59	59
	90th	106	107	109	111	113	114	116	70	70	71	72	73	74	74
	95th	110	111	113	115	117	118	119	74	74	75	76	77	78	78
	99th	117	118	120	122	124	125	126	82	82	83	84	85	86	86
8	50th	94	95	97	99	100	102	102	56	57	58	59	60	60	61
	90th	107	109	110	112	114	115	116	71	72	72	73	74	75	76
	95th	111	112	114	116	118	119	120	75	76	77	78	79	79	80
	99th	119	120	122	123	125	127	127	83	84	85	86	87	87	88
9	50th	95	96	98	1200	102	103	104	57	58	59	60	61	61	62
	90th	109	110	112	114	115	117	118	72	73	74	75	76	76	77
	95th	113	114	116	118	119	121	121	76	77	78	79	80	81	81
	99th	120	121	123	125	127	128	129	84	85	86	87	88	88	89
10	50th	97	98	100	102	103	105	106	58	59	60	61	61	62	63
	90th	111	112	114	115	117	119	119	73	73	74	75	76	77	78
	95th	115	116	117	119	121	122	123	77	78	79	80	81	81	82
	99th	122	123	125	127	128	130	130	85	86	86	88	88	89	90

(*Continued*)

Table 29.1 (*Continued*)

Age (year)	BP Percentile ↓	Systolic BP (mmHg) ← Percentile of Height →							Distolic BP (mmHg) ← Percentile of Height →						
		5th	10th	25th	50th	75th	90th	95th	5th	10th	25th	50th	75th	90th	95th
11	50th	99	100	102	104	105	107	107	59	59	60	61	62	63	63
	90th	113	114	115	117	119	120	121	74	74	75	76	77	78	78
	96th	117	118	119	121	123	124	125	78	78	79	80	81	82	82
	99th	124	125	127	129	130	132	132	86	86	87	88	89	90	90
12	50th	101	102	104	106	108	109	110	59	60	61	62	69	63	64
	90th	115	116	118	120	121	123	123	74	75	75	76	77	78	79
	96th	119	120	122	123	125	127	127	78	79	80	81	92	82	83
	99th	126	127	129	131	133	134	135	86	87	88	89	90	90	91
13	50th	104	105	106	108	11	111	112	60	60	61	62	63	64	64
	90th	117	118	120	122	124	125	126	75	75	76	77	78	79	79
	96th	121	122	1247	126	128	129	130	79	79	80	81	82	83	83
	99th	128	130	131	133	135	136	137	87	87	88	89	90	91	91
14	50th	106	107	109	111	113	114	115	60	61	62	63	64	65	65
	90th	120	121	123	125	126	128	128	75	76	77	78	79	79	80
	96th	124	125	127	128	130	132	132	80	80	81	82	83	84	84
	99th	131	132	134	136	138	139	140	87	88	89	90	91	92	92
15	50th	109	110	112	113	115	117	117	61	62	63	64	65	66	66
	90th	122	124	125	127	129	130	131	76	77	78	79	80	80	81
	96th	126	127	129	131	133	134	135	81	81	82	83	84	85	85
	99th	134	135	136	138	140	142	142	88	89	90	91	92	93	93
16	50th	111	112	114	116	118	119	120	63	63	64	65	66	67	67
	90th	125	126	128	130	131	133	134	78	78	79	80	81	82	82
	96th	129	130	132	134	135	137	137	82	83	83	84	85	86	87
	99th	136	137	139	141	143	144	145	90	90	91	92	93	94	94
17	50th	114	115	116	118	120	121	122	66	66	66	67	68	69	70
	90th	127	128	130	132	134	135	136	80	80	81	82	83	84	84
	96th	131	132	134	136	138	139	140	84	85	86	87	87	88	89
	99th	139	140	141	143	145	146	147	92	93	83	94	95	96	97

any given child. The basic tenet is that the BP cuff should completely encircle the arm, the inflatable bladder should cover 40% of the arm circumference midway between the olecranon and acromion, and the bladder length should cover at least 80–100% of the arm circumference. The systolic BP is indicated by the first Korotkoff sound. The diastolic BP is indicated by the fifth Korotkoff sound or its disappearance. Palpation is useful for rapid determination of systolic BP but it tends to underestimate the auscultated BP by 10 mmHg or so. Doppler is very accurate in determining systolic BP but less so for diastolic BP.

Clinical presentation and etiology

Children and adolescents with hypertension are typically asymptomatic. The majority of affected children (80%) are receiving follow-up care for diseases known to be associated with hypertension, such as renal diseases. About 10–15% of hypertensive children are detected on evaluations performed routinely and not associated with symptoms. Five percent present in hypertensive crisis. A hypertensive crisis is characterized by extreme elevation

Table 29.2 Blood pressure levels for girls by age and height percentile. (Courtesy of the US National Heart Lung and Blood Institute, http://www.nhlbi.nih.gov/guidelines/hypertension/child_tbl.htm)

Age (year)	BP Percentile ↓	Systolic BP (mmHg) ← Percentile of Height →							Distolic BP (mmHg) ← Percentile of Height →						
		5th	10th	25th	50th	75th	90th	95th	5th	10th	25th	50th	75th	90th	95th
1	50th	83	84	85	86	88	89	90	38	39	39	40	41	41	42
	90th	97	97	98	100	101	102	103	52	53	53	54	55	55	56
	95th	100	101	102	104	105	106	107	55	57	57	58	59	59	60
	99th	108	108	109	111	112	113	114	64	64	65	65	66	67	67
2	50th	85	85	97	88	89	91	91	43	44	44	45	46	46	47
	90th	98	99	100	101	103	104	106	57	58	58	59	60	61	61
	95th	102	103	104	105	107	108	109	61	62	62	63	64	66	65
	99th	109	110	111	112	114	115	116	69	69	70	70	71	72	72
3	50th	86	97	88	89	91	92	93	47	48	48	49	50	60	51
	90th	100	100	102	103	104	106	106	61	62	62	63	64	64	65
	95th	104	104	105	107	108	109	110	65	66	66	67	58	68	69
	99th	111	111	113	114	115	116	117	73	73	74	74	75	76	76
4	50th	89	88	90	91	92	94	94	50	50	51	52	52	53	54
	90th	101	102	103	104	106	107	108	64	64	65	66	67	67	68
	95th	105	106	107	108	110	111	112	68	68	69	70	71	71	72
	99th	112	113	114	115	117	118	119	76	76	76	77	78	79	79
5	50th	89	90	91	93	94	95	96	52	53	53	54	55	55	56
	90th	103	103	105	106	107	109	109	66	67	69	68	69	69	70
	95th	107	107	108	110	111	112	113	70	71	71	72	73	73	74
	99th	114	114	116	117	118	120	120	78	78	79	79	80	81	81
6	50th	91	92	93	94	86	97	98	54	54	56	56	66	57	58
	90th	104	105	106	108	109	110	111	68	68	69	70	70	71	72
	95th	108	109	110	111	113	114	115	72	72	73	74	74	75	76
	99th	115	116	117	109	120	121	122	80	80	80	81	82	83	83
7	50th	93	93	95	96	97	99	99	55	56	56	57	58	58	59
	90th	106	107	108	109	111	112	113	69	70	70	71	72	72	73
	95th	110	111	112	113	115	116	116	73	74	74	75	76	76	77
	99th	117	118	119	120	122	123	124	81	81	82	82	83	84	84
8	50th	95	95	96	98	99	100	101	57	57	57	58	59	60	60
	90th	108	109	110	111	113	114	114	71	71	71	72	73	74	74
	95th	112	112	114	115	116	118	118	75	75	75	76	77	78	78
	99th	119	120	121	122	123	125	125	82	82	83	83	84	85	86
9	50th	96	97	98	100	101	102	103	58	58	58	59	60	61	61
	90th	110	110	112	113	114	116	116	75	72	72	73	74	75	75
	95th	114	114	115	117	118	119	120	76	76	76	77	78	79	79
	99th	121	121	123	124	125	127	127	83	83	84	84	85	86	87
10	50th	98	99	100	102	103	1047	106	59	59	59	60	61	62	62
	90th	112	112	114	115	116	118	118	73	73	73	74	75	76	76
	95th	116	116	117	119	120	121	122	77	77	77	78	79	80	80
	99th	123	123	125	126	127	129	129	84	84	85	86	86	87	88

(Continued)

Table 29.2 (*Continued*)

Age (year)	BP Percentile ↓	Systolic BP (mmHg) ← Percentile of Height →							Distolic BP (mmHg) ← Percentile of Height →						
		5th	10th	25th	50th	75th	90th	95th	5th	10th	25th	50th	75th	90th	95th
11	50th	100	101	102	103	105	106	107	60	60	60	61	62	63	63
	90th	114	114	116	117	118	119	120	74	74	74	75	76	77	77
	96th	118	118	119	121	122	123	124	78	78	78	79	90	81	81
	99th	125	125	126	128	129	130	131	85	85	86	87	87	88	89
12	50th	102	103	104	106	107	108	109	61	61	61	62	63	64	64
	90th	116	116	117	119	120	121	122	75	75	75	76	77	78	78
	96th	119	120	121	123	124	125	126	79	79	79	80	81	82	82
	99th	127	127	128	130	13	132	133	86	86	87	88	88	89	90
13	50th	104	105	106	107	109	110	110	62	61	62	63	64	65	65
	90th	117	118	119	121	122	123	124	76	76	76	77	78	79	79
	96th	121	122	123	124	126	127	128	80	80	80	81	82	83	83
	99th	128	129	130	132	133	134	135	87	87	88	89	89	90	91
14	50th	106	106	107	109	110	111	112	63	63	63	64	65	66	66
	90th	119	120	121	122	124	125	125	77	77	77	78	79	80	80
	96th	123	123	125	126	127	129	129	81	81	81	82	83	84	84
	99th	130	131	132	133	135	136	136	88	88	89	90	90	91	92
15	50th	107	108	109	110	111	113	113	64	64	64	65	66	67	67
	90th	120	121	122	123	125	126	127	78	78	78	79	80	81	81
	96th	124	125	126	127	129	130	131	82	82	82	83	94	85	85
	99th	131	132	133	134	136	137	138	89	89	90	91	91	92	93
16	50th	108	108	110	111	112	114	114	64	64	65	65	66	67	68
	90th	121	122	123	124	126	127	128	78	78	79	80	81	81	82
	96th	125	126	127	128	130	131	132	82	82	83	84	85	85	86
	99th	132	133	134	135	137	138	139	90	90	90	91	92	93	93
17	50th	108	109	110	111	113	114	115	64	66	65	66	67	67	68
	90th	122	122	123	125	126	127	128	78	79	79	80	81	81	82
	96th	125	126	127	129	130	131	132	82	83	83	84	85	85	86
	99th	133	133	134	136	137	138	139	90	90	91	91	92	93	93

of BP with systolic BP of 180 mmHg or higher and diastolic BP of 110 mmHg or higher. Also, symptoms including headache, vomiting, altered mental status, congestive heart failure, and pulmonary edema may complicate the presentation.

Symptoms associated with hypertension include:
- **Headache:**
  ◦ An important but inconsistent symptom in the pediatric age group
  ◦ Reported as a presenting symptom in 5–30% of children and is more likely to be present in those with severe or rapid elevation of BP.

- **Irritability:** May be an indication of a headache in an infant with hypertension.

Uncommon modes of presentation are:
- Abdominal pain;
- Visual disturbances;
- Failure to thrive;
- Bell's palsy;
- Chest pain;
- Decreased exercise tolerance;
- Neonates and infants may present with congestive heart failure;
- Epistaxis.

Causes of hypertension

Primary or essential hypertension

- No known cause

Secondary causes

- **Renal:** Glomerulonephritis, pyelonephritis, polycystic or dysplastic kidneys, hydronephrosis, hemolytic uremic syndrome, collagen vascular disease, nephrotoxic medications, radiation, renal artery stenosis, renal artery or vein thrombosis
- **Cardiovascular:** Coarctation of the aorta, patent ductus arteriosus
- **Endocrine:** Hyperthyroidism, pheochromocytoma, neuroblastoma, congenital adrenal hyperplasia, Cushing syndrome, hyperaldosteronism, hyperparathyroidism
- **Neurogenic:** Increased intracranial pressure, dysautonomia
- **Drugs:** Sympathomimetic drugs, amphetamines, steroids, oral contraceptives, heavy metal poisoning, cocaine
- **Miscellaneous:** Obesity, sickle cell anemia, Williams syndrome, Turner syndrome

Essential hypertension is rare in the young pediatric patient but may account for 12–18% of all pediatric hypertension.

Laboratory investigations

Laboratory investigations are directed at uncovering common causes of secondary hypertension (see above). A child under 10 years of age should have a complete evaluation, while an obese adolescent with mild hypertension can be approached first through weight management. The initial evaluation should include a thorough history, family history for cardiovascular diseases, physical examination with four extremity BPs, inspection for café-au-lait spots or other signs of a syndrome, fundoscopic examination, palpation of peripheral pulses, palpation to detect abdominal masses, and auscultation for abdominal bruits. CXR, EKG or echocardiogram may be obtained to

Table 29.3 Oral antihypertensives

Drug	Dose (mg/kg)	Frequency (hours)
Diuretics		
Hydrochlorothiazide	1–2	12–24
Chlorothiazide	0.5–2	24
Furosemide	1–2	6–12
Arterial dilators		
Hydralazine	1–5	12–8
Minoxidil	0.1–1	12
Adrenergic inhibitors		
Propranolol	1–3	8
Atenolol	1–2	12–24
Methyldopa	5–10	12
ACE inhibitors		
Captopril:		
<2 months	0.05–0.1	6–24
Infants and children	0.15–0.5	8–12
Older children and adolescents	6.25–12.5	8–12
Enalapril:		
Children	0.2–1	12–24
Adolescents	2.5–5 (max 40 mg)	12–24
Calcium channel blockers		
Nifedipine SR	30–120 mg total dose	24
Amlodipine	2.5–10 mg total dose	12–24

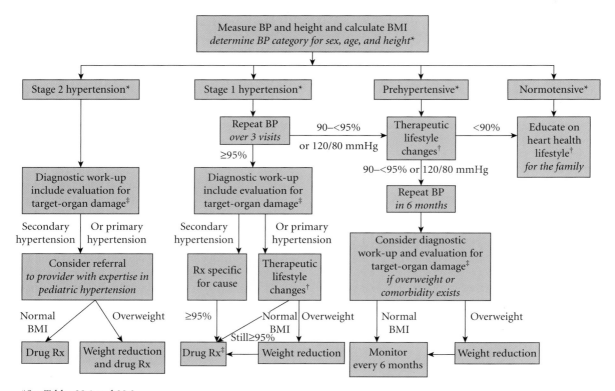

*See Tables 29.1 and 29.2
†Diet modification and physical activity.
‡Especially if younger, very high BP, little or no family history, diabetic, or other risk factors.

Figure 29.1 Management algorithm. BMI, body mass index; BP, blood pressure; Rx, prescription. (Courtesy of the US National Heart Lung and Blood Institute, http://www.nhlbi.nih.gov/health/prof/heart/hbp/hbp_ped.htm)

determine the presence of coarctation of the aorta, or a patent ductus arteriosus, or the effects of long-standing hypertension on the heart. Laboratory evaluation should include complete blood count, serum electrolytes, BUN (urea) and creatinine, serum cholesterol, plasma renin activity, drug screen, urinalysis, and urine culture. Renal ultrasound and radionuclide scan are useful in detecting anatomic and perfusion abnormalities.

Treatment

The approach to therapy is based on the cause and the severity of the hypertension. In an obese adolescent with hypertension, a change in lifestyle focusing on diet and regular exercise is a reasonable first step. The goal is to achieve BPs consistently below the 95th percentile. Medication is reserved for the child who does not respond to non-pharmacologic therapy or a child in whom there is evidence of end-organ damage or additional risk factors such as hyperlipidemia. The management algorithm recommended by the Fourth Report on the Diagnosis, Evaluation and Treatment of High Blood Pressure in Children and Adolescents is shown in Figure 29.1.

Acceptable drug classes for use in children include diuretics, ACE-Is, calcium channel blockers, angiotensin-receptor blockers, and beta-blockers (Table 29.3). Though some diuretics and beta-blockers have a long clinical history of safety and efficacy in children, the choice of agent is the preference of the treating physician. Medication can assist in controlling secondary hypertension during the evaluation of the primary cause.

Immediate parenteral treatment of hypertensive crisis is required to lower the BP. Diazoxide and nitroprusside are the medications of choice.

Further reading

Kher KK. Hypertension. In: Kher KK, Makker SP, eds. *Clinical Pediatric Nephrology*. New York: McGraw-Hill Inc., 1992, p. 329.

National High Blood Pressure Education Program Working Group on High Blood Pressure in Children and Adolescents. The fourth report on the diagnosis, evaluation, and treatment of high blood pressure in children and adolescents. http://www.nhlbi.nih.gov/health/prof/heart/hbp/hbp_ped.pdf

Staessen JA, Wang J, Bianchi G, Birkenhäger WH. Essential hypertension. *Lancet* 2003;361:1629–1641.

Sinaiko AR, Gomez-Martin O, Prineas RJ. Prevalence of "significant" hypertension in junior high school-aged children: the children and adolescent blood pressure program. *J Pediatr* 1989;114:664–669.

Sorof JM, Lai D, Turner J, Poffenbarger T, Portman RJ. Overweight, ethnicity, and the prevalence of hypertension in school-aged children. *Pediatrics* 2004;113:475–482.

30 Fetal cardiology

Helena M. Gardiner

Imperial College, London, UK

Why do we screen for congenital heart disease in the fetus?

Congenital heart disease is both common and important. It affects almost 1% of all fetuses and major heart disease is present in about 3.5 per 1000 live births.

There are several advantages in knowing that a fetus has a cardiac defect as the place and timing of delivery can be discussed in advance and the baby delivered to the cardiac surgeons in the best possible condition. It is also important to recognize that approximately one-third of fetuses with heart defects will have an extracardiac malformation or abnormal chromosomes (aneuploidy). An early diagnosis allows the parents the chance to discuss these associated abnormalities with experts in the field and to decide upon the future of the pregnancy.

All newborn babies have a clinical examination before discharge home, but studies have found that fewer than half of them who are later found to have heart disease are detected at this stage. Some major heart defects depend on patency of the arterial duct to support the systemic or pulmonary circulation and, if the arterial duct closes when the baby is at home, cardiovascular collapse and death or serious brain injury prior to surgery may result.

When do we screen?

The heart is fully formed by 6–8 weeks, but is difficult to image using current ultrasound technologies. Traditionally the fetal heart has been examined at the fetal anomaly scan, which is usually performed at about 20 weeks of gestation. This screening ultrasound examination is designed to measure fetal biometry and thus assess whether growth has been appropriate for estimated gestational age and whether there are any structural defects in any of the organ systems. Examination of the fetal heart was introduced into this scan in the form of assessment of the four chambers of the heart in the 1980s. Standards in the United Kingdom have since been updated to include views of the great arterial cross-over (also known as the outflow tracts) and the pulmonary trunk and its branches (the three-vessel view). The final view, that showing the transverse aortic and ductal arches and superior caval vein and their relationship to the trachea (the three-vessel and tracheal view), has yet to be formally incorporated into this screening program.

Nuchal translucency screening was universally introduced in the United Kingdom in 2007 to detect aneuploid fetuses early. It is recognized that an increased nuchal translucency is associated with a structural heart defect in some and these pregnancies ideally require a detailed fetal cardiac scan at 14 weeks of gestation.

Whom do we screen?

The population thought to be at increased risk for congenital heart disease, previously termed the "high-risk" population, comprises:
• Pregnancies where there is a family history of congenital heart disease in a first-degree relative;
• Mothers who have type I or type II diabetes;
• Mothers with systemic disease, such as systemic lupus erythematosus or Sjögren, who have Anti-Ro antibodies that may cross the placenta;
• Mothers receiving drugs for conditions such as epilepsy where the drug may have teratogenic effects.

Pediatric Heart Disease: A Practical Guide, First Edition. Piers E. F. Daubeney, Michael L. Rigby, Koichiro Niwa, and Michael A. Gatzoulis. © 2012 Blackwell Publishing Ltd. Published 2012 by Blackwell Publishing Ltd.

However, the 10% of mothers in this group have a slightly increased risk, usually not greater than 3%, compared with the normal population risk of 1%. The vast majority of babies born with congenital heart disease are born to mothers with no identifiable risk factors, hence the importance of improving the antenatal cardiac screening of the whole population.

How do we screen for congenital heart disease in the fetus?

Ultrasound imaging is the primary screening tool to detect cardiac malformations. The heart lies horizontally in the fetal thorax and so five transverse planes through the fetal abdomen and thorax provide a series of views similar to those seen on MRI that will detect virtually all major cardiac malformations. The practical sequence is to establish fetal lie and sweep up the fetal chest imaging abdominal situs, the four chamber view, the outflow tracts (aortic root and great arterial cross-over), and the three-vessel and tracheal view (transverse aortic and ductal arch and superior caval vein, with trachea). With training these views can be easily incorporated into the fetal anomaly screening scan at 20 weeks.

Cardiac details

At each level the cardiac structures are assessed for symmetry, the characteristic features of left- or right-sided morphology, the cardiac connections, and the presence of septal defects (Figure 30.1). Defects can be identified readily using the five transverse views. Color Doppler can be a useful tool for recognizing reversal of flow, especially in the three-vessel and tracheal view.

If a cardiac defect is found, extracardiac malformations should be sought, including ultrasound evidence of a chromosomal defect such as trisomy 21, 13 or 18.

Referral to the fetal cardiologist

The fetal cardiologist will see cases referred for suspected ultrasound abnormality and, in general, more than 90% of them are true positives. They may also see some of the women identified at their booking scan to fall into the high-risk groups, although most are now seen by fetal medicine specialists and only referred for suspected cardiac anomaly.

Referral criteria for fetal echocardiography

Fetal factors

- Extracardiac anomalies
- Aneuploidy
- Monochorionic fetal pregnancy
- Fetal cardiac arrhythmia

Maternal factors

- Family history/maternal congenital heart disease
- Pre-existing type I or II diabetes mellitus
- Autoimmune antibodies (connective tissue disease)
- Teratogenic drugs (e.g. lithium)

Ultrasound findings

- Raised nuchal translucency (>3.5 mm*)
- Suspicious or "non-diagnostic" cardiac scan

*Fetuses with a raised nuchal less than this may have a two-fold increased risk of congenital heart disease, but in most centers there is insufficient capacity to offer these mothers a detailed cardiac scan.

Fetal Heart Screening in 5 Transverse Views

A systematic examination of the heart, including orientation, connections and relationships

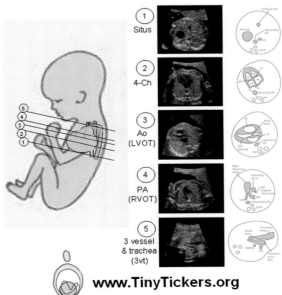

www.TinyTickers.org

Figure 30.1 Training poster showing the five transverse views used in the systematic examination of the fetal heart. (Reproduced with permission from Tiny Tickers, the congenital heart disease charity (www.tinytickers.org).)

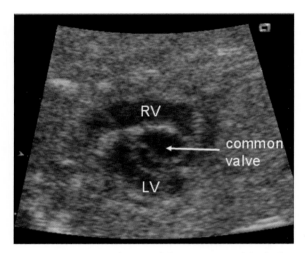

Figure 30.2 Ultrasound image of short axis view of the fetal heart confirming a common atrioventricular valve associated with trisomy 21. LV, left ventricle; RV, right ventricle.

If a cardiac abnormality is confirmed, the diagnosis is further refined by use of additional planes such as short axis and longitudinal planes (Figure 30.2). Color flow mapping and Doppler are used to assess flow and function not only in the heart, but also in the arterial and venous ducts, pulmonary veins, isthmus, and the middle cerebral artery in left heart obstructive disease.

Extracardiac malformations and aneuploidy

If extracardiac malformations are suspected, the fetal medicine team will also check for these and confirm fetal growth and amniotic fluid index. The parents ideally should be counseled jointly by a team that initially will include the fetal cardiologist and fetal medicine consultant, and also involve the early input of the cardiac liaison nurse. Additional appointments may be organized with the genetic counselors, cardiac and pediatric surgeons, adult congenital cardiologists, and other specialists such as hematologists where appropriate. It may be that a cardiac lesion such as an interrupted aortic arch will be the first sign of 22q11 deletion in an already affected family. The skills of the multidisciplinary team are essential in managing these challenging situations.

Preparation for delivery

Following the diagnosis of a structural heart defect, the fetus is observed throughout pregnancy using serial ultrasound and Doppler. This is to check for changes in heart morphology, growth, and function, as well as to measure fetal growth and check well-being. Serial diameters and Doppler velocities and assessment of ventricular function may be helpful in determining whether a heart defect is likely to be suitable for a one- or two-ventricle surgical pathway after birth. Close liaison with the other specialists involved is critical to successful perinatal transition. These will include the local obstetricians, neonatologists, cardiac intensive care and specialist nurses. Regular multidisciplinary planning meetings before delivery are helpful in ensuring good communication and delivering the new baby to the surgeons in the best possible state.

Serial assessment of placental function and fetal growth is important, particularly towards the end of pregnancy, in order to plan the timing of delivery. Near to term, fetal lie will be reassessed to determine whether the baby is in a cephalic or breech position as this may guide the mode of delivery. If the fetus is to be delivered early, steroids will be given to the mother in order to mature the fetal lungs and minimize the associated problems of respiratory disease. Clearly there needs to be close liaison with the neonatal unit receiving the baby.

Delivery

Most babies can be delivered vaginally and only those with hydrops, poor ventricular function, and bradyarrhythmias will require delivery by cesarean section. The decision to maintain ductal patency using prostaglandin is important in cases with a duct-dependent systemic or pulmonary circulation. The need for this is usually clear from scans made during the pregnancy and can be documented in the neonatal notes to avoid any confusion. The timing of surgery for extracardiac malformations will require planning and coordination of appropriate equipment and expertise.

Helping the family

Some families will live remote from their nearest cardiac center and therefore the place and timing of delivery for these families will be critical. They may have other children and will require help in planning for the delivery of the affected child. Most cardiac centers have facilities for families to stay, and play specialists who are expert in introducing the other children to concepts of cardiac disease in their new sibling and preparing them for future visits to hospital.

Fetal therapy

Arrhythmia: diagnosis and treatment

One of the important aims in tachyarrhythmia assessment is to make the diagnosis (one-to-one conduction or not) and identify the mechanism correctly (long or short RP [the interval between the electrical signal of ventricular (R) and atrial (P) activation] tachycardia) so that the most effective drug can be administered to the fetus and time is not lost in achieving control. Doppler methods may be used to differentiate these mechanisms but require skill and experience.

Non-invasive fetal EKG and magnetocardiography are under development; one of their potential advantages is that the recording is an electrical, rather than mechanical, record of the arrhythmia. Usually it can be made by personnel unskilled in Doppler ultrasound.

Certain high-risk groups such as mothers with anti-Ro or La antibodies require evaluation as their fetuses have a 3% risk of developing complete heart block, increasing to 15% in families in whom a previous case has been identified. Although there is to date no clear benefit from prophylactic maternal therapy, such as plasmaphoresis or immunoglobulin administration to prevent transmission of antibodies, nor has the use of steroids conclusively prevented progression of second-degree heart block, hopefully newer technologies will enable a more robust study of the natural history of this disease and guide us towards the optimal therapeutic strategy for the individual patient.

Fetal pacing may have a limited role for fetuses with hydrops and/or a heart rate of below 55 bpm who present in the second trimester when delivery is not an option. There have been occasional reports of pacing in humans, but there is usually important cardiomyopathy in fetuses requiring this type of intervention and cases are rare. We will have to await the results of clinical studies to assess any future role of pacing in patient management.

Fetal cardiac surgery

Fetal cardiac surgery represents a new challenge in fetal therapy over and above current experience of surgery in the low birth weight population. Both open surgery on cardiopulmonary bypass and the less "invasive" catheter techniques have been used. The rationale underlying *in utero* surgical procedures is to prevent extracardiac secondary damage resulting from the malformation.

Conditions where open fetal surgery may prove beneficial include absent pulmonary valve syndrome, which is often associated with tracheobronchial compression; Ebstein malformation associated with significant lung hypoplasia; and small central pulmonary arteries and major collateral vessels, in order to promote pulmonary arborization and growth.

Fetal surgery on bypass is challenging, particularly because the placental vasculature is much more reactive than the lung vasculature and manipulation may result in fetal death. However, there is now a 90% survival in animal models using a hemo-pump to maintain placental flow. One hour of bypass time is technically feasible, making this more attractive in selected cases.

Fetal catheter interventions

These same principles guide the use of catheter interventions in the fetus. Catheter interventions have been performed by several groups in the United States and Europe to treat severe aortic and pulmonary stenosis or atresia and to open a closed or restrictive interatrial communication. The underlying rationale is to promote growth of the supporting ventricle to achieve a two-ventricle circulation, prevent secondary damage to the myocardium and lungs in particular, and improve the fetal circulation in cases of hydrops. These programs have shown technical success but failure of the left ventricle to grow, and a study is required to assess outcome compared with contemporaneous natural history. However, to attempt a two-ventricle circulation repair in borderline cases may lead to demise, whereas a one-ventricle circulation may, in some cases, provide a good outcome with a satisfactory quality of life.

Antenatal surgery may, by its complex nature, utilizes more resources initially, but if it proves successful for the sickest fetuses it may improve eventual outcome because the fetus remains connected to the placenta and is nursed postoperatively within the mother. If successful, this may reduce mortality and morbidity for babies who normally require extensive expertise and resources postoperatively.

Conclusions

Fetal cardiology has been advanced by earlier detection of congenital heart disease and technologic advances enabling us to provide high-level non-invasive assessment and in some cases therapy. There are now realistic opportunities for better understanding of the development of the cardiovascular system before birth and for examining further different therapeutic strategies.

Further reading

Clur SA, Ottenkamp J, Bilardo CM. The nuchal translucency and the fetal heart: a literature review. *Prenat Diagn* 2009;29: 739–748.

Fouron JC. Fetal arrhythmias: the Saint-Justine hospital experience. *Prenat Diagn* 2004;24:1068–1080.

Gardiner HM. Fetal echocardiography: 20 years of progress. *Heart* 2001;86 (Suppl II):ii12–ii22.

McElhinney DB, Marshall AC, Wilkins-Haug LE, *et al.* Predictors of technical success and postnatal biventricular outcome after in utero aortic valvuloplasty for aortic stenosis with evolving hypoplastic left heart syndrome. *Circulation* 2009;120:1482–1490.

Richmond S, Wren C. Early diagnosis of congenital heart disease. *Semin Neonatol* 2001;6:27–35.

Tulzer G, Arzt W, Franklin RC, Loughna PV, Mair R, Gardiner HM. Fetal pulmonary valvuloplasty for critical pulmonary stenosis or atresia with intact septum. *Lancet* 2002;360:1567–1568.

Wimalasundera RC, Gardiner HM. Congenital heart disease and aneuploidy. *Prenat Diagn* 2004;24:1116–1122.

31 Adult congenital heart disease

Anselm Uebing[1,2] and Michael A. Gatzoulis[1,3]

[1]Royal Brompton Hospital, London, UK
[2]University Hospital of Schleswig-Holstein, Kiel, Germany
[3]National Heart and Lung Institute, Imperial College, London, UK

General principles

Continuous improvement of medical and surgical therapy over the past five decades has led to more than 85% of children with congenital heart lesions surviving into adulthood. There are in fact more than 250 000 adults with congenital heart disease currently living in the United Kingdom and this number continues to grow. However, treatment of congenital heart disease can rarely be considered as being curative and about half of adults with congenital heart disease face the prospect of further surgery or non-surgical intervention, arrhythmia, heart failure, and – if managed inappropriately – premature death (Figure 31.1). As patients with congenital heart disease grow older, acquired heart or general health problems impose on the underlying cardiac anomaly. This becomes an increasing problem as the patient population ages (Figure 31.2).

Patients with congenital heart disease may present in adulthood with mild unrepaired lesions, undetected defects (often during pregnancy) or residua or sequelae from surgical repair.

Groups who need to attend a specialized center

- Assessment of patients if congenital heart disease is suspected
- Follow-up and continuous care for patients with congenital heart disease
- Further surgery or non-surgical interventions
- Risk assessment and counseling on non-cardiac surgery
- Risk assessment and counseling on pregnancy
- Counseling on contraception

Tertiary adult congenital heart disease centers provide optimal care for patients with congenital heart disease, reducing errors and avoiding crisis management. But tertiary care is not possible for every patient all the time for many reasons, including geography, lack of capacity, and need for local emergency care. It is therefore essential that tertiary centers offer educational resources to patients and a broader professional audience, including not only pediatric and adult cardiologists but also family physicians, obstetricians, surgeons, and anesthetists. Education is in fact the key to improving the care of adults with congenital heart disease.

Transition of care from pediatric cardiology to adult congenital heart disease

Pediatric cardiology centers play a key role in securing appropriate lifelong care for patients with congenital heart disease. Not only do these centers often form the nucleus for adult congenital heart units, but they also have to transfer care to the adult unit when patients reach adulthood. Transition pathways need to be identified and should take place in a structured way. A transition clinic run jointly with the pediatric cardiologist and the specialist in adult congenital heart disease would be an ideal model. Patients need to be prepared and educated regarding their diagnosis and specific health behaviors prior to transition, and this needs to be reinforced during transition. Comprehensive information, including diagnosis, previous surgical and/or catheter interventions, medical therapy, investigations, current outpatient clinic reports and medication should be copied to the patient and be provided to the adult congenital heart disease facility.

Pediatric Heart Disease: A Practical Guide, First Edition. Piers E. F. Daubeney, Michael L. Rigby, Koichiro Niwa, and Michael A. Gatzoulis.
© 2012 Blackwell Publishing Ltd. Published 2012 by Blackwell Publishing Ltd.

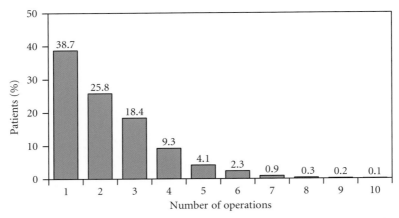

Figure 31.1 Cardiac operations performed at the Adult Congenital Heart Disease Unit at the Mayo Clinic from 1987 to 2003. More than 30% of the patients had three operations or more. (Modified from Warnes CA. The adult with congenital heart disease: born to be bad? *J Am Coll Cardiol* 2005;46:1–8.)

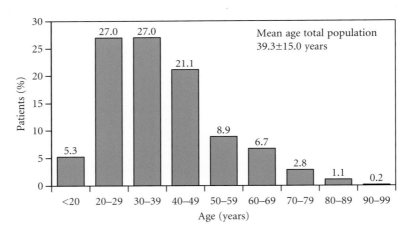

Figure 31.2 Age of the patient population seen at the Adult Congenital Heart Disease Unit, Royal Brompton Hospital, London, UK. More than 40% of patients are older than 40 years.

Furthermore, to facilitate care, it is essential to share this information with local general cardiologists and family physicians.

Pregnancy in congenital heart disease

Pregnancy carries an increased risk of adverse maternal and fetal outcome in patients with congenital heart disease. Timely pre-pregnancy counseling should therefore be offered to all women with congenital heart disease to prevent avoidable risks and crisis management, and to allow patients to plan their lives. Adequate care during pregnancy, delivery, and the postpartum period requires close cooperation between cardiologists, obstetricians, and anesthesiologists. Successful pregnancy is feasible for most women with congenital heart disease at relatively low risk when appropriate counseling and optimal care are provided.

Maternal and fetal risk associated with pregnancy

Maternal risk factors

The risk for the mother with congenital heart disease of having adverse cardiovascular events (arrhythmia, stroke, heart failure, death) during pregnancy or the postpartum increases with:

- Poor functional class before pregnancy (NYHA > II)
- Cyanosis
- Left heart obstruction (mitral valve area < 2 cm², aortic valve area < 1.5 cm², left ventricular outflow tract gradient > 30 mmHg before pregnancy)
- Impaired systemic ventricular function (ejection fraction < 40%)
- Impaired function of the subpulmonary ventricle
- Severe pulmonary regurgitation
- Preconception history of adverse cardiac events such as arrhythmia, stroke, and heart failure

Fetal risk factors

Additional risk to fetus arises from:

- Maternal smoking
- Maternal age < 20 or >35 years
- Treatment with anticoagulants

Different congenital heart lesions carry specific risks based on their morphologic features, previous operations, and current hemodynamic status. Potential hazards during pregnancy and recommendations regarding treatment during pregnancy and the peripartum are summarized in Table 31.1.

Conditions such as pulmonary hypertension, Eisenmenger syndrome, or Marfan syndrome with aortic root dilatation > 4 cm carry a prohibitively high risk for maternal death. These women should be discouraged from pregnancy and therapeutic termination should be offered. The need for thorough assessment of patients with congenital heart disease **before** pregnancy cannot be overemphasized. It forms the basis for risk stratification, advice, and decision-making.

Contraception and termination of pregnancy

Most women with congenital heart disease will be participating in lifestyles and sexual activities similar to their peers. For this reason, contraceptive counseling must be part of their healthcare plan and discussions about contraception should begin in early adolescence to avoid unplanned pregnancies.

A variety of contraceptive methods is available but unfortunately no method is perfect. "Natural methods" (abstinence, withdrawal, safe period) and "barrier methods" (condoms, diaphragm) have unacceptably high failure rates and cannot be recommended for women in whom any unplanned pregnancy carries a substantial risk.

Combined oral contraceptives should be avoided in patients at risk of thromboembolism (cyanosis, impaired cardiac function, atrial arrhythmias, Fontan-type circulation, prosthetic heart valves) because of the thrombophilic properties of estrogen. For these patients, the use of warfarin to counteract the effects of the combined pill is one option (although it carries all the risks of warfarin administration), while another is to use progestagens only. The "mini pill" or "progestagen-only pill" has few serious side effects but its failure rate is higher than that of the combined pill, and irregular uterine bleeding can be a problem. "Depot" injections of progestagen are an alternative to the "mini pill," especially for adolescents who find it difficult to remember to take a pill or for whom compliance is a concern.

The recent introduction of an intrauterine coil impregnated with progestagen has been an important advance in contraception for patients with high risk of pregnancy-related complications and thromboembolism. Mirena® coils are highly effective and safe. They reduce menstrual bleeding (causing amenorrhea in 80%) and carry a very low risk of infection and ectopic pregnancy. As vagal bradycardia with hypotension can occur during insertion, these coils should be inserted in an operating theater with appropriate anesthetic staff in attendance. Antibiotic prophylaxis at insertion is advisable.

Sterilization (laparoscopic tubal occlusion) should be considered only for women in whom pregnancy would carry a high risk, such as those with Eisenmenger syndrome, or if a couple decide that they never want to have children. Sterilization has the advantage of being permanent, although there is still a 1 in 200 pregnancy rate, and there are surgical risks associated with the procedure. Use of the Mirena® coil may well be safer overall.

Careful and adequate contraception is essential for women with congenital heart disease, especially as termination of pregnancy itself is not without risks, and the emotional impact of termination on women and their families when they actually want a child but feel they cannot take the risk is considerable.

Table 31.1 Pregnancy-related risks for women with congenital heart disease by specific lesion. (Reproduced from Uebing A, Steer PJ, Yentis SM, Gatzoulis MA. Pregnancy and congenital heart disease. *BMJ* 2006;332:401–406 with permission from BMJ Publishing Group Ltd.)

Relative risk	Lesion	Exclude before pregnancy	Potential hazards	Recommended treatment during pregnancy and peripartum
Low	Ventricular septal defect (VSD)	Pulmonary arterial hypertension	Arrhythmias Endocarditis (unoperated or residual VSD)	Antibiotic prophylaxis for unoperated or residual VSD
	Atrial septal defect (unoperated)	Pulmonary arterial hypertension Ventricular dysfunction	Arrhythmias Thromboembolic events	Thromboprophylaxis if bed rest is required Consider low-dose aspirin during pregnancy
	Coarctation (repaired)	Recoarctation Aneurysm formation at the site of repair (MRI) Associated lesion such as bicuspid aortic valve (+aortic stenosis and/or aortic regurgitation), ascending aortopathy Systemic hypertension Ventricular dysfunction	Pre-eclampsia Aortic dissection Congestive heart failure Endarteritis	Beta-blockers if necessary to control systemic blood pressure Consider elective cesarean section before term in case of aortic aneurysm formation or uncontrollable systemic hypertension Antibiotic prophylaxis
	Tetralogy of Fallot	Severe right ventricular outflow tract obstruction Severe pulmonary regurgitation Right ventricular dysfunction DiGeorge syndrome (present in up to 15% of patients)	Arrhythmias Right ventricular failure Endocarditis	Consider preterm delivery in the rare case of right ventricular failure Antibiotic prophylaxis
Moderate	Mitral stenosis	Severe stenosis Pulmonary venous hypertension	Atrial fibrillation Thromboembolic events Pulmonary edema	Beta-blockers Low-dose aspirin Consider bed rest during the third trimester with additional thromboprophylaxis Antibiotic prophylaxis

	Lesion	Risk factors	Complications	Management
	Aortic stenosis	Severe stenosis (peak pressure gradient on Doppler > 80 mmHg, ST segment depression, symptoms) Left ventricular dysfunction	Arrhythmias Angina Endocarditis Left ventricular failure	Bed rest during third trimester with thromboprophylaxis Consider balloon aortic valvotomy (for severe symptomatic valvar stenosis) or preterm cesarean section if cardiac decompensation ensues (bypass surgery carries a 20% risk of fetal death) Antibiotic prophylaxis
	Systemic right ventricle: TGA after atrial switch procedure ccTGA	Ventricular dysfunction Severe systemic AV valve regurgitation Arrhythmias (brady- and tachy-arrhythmias) Heart failure (NHYA > II) Obstruction of venous pathways after atrial switch as venous blood flow significantly increases during pregnancy	Right ventricular dysfunction (potentially persisting after pregnancy) Heart failure Arrhythmias Thromboembolic events Endocarditis	Regular monitoring of heart rhythm Restore sinus rhythm in case of atrial flutter (DC cardioversion usually effective and safe) Alter afterload reduction therapy (stop ACE inhibitors; consider beta-blockers) Low-dose aspirin (75mg) Antibiotic prophylaxis
	Cyanotic lesions *without* pulmonary hypertension	Ventricular dysfunction	Hemorrhage (bleeding diathesis) Thromboembolic events Increased cyanosis Heart failure Endocarditis	Consider bed rest and oxygen supplementation to maintain oxygen saturation and promote oxygen tissue delivery (thromboprophylaxis with low molecular weight heparin) Antibiotic prophylaxis
	Fontan-type circulation	Ventricular dysfunction Arrhythmias Heart failure (NYHA > II)	Heart failure Arrhythmias Thromboembolic complications Endocarditis	Consider anticoagulation with low molecular weight heparin and aspirin throughout pregnancy Maintain sufficient filling pressures and avoid dehydration during delivery Antibiotic prophylaxis
High	Marfan syndrome	Aortic root dilatation > 4 cm	Type A dissection of the aorta	Beta-blockers in all patients Elective cesarean section when aortic root > 45 mm (~35 weeks of gestation)
	Eisenmenger syndrome; other pulmonary arterial hypertension	Ventricular dysfunction Arrhythmias	30–50% risk of death related to pregnancy Arrhythmia Heart failure Endocarditis for Eisenmenger syndrome	Therapeutic termination should be offered If pregnancy continues close cardiovascular monitoring, early bed rest, pulmonary vasodilator therapy with supplemental oxygen should be considered Close monitoring necessary for 10 days postpartum

The risk of termination increases with increasing gestational age. Once the decision to terminate has been made, it should therefore be performed as early as possible, preferably in the first trimester. Suction curettage under local anesthesia is the preferred method. Medical abortion with oral antiprogesterones and vaginally administered prostaglandins is probably contraindicated as the hemodynamic effects of the drugs used are unpredictable and the 5% incidence of heavy bleeding and/or retained products with infection is a worry.

Specific congenital heart lesions

Patients with congenital heart disease require life-long follow-up. The most common congenital heart lesions will briefly be reviewed to support this thesis.

Left-sided obstructive lesions

Aortic valve stenosis/bicuspid valve (see also Chapter 11)
Patients can present with exercise intolerance, dyspnea, chest pain, presyncope, or syncope and are at risk for endocarditis and sudden cardiac death (severe cases). Aortic root enlargement from cystic media changes is often seen in these patients. The lesion can progress with age.

Management
Therapy is indicated when the peak pressure gradient across the valve is > 60 mmHg or > 50 mmHg in a symptomatic patient. Balloon valvuloplasty is an option in selected patients (aortic valve not calcified) but must be considered as a palliative procedure. Aortic valve replacement is considered a more definitive treatment. Pulmonary autograft aortic valve replacement (Ross procedure) has become the surgical procedure of choice in young adults and women of reproductive age as no permanent anticoagulation is needed.

Key clinical points
- Progression of aortic stenosis with age
- High prevalence of aortic root enlargement in patients with bicuspid aortic valve
- Indication for treatment if the peak pressure gradient is > 60 mmHg or > 50 mmHg in a symptomatic patient
- Ross procedure treatment of choice in women of reproductive age (no need for anticoagulation)

Subaortic stenosis (see Chapter 11)
Patients with a discrete fibromuscular subaortic stenosis have usually undergone surgery in childhood. But this lesion has a tendency for regrowth (~30% at 10 years after repair). Predictors for recurrence are a preoperative gradient > 40 mmHg, a postoperative gradient > 10 mmHg, and young age at repair. Aortic regurgitation resulting from long-standing turbulent blood flow in the left ventricular outflow tract may develop with this lesion.

Management
Surgical therapy (resection of fibrous tissue plus myomectomy) is indicated in a symptomatic patient if the peak pressure gradient is > 60 mmHg or aortic regurgitation occurs.

Aortic regurgitation
Aortic regurgitation can result from several congenital conditions:
- Congenitally abnormal aortic valve (bicuspid valve with dilatation of the ascending aorta, congenital aortic stenosis after balloon valvuloplasty, tetralogy of Fallot with dilatation of the aortic root);
- Subaortic stenosis damaging the aortic valve;
- Aortic cusp prolapse from a perimembranous ventricular septal defect (VSD);
- Aortic root dilatation from connective tissue disorder (Marfan);
- Endocarditis (acute onset of aortic regurgitation).

Management
Timely surgery to replace or repair the aortic valve has a good long-term outlook. To identify patients with early symptoms of left ventricular dysfunction is therefore crucial in the management of these patients. All patients with aortic regurgitation need regular follow-up. Vasodilator therapy (ACE inhibitors, calcium antagonists) is commonly used in patients with moderate or severe aortic regurgitation and may reduce the need for operation.

Indications for aortic valve replacement are:
- Symptoms such as dyspnea, chest pain or heart failure;
- Left ventricular dilatation (end-diastolic left ventricular dimension > 70 mm; end-systolic left ventricular dimension > 55 mm);
- Left ventricular dysfunction (ejection fraction < 50%).

Coarctation (see Chapter 12)
Coarctation of the aorta is usually postoperative in adulthood, but adult patients with unrepaired coarctation present as well. Life expectancy is reduced in coarctation

patients mainly because the majority of repaired patients will develop systemic hypertension (irrespective of age at repair or presence of a residual gradient). Early atherosclerotic disease is therefore common and accounts for morbidity and mortality.

Complications after coarctation repair

- Systemic hypertension
- Re-coarctation
- Aneurysm formation at the site of repair and aortic dissection
- Progressive aortic valve disease
- Cerebral stroke from a ruptured berry aneurysm
- Heart failure from long-standing left ventricular pressure load

---

Key clinical and investigation findings

- Upper limb hypertension and differential arm–leg pulses (a pressure difference of ≥ 20 mmHg would suggest significant coarctation)
- Continuous murmur in the back
- **EKG:** Left ventricular hypertrophy
- **CXR:** "3 sign" caused by narrowing of the aorta at the site of coarctation with dilatation of the vessel before and after the coarctation), "rib notching"
- **MRI:** Useful to delineate the exact anatomy of the coarctation, possible aneurysm formation, and, using contrast magnetic resonance angiography, to visualize the arch geometry and collaterals. Flow velocity mapping can assess the degree of stenosis

---

Management

- Meticulous treatment of systemic hypertension (beta-blockers, ACE inhibitors).
- If pressure peak-to-peak gradient across the coarctation is > 20 mmHg and/or proximal hypertension, surgical repair or stenting of the coarctation is indicated.
- Interventional implantation of an endovascular stent graft can be offered in specialized centers to seal aneurysms at the site of coarctation.

Left-to-right shunt lesions

Ventricular septal defect (see Chapter 9)

Most patients with a VSD will have been repaired by adulthood, but adult patients can present with:

- A restrictive VSD (native or residual) that produces a significant pressure gradient between the left and right ventricle and usually a small but not significant left-to-right shunt, sometimes with mild enlargement of the left atrium and ventricle;
- A moderately restrictive (native or residual) VSD with a moderate shunt and left atrial and ventricular enlargement;
- A non-restrictive VSD or Eisenmenger VSD with pulmonary hypertension and cyanosis.

Complications in adulthood
- Endocarditis
- Atrial or ventricular arrhythmia from atrial and ventricular enlargement
- Complete heart block from previous surgery with damage to the AV node
- Pulmonary hypertension can progress in patients even after successful closure of the defect late in childhood (> 6 months of age)
- Aortic regurgitation from prolapse of the aortic valve (if the defect is perimembranous or doubly-committed)
- Heart failure resulting from left-to-right shunting or aortic regurgitation
- Pulmonary artery stenosis (from previous pulmonary artery banding)

Management
Patients with a restrictive VSD and those after successful closure have an excellent long-term outcome. Their life expectancy is close to normal.

Patients with moderately restrictive and non-restrictive VSDs need timely surgery. When pulmonary hypertension is present, closure is considered a high-risk procedure and can only be considered if there is still a predominantly left-to-right shunt (Qp:Qs > 1.5), response of the pulmonary vasculature to a vasodilator, or evidence from lung biopsy that the pulmonary artery changes resulting from hypertension are reversible.

Key clinical points

- Assess hemodynamic importance of the defect (left atrial and ventricular enlargement indicates significant shunting)
- Exclude pulmonary hypertension when closure of a VSD is consideredExclude aortic regurgitation in a restrictive perimembranous VSD

Atrial septal defect (see Chapter 9)

Adult patients with an unclosed atrial septal defect (ASD) can present with:

- Dyspnea on exertion;
- Palpitations due to atrial tachyarrhythmia;
- Cardiomegaly on CXR;
- Cerebrovascular events from paradoxical embolism;
- Heart failure.

Management

An ASD that results in right atrial and ventricular enlargement with a mean pulmonary artery pressure of less than 50% of systemic arterial pressure should be closed irrespective of symptoms.

Patients who had ASD closure before the age of 25 years have a normal long-term survival. Patients who underwent closure at an older age and those with elevated pulmonary artery pressure before closure have lower long-term survival rates. However, even patients who present at an age older than 40 years benefit from ASD closure in that it improves survival, functional class, and exercise tolerance, and reduces the risk of heart failure and pulmonary hypertension. The risk of arrhythmia remains high in these patients.

Atrioventricular septal defect (see Chapter 9)

The physiologic consequences of an atrioventricular septal defect (AVSD) are similar to a VSD and ASD. Adult patients with repaired AVSDs can present with:
- Complete heart block;
- Atrioventricular valve regurgitation or stenosis;
- Pulmonary hypertension;
- Left ventricular outflow tract obstruction.

Patients with unrepaired AVSDs with a large ventricular component present with Eisenmenger syndrome. These are often patients with Down syndrome, some of whom were not offered repair during the earlier years of open heart surgery.

Cyanotic congenital defects
Tetralogy of Fallot (see Chapter 15)

The majority of adults with tetralogy of Fallot will have undergone complete repair in childhood, often with transannular patch enlargement of the right ventricular outflow tract or implantation of a conduit from the right ventricle to the pulmonary arteries. Many patients will also have had a prior systemic-to-pulmonary artery shunt (i.e. Blalock–Taussig, Waterston, Potts shunts) to increase pulmonary blood flow in severe cases of pulmonary stenosis or pulmonary atresia.

Potential residua from previous surgery
- Branch pulmonary artery stenosis from previous shunt procedure (especially Waterston shunts)

- Right ventricular outflow tract obstruction (subvalvar, valvar or supravalvar pulmonary stenosis)
- Pulmonary regurgitation is almost always present when transannular patch enlargement of the right ventricular outflow tract was performed at repair
- Residual VSD

Long-term complications after tetralogy repair
- **Pulmonary regurgitation:** If mild or moderate, is usually well-tolerated. Severe pulmonary regurgitation has deleterious long-term effects. It is related to **right ventricular dilatation, right ventricular dysfunction, tricuspid valve regurgitation.**
- **Aortic regurgitation:** Can result from damage to the valve during VSD closure or secondary to an intrinsic abnormality of the aortic root ("cystic media necrosis").
- **Left ventricular dysfunction:** Can be associated with severe right ventricular enlargement and dysfunction, the latter often resulting from long-standing pulmonary regurgitation. Long-standing cyanosis, repeated cardiac surgery or chronic volume overload of the left ventricle (residual VSD, long-standing palliative shunt before repair, aortic regurgitation) can cause left ventricular dysfunction as well.
- **Atrial arrhythmia:** Common late after repair of tetralogy (atrial flutter or atrial fibrillation), occurring in about 30% of adult patients.
- **Ventricular tachycardia:** Less common than atrial tachycardia. It is associated with right ventricular dilatation and dysfunction. The QRS duration of the surface EKG has been shown to correlate with right ventricular size and a QRS duration of greater than 180 ms is a highly sensitive marker for sustained VT and **sudden death.**
- **Sudden death:** Reported to occur with an incidence of between 0.5% and 6% over a period of 30 years after repair.

Key findings on routine investigations
- **EKG:** Complete right bundle branch block, QRS prolongation
- **CXR:** Cardiomegaly, dilatation of the ascending aorta

Management

For patients with severe pulmonary regurgitation and right ventricular dilatation, pulmonary valve replacement should be considered. In the long-term, the development of clinical arrhythmias, such as ventricular tachycardia and atrial flutter/fibrillation, warrants both full electrophysiologic assessment and thorough review of the hemodynamics. Target lesions should be repaired.

Tetralogy of Fallot can be part of DiGeorge syndrome (present in 15% of tetralogy patients). Genetic testing should be offered to any tetralogy patient of reproductive age as the recurrence risk of DiGeorge syndrome is 50%.

Complete transposition of the great arteries (see Chapter 14)

After "atrial switch operation"
Most adult patients with complete transposition of the great arteries will have had an "atrial switch operation" (Mustard or Senning operation) in childhood. The right ventricle remains the systemic ventricle in this situation. Although most of these patients do well for many years, life expectancy is clearly limited.

> **Key clinical and routine investigation findings**
> - Systolic heart murmur from tricuspid regurgitation
> - Heart failure
> - Peripheral edema and ascites from systemic venous congestion
> - **EKG:** Right axis deviation, right ventricular hypertrophy, abnormal atrial rhythm
> - **CXR:** Narrow vascular pedicle, cardiomegaly, pulmonary congestion

Long-term complications
- **Atrial arrhythmia (atypical atrial flutter/fibrillation):** Occurs in 20% of patients by the age of 20 years as a result of extensive atrial surgery.
- **Sinus node dysfunction with junctional escape rhythm:** Common, also as a result of atrial surgery. Sixteen years after atrial switch only 18% of patients remain in permanent sinus rhythm. Patients often need permanent pacing.
- **Right (systemic) ventricular dysfunction:** Common, as the right ventricle is not designed to support the systemic circulation.
- **Tricuspid regurgitation:** Can accompany right heart failure.
- **Obstruction of the atrial pathways ("baffle obstruction"):** Can lead to systemic or pulmonary venous congestion and is associated with an increased risk of sudden cardiac death.

Management
Thorough assessment of right ventricular function, tricuspid valve function, heart rhythm, and the function of the

intra-atrial venous pathways is paramount. Therapeutic options include catheter procedures such as balloon dilatation and stenting for pathway obstruction, surgical procedures such as tricuspid valve replacement, or even conversion to the arterial switch operation. This would only be appropriate for selected patients and would require banding of the pulmonary artery in the first instance to retrain the left (subpulmonary) ventricle. The end of the therapeutic spectrum is heart transplantation. Transvenous pacing for bradyarrhythmia is highly specialized as placement of the leads within the atria and left ventricle can be troublesome due to the abnormal cardiac connections.

> **Key clinical points**
> - Atrial tachycardia and/or bradycardia often develop early in adulthood.
> - Right (systemic) ventricular failure and systemic (tricuspid) atrioventricular valve regurgitation may need valve replacement (if ventricular function is adequate). In cases of severe impairment of right (systemic) ventricular function, heart transplantation or late anatomic correction (arterial switch with previous banding of the pulmonary artery) must be considered.

After "arterial switch operation"
In this decade the number of adults who have survived the arterial switch procedure ("Jatene operation") will increase. Arrhythmias are less common in these patients and ventricular function is usually well preserved.

Long-term complications
- The arterial switch procedure carries the need for suture lines in the pulmonary trunk, which can cause **pulmonary trunk stenosis**.
- The procedure brings the pulmonary bifurcation into a position anterior to the ascending aorta, which can cause **peripheral pulmonary artery stenosis**.
- **Progressive dilatation of the aortic root** (former pulmonary root) can cause **aortic regurgitation**.
- As the arterial switch operation includes coronary artery reimplantation, there is the potential for **coronary stenosis** and ischemia.

> **Key clinical and routine investigation findings**
> - Ejection systolic heart murmur from pulmonary artery stenosis
> - Diastolic heart murmur from aortic regurgitation
> - **EKG:** Signs of myocardial ischemia and right ventricular hypertrophy may be present

Management

The main issue in the care of patients after arterial switch operation is to exclude significant pulmonary artery stenosis, myocardial ischemia, and aortic valve regurgitation. All these situations may warrant intervention.

Congenitally corrected transposition of the great arteries (see Chapter 14)

Patients with congenitally corrected transposition of the great arteries (ccTGA) may not be diagnosed before adulthood. ccTGA is often associated with other heart lesions such as systemic (tricuspid) atrioventricular valve abnormalities with valve insufficiency, VSD, subpulmonary stenosis, complete heart block, and Wolff–Parkinson–White syndrome (see Chapter 24). ccTGA can occur with dextrocardia. Patients may have been operated on for their associated lesions. Common procedures are VSD closure, implantation of a conduit from the left ventricle to the pulmonary artery, and systemic (tricuspid) atrioventricular valve replacement. A "corrective procedure" would be the "double-switch operation" (combination of an atrial and arterial switch operation). Atrial arrhythmia is common after "double switch," as it is after atrial switch for complete transposition of the great arteries.

Long-term complications

• **Progressive right (systemic) ventricular dysfunction:** Common as the right ventricle is not designed to support the systemic circulation.
• **Progressive systemic (tricuspid) atrioventricular valve regurgitation:** Can manifest and aggravate heart failure.
• ccTGA patients are at risk of developing both **bradyarrhythmia** (complete AV block develops in 2% of patients per year) and **tachyarrhythmia** (atrial arrhythmia or supraventricular tachycardia secondary to Wolff–Parkinson–White syndrome).
• Patients with a VSD and pulmonary stenosis can have **cyanosis**.

Key clinical and routine investigation findings

• Systolic heart murmur (ventricular septal defect, pulmonary stenosis or tricuspid regurgitation may be difficult to differentiate)
• **EKG:** Arrhythmia (complete atrioventricular block, atrial arrhythmia)
• **CXR:** Dextrocardia (20% of patients), cardiomegaly

Management

Preservation of systemic (right) ventricular function is crucial. Tricuspid (systemic) valve regurgitation has to be treated surgically before ventricular dysfunction becomes irreversible. Valve replacement is usually necessary because of the abnormal, often "Ebstein-like," anatomy of the tricuspid valve. Complete atrioventricular block may require pacemaker implantation.

Single ventricle and Fontan circulation (see Chapters 16 and 34)
Single ventricle

• Hearts with an "anatomically" or "functionally" single ventricle receive the systemic and pulmonary venous blood in "one" ventricle and are therefore **cyanotic**. The single ventricle pumps blood into the pulmonary artery (when not atretic) and the aorta.
• The single ventricle can be predominantly of left or right ventricular morphology.
• In the case of an "ideal" anatomy, blood flow into the single ventricle is unrestricted, and if ventricular function is good, an adequate and equivalent amount of blood should be delivered to the lungs and into the body. Invariably in this "well-balanced" situation, excessive pulmonary blood flow is avoided by an obstruction to the pulmonary outflow tract.
• If pulmonary outflow tract obstruction is not present, excessive blood flow into the lungs will lead to **pulmonary hypertension** and the **Eisenmenger syndrome**.
• Severe pulmonary outflow tract obstruction with reduced pulmonary blood flow causes **severe cyanosis**.
• **Surgery in patients with single ventricles is always palliative** and aims to secure adequate pulmonary and systemic blood flow and maintain systemic ventricular function.

Management

• **Systemic-to-pulmonary shunts** (e.g. Blalock–Taussig): Commonly performed in early infancy to improve pulmonary blood flow.
• **Pulmonary artery banding:** Performed to protect patients from pulmonary hypertension when pulmonary blood flow is unobstructed.
• Systemic venous-to-pulmonary artery connections like the cavopulmonary anastomosis (**Glenn shunt**) or the total cavopulmonary connection (**Fontan operation**) are performed as definitive palliations to improve pulmonary blood flow and separate the pulmonary from the systemic circulation while unloading the systemic ventricle (see Chapter 34).

After the Fontan operation (total cavopulmonary connection

Many adult patients with a single ventricle have undergone Fontan operations as definitive palliation (see Chapter 34). Long-term survival is clearly reduced in these patients. The 10-year survival rate is about 70%. Following this operation, all systemic venous return is diverted to the pulmonary circulation without employing a subpulmonary ventricle. Blood flow to the lungs is only driven by systemic venous pressure. "Fontan patients" are at risk of various complications related to surgery and/or the abnormal circulatory physiology persisting after surgery.

Long-term complications
• **Atrial flutter/fibrillation** related to scarring from surgery or to atrial distension from high venous pressure. Atrial arrhythmias in Fontan patients need **prompt treatment** as they can cause profound hemodynamic deterioration.
• **Sinus node dysfunction:** May warrant pacemaker implantation.
• **Thromboembolism:** Can be associated with sluggish venous blood flow in dilated systemic venous pathways.
• **Protein-losing enteropathy (PLE):** Occurs in 10% of "Fontan patients" and is characterized by intestinal protein loss leading to low serum protein levels and subsequently to peripheral edema and ascites. The condition is associated with a poor prognosis.
• **Deterioration of ventricular function:** Part of the "natural" history, especially if the ventricle is of right ventricular morphology.
• **Hepatic dysfunction:** Resulting from high hepatic venous pressure.
• **Cyanosis:** Often results from persistent systemic-to-pulmonary venous connections or intrapulmonary arteriovenous malformations leading to right-to-left shunting.

Key clinical and routine investigation findings
• A good "Fontan patient" has no murmurs with a single second heart sound (systolic murmurs can indicate atrioventricular valve incompetence)
• Peripheral edema can result from heart failure or PLE or a combination of both
• **EKG:** Arrhythmia (tachy- and brady-arrhythmia)
• **CXR:** Cardiomegaly, atrial enlargement
• **Laboratory findings:** Abnormal liver function tests, low protein/albumin suggestive of PLE

Management
"Fontan patients" are one of the most challenging groups of patients in cardiology and require close follow-up (every 6–12 months). Treatment aims to maintain optimal pulmonary and systemic circulation and to preserve ventricular function. Therefore, the complications listed above need to be treated promptly.

Conversion of an atriopulmonary anastomosis type of Fontan to a total cavopulmonary connection with concomitant arrhythmia surgery is an option for patients with a "failing Fontan circulation" (arrhythmia, ventricular dysfunction, PLE, thrombus formation) and can improve clinical status and exercise tolerance, and reduce arrhythmia propensity.

Cyanosed patient
Cyanosis is common in adults with congenital heart disease secondary to right-to-left shunting or decreased pulmonary blood flow. Cyanosis results in hypoxemia and adaptive mechanisms ensue to increase oxygen delivery to the tissue. These include a rightward shift in the oxyhemoglobin binding curve and in hemoglobin (secondary erythrocytosis and **not** polycythemia).

Symptoms related to cyanosis/hypoxia
• Shortness of breath at rest or on exertion
• Chest pain
  Chronic cyanosis affects multiple organ systems.

Multiorgan consequences of cyanosis
• **Hematology:**
  ○ Secondary erythrocytosis
  ○ Iron deficiency often results from an increased demand and inappropriate iron uptake or repeated inappropriate venesections
  ○ Coagulopathy with bleeding diathesis results from thrombocytopenia and impaired clotting function
• **Neurology:**
  ○ Brain injury from paradoxical embolism, hemorrhage, abscesses
• **Renal:**
  ○ Hypoxemia-induced glomerulopathy (hematuria, proteinuria)
  ○ Nephrolithiasis (uric acid)
• **Rheumatology:**
  ○ Gout
  ○ Osteoarthropathy

Management

• **Venesection** in cyanosed patients is only indicated **if** the patient has severe symptoms from "**hyperviscosity syndrome**" (after correcting for dehydration), such as headache, dizziness, fatigue, visual disturbance, tinnitus or myalgia (not common in patients with stable, compensated secondary erythrocytosis) and the hematocrit is > 65% or **if** surgery is planned and the hematocrit is > 65%. No more than 250–500 mL of blood should be to be removed over a period of 45 min and replaced with **dextrose.** Intravenous "air filters" must be used.

• **Iron deficiency:** Needs to be treated by oral or intravenous iron supplements.

• **Anticoagulation:** No general consensus on routine anticoagulation exists.

Further reading

Baumgartner H, Bonhoeffer P, De Groot NM, *et al.* ESC Guidelines for the management of grown-up congenital heart disease (new version 2010). *Eur Heart J* 2010;31(23):2915–2957.

Bonow RO, Carabello B, de Leon AC Jr, *et al.* Guidelines for the management of patients with valvular heart disease: executive summary. A report of the American College of Cardiology/American Heart Association Task Force on Practice Guidelines (Committee on Management of Patients with Valvular Heart Disease). *Circulation* 1998;98:1949–1984.

Gatzoulis MA. Adult congenital heart disease: education, education, education. *Nat Clin Pract Cardiovasc Med* 2006;3:2–3.

Gatzoulis MA, Swan L, Therrien J, Pantely GA, eds. *Adult Congenital Heart Disease: A Practical Guide.* Oxford: BMJ Publishing Group, Blackwell Publishing Ltd, 2005.

Murphy DJ Jr. Transposition of the great arteries: long-term outcome and current management. *Curr Cardiol Rep* 2005;7: 299–304.

Uebing A, Steer PJ, Yentis SM, Gatzoulis MA. Pregnancy and congenital heart disease. *BMJ* 2006;332:401–406.

van den Bosch AE, Roos-Hesselink JW, Van Domburg R, Bogers AJ, Simoons ML, Meijboom FJ. Long-term outcome and quality of life in adult patients after the Fontan operation. *Am J Cardiol* 2004;93:1141–1145.

Warnes CA. The adult with congenital heart disease: born to be bad? *J Am Coll Cardiol* 2005;46:1–8.

Wren C, O'Sullivan JJ. Survival with congenital heart disease and need for follow up in adult life. *Heart* 2001;85:438–443.

32 Principles of medical management

Zdenek Slavik

Royal Brompton Hospital, London, UK

The major circumstances requiring drug treatment of heart disease pertain to arrhythmias (see Chapters 23 and 24), circulatory failure, and hypoxia. The circulation provides a mechanism for the delivery of oxygen and metabolites to the various tissues of the body to maintain cellular integrity, specialized function, and growth.

Intrinsic control of cardiac output is predominantly by:
- The Frank–Starling mechanism;
- Autoregulation of peripheral vascular tone.

Extrinsic control is mainly through:
- Neural regulation of heart rate;
- Atrioventricular conduction;
- Peripheral vascular resistance (afterload);
- Peripheral venous capacitance (preload).

The fundamental determinants of stroke volume are:
- Preload;
- Afterload;
- Intrinsic myocardial contractility.

The availability and efficacy of compensatory mechanisms maintaining adequate cardiac output differ depending on age and the underlying heart disease.

Cardiac output, the product of myocardial stroke volume and heart rate, is particularly heart-rate dependent in early infancy so that in the presence of significant heart disease, bradycardia may be poorly tolerated. The atrioventricular (AV) node is less rate limiting and heart rates up to 200 bpm are well tolerated in infancy. Myocardial contractility is mainly under adrenergic control; in infancy the myocardium is particularly sensitive to negative inotropic factors:

- Hypoxia;
- Acidosis;
- Hypocalcemia;
- Hypoglycemia.

Regional blood flow distribution is under neural and autoregulatory or local control, so that when cardiac output falls, blood flow to organs with greatest metabolic demand (heart and brain) is preferentially maintained. When cardiac output is inadequate, increased adrenergic neurohumoral tone reduces blood flow to the skin, kidneys, and gastrointestinal tract, and increases heart rate. This accounts for the usual clinical signs in severe cases of tachycardia, pallor, cold skin, pyrexia, and oliguria. Circulatory failure, however, in the presence of fever, sepsis or anemia may be associated with normal cardiac output. The early physical signs of circulatory failure are anxiety, restlessness, and tachycardia with cool and pale extremities. Early decompensation is characterized by tachypnea, metabolic acidosis, oliguria; finally impaired consciousness, hypotension, and periodic breathing develop.

Acute heart failure

Acute heart failure presents most frequently in neonates and young infants. It is not unusual for mild circulatory failure to precede the acute episode especially, but not exclusively, in anomalies associated with left-to-right shunting. Dehydration, hypovolemia, anemia, and sepsis may be a primary cause or make existing heart failure worse.

Pediatric Heart Disease: A Practical Guide, First Edition. Piers E. F. Daubeney, Michael L. Rigby, Koichiro Niwa, and Michael A. Gatzoulis.
© 2012 Blackwell Publishing Ltd. Published 2012 by Blackwell Publishing Ltd.

Common causes of acute heart failure

- Severe ("critical") aortic stenosis (see Chapter 11)
- Coarctation of the aorta (see Chapter 12)
- Aortic interruption (see Chapter 12)
- Hypoplastic left heart syndrome (see Chapter16)
- Obstructed total anomalous pulmonary venous connection (see Chapter 16)
- Persistent pulmonary hypertension (see Chapter 21)
- Cardiac surgery (see Chapter 34)
- Large ventricular septal defect (see Chapter 9)
- Complete atrioventricular septal defect (see Chapter 9)
- Myocarditis or heart muscle disease (see Chapter 19)
- Anomalous origin of left coronary artery from the pulmonary trunk (see Chapter 13)
- Arrhythmias (see Chapters 23 and 24)

The mechanisms of acute circulatory failure are varied and complex and depend on the primary etiology. These mechanisms include left ventricular systolic and diastolic dysfunction, an elevated left atrial and/or pulmonary venous pressure, raised pulmonary artery pressure and pulmonary vascular resistance, and right ventricular systolic and/or diastolic dysfunction. Right heart failure with hepatic congestion occurs in the majority and the emergency management is similar in most groups of patients.

- Initial management comprises rapid endotracheal intubation, artificial ventilation with increased inspired oxygen fraction, and intravenous sedatives (see below), opiates, and muscle relaxants.
- Where there is uncertainty about the presence of congenital heart disease in the newborn period, an intravenous infusion of prostaglandin E is warranted to keep the arterial duct open and maintain systemic blood flow from the pulmonary artery to the aorta; a secondary effect is a reduction in pulmonary arterial resistance.
- For neonates with persistent pulmonary hypertension, inhaled nitric oxide, high inspired oxygen levels, and maintenance of low–normal systemic arterial carbon dioxide are required; very few will require extracorporeal membrane oxygenation support.
- For patients with persistent congestive cardiac failure, the choice of inotropic agent remains controversial with dopamine or dobutamine used most frequently. Caution should be exercised in the use of large intravenous fluid volumes in the initial resuscitation because of the risk of aggravating the heart failure.

- The return of spontaneous urine output and resolution of metabolic acidosis represent signs of therapeutic success, but some patients will require intravenous diuretics by bolus or continuous infusion.
- The combination of fluid restriction with diuretics carries the risk of dehydration and should be used with caution.
- After initial resuscitation and the achievement of relative stability, urgent treatment of the underlying heart malformation is essential.

Low cardiac output immediately following cardiac surgery

In the absence of residual malformations, a postoperative low cardiac output state is likely to result from impaired systolic and/or diastolic myocardial function, which cannot usually be attributed to a single cause. A combination of factors is often responsible, including:

- Preoperative congenital heart disease leading to myocardial dysfunction;
- Impaired perioperative myocardial protection;
- Reperfusion injury;
- Postoperative inflammatory response with increased capillary permeability leading to generalized tissue edema.

The preoperative administration of steroids and use of modified ultrafiltration at the end of cardiopulmonary bypass, coupled with restriction of crystalloid intake (20–40 mL/kg/day) in the early postoperative period, limit the negative impact of the postoperative inflammatory response and increased capillary permeability. There is also favorable evidence for the short-term use of steroids in postoperative low cardiac output states.

Drug treatment of low cardiac output

- **Sedatives and opiates:**
  - Used with caution, with doses titrated to clinical effect
  - Metabolism is likely to be impaired by hepatic and renal dysfunction
  - Potential side effects include myocardial dysfunction (midazolam) and systemic hypotension
  - Advantageous effects include a reduction in sympathetic drive and tissue oxygen demand
- **Muscle relaxants:**
  - Should be reserved mainly for patients with delayed postoperative sternal closure or recurrent pulmonary hypertensive episodes
  - "Drug holidays" should be considered to avoid accumulation if long-term paralysis is needed

- **Inotropes:**
  - Epinephrine (adrenaline), dopamine, and dobutamine have traditionally been used in children with low cardiac output states. Catecholamines, however, lead to an increase in myocardial oxygen consumption
  - The potential to impair ventricular function can be avoided by the use of inodilators which have inotropic and vasodilating effects
  - Milrinone, a phosphodiesterase inhibitor and inodilator, not only improves postoperative low cardiac output state in all age groups, but may also shorten the time to hospital discharge
- **Mild hypothermia:** A body temperature of 35 °C can improve the oxygen delivery/utilization balance in low output postoperative states

Treatment in special situations

- **Pulmonary hypertension:** When a fixed or fluctuating raised pulmonary vascular resistance causes acute right ventricular failure the following treatments can be used successfully:
  - Inhaled nitric oxide
  - Inodilators (milrinone, enoximone) which reduce the need for peripheral venous and arterial vasodilators such as sodium nitroprusside and glyceryl trinitrate
  - Intravenous prostacycline.
- **Systemic hypertension:** Hypertension encountered following cardiac surgery will respond to sodium nitroprusside, ACE inhibitors, and beta blockers, although the latter should be avoided if ventricular function is impaired. Glyceryl trinitrate will also increase coronary blood flow.
- **Junctional ectopic tachycardia:** An important and potentially life-threatening but transient cause of early postoperative low cardiac output. Although it is poorly responsive to antiarrhythmic drugs, it may respond to amiodarone or mild hypothermia with a reduction in heart rate which then allows sequential atrioventricular pacing.
- **Renal failure:** Low urine output may respond to treatment with intravenous diuretics with or without aminophylline. In some cases a short period of peritoneal dialysis or hemofiltration is helpful.
- **Mechanical support:** Rarely patients with extremely low cardiac output may benefit from temporary mechanical support of cardiac or cardiorespiratory function with a ventricular assist device or extracorporeal membrane oxygenation.

- **Newer developments:** There are new, promising avenues in the treatment of low cardiac output states, including strict postoperative control of blood glucose levels, the use of levosimendan, a calcium sensitizer and potassium channel opener with inodilating properties, and the use of natriuretic peptide B.

Acute myocardial failure due to myocarditis (see Chapter 19)

A small minority, but more common in small children over the age of 1 year, of cases of viral myocarditis present with severe symptoms of low cardiac output. Conventional treatment comprises diuretics, short-term intravenous infusion of dobutamine and/or milrinone and non-invasive positive pressure ventilation. Full artificial ventilation with sedation may be necessary in more severe forms of myocardial failure. Some centers advocate immunoglobulin, steroid or immunosuppressive therapy with or without preceding myocardial biopsy. Temporary mechanical support using a ventricular assist device, artificial heart (e.g. Berlin Heart) or extracorporeal membrane oxygenation is reserved for the small minority of cases resistant to less invasive treatment interventions. They should be viewed as a bridge to myocardial recovery or heart transplantation.

Treatment of arrhythmia (see Chapter 24)

Unrecognized, recurrent, and protracted episodes of supraventricular tachycardia, including neonatal atrial flutter, may cause left ventricular dysfunction and acute myocardial failure in early infancy. Intravenous bolus administration of adenosine is the first-line treatment for supraventricular tachycardia. Neonatal atrial flutter or a failure to respond to adenosine are indications for DC cardioversion. Some antiarrhythmic drugs, such as flecainide or beta-blockers, may have a negative inotropic effect and should be administered with great care.

Chronic heart failure

Chronic heart failure refers to a situation where symptoms such as failure to thrive, breathlessness or effort intolerance are improved or remain stable with drug treatment. Chronic heart failure caused by an uncorrectable underlying condition can lead to acute circulatory collapse at any time. Many of those infants or children with short-lived chronic heart failure are best managed by surgical treatment of their underlying condition.

Common causes of chronic heart failure
• Excessive pulmonary blood flow
• Ventricular volume overload caused by semilunar or atrioventricular valvar incompetence
• Recurrent or incessant arrhythmias
• Primary myocardial failure

Congenital heart defects are the leading cause amongst children in the developed world, whereas rheumatic heart disease predominates in some developing countries.

Etiology

Acyanotic conditions with a left-to-right shunt
• Complete atrioventricular septal defect (AVSD) (see Chapter 9)
• Moderate-to-large ventricular septal defect (VSD) (see Chapter 9)
• Moderate-to-large patent ductus arteriosus (PDA) (see Chapter 9)

These are the commonest causes of congestive heart failure during the first 6 months of life. The onset of symptoms is usually from 4 to 6 weeks of age, coinciding with the gradual fall in pulmonary vascular resistance (PVR) from birth. The onset is earlier in premature infants who display a much more rapid fall in PVR. The consequences of a high pulmonary blood flow include left atrial and ventricular volume loading, pulmonary venous congestion, pulmonary edema, and dilated pulmonary arteries.

Valve insufficiency
• Aortic regurgitation (see Chapter 11)
• Mitral regurgitation (see Chapter 11)
• Atrioventricular valve regurgitation in AVSD (see Chapter 9)

Aortic regurgitation is frequently encountered in rheumatic heart disease. Congenital aortic regurgitation is usually associated with a bicuspid aortic valve. An ascending aortopathy found in Marfan syndrome often gives rise to insufficiency. Mitral insufficiency, common in rheumatic heart disease and patients with dilated cardiomyopathy, may also be congenital. Various causes are encountered, including dysplastic valve leaflets, mitral prolapse, isolated cleft of the anterior leaflet, and an "arcade" lesion. Some degree of insufficiency is frequent in all types of AVSD and can be extremely severe, e.g. giving rise to heart failure when there is an isolated primum defect.

Cyanotic conditions without pulmonary stenosis or atresia
• Common arterial trunk (see Chapter 16)
• Double outlet right ventricle (DORV) with subaortic or subpulmonary VSD (see Chapter 15)
• Transposition with large VSD (see Chapter 14)
• Hearts with univentricular atrioventricular connection (see Chapter 16)
• Total anomalous pulmonary venous connection (see Chapter 16)

In this group, cyanosis is usually mild; pulmonary blood flow increases as pulmonary vascular resistance gradually falls after birth so that symptoms begin at 4–6 weeks.

Acquired heart disease
• Acute rheumatic carditis (see Chapter 25)
• Rheumatic heart disease (predominantly aortic and/or mitral insufficiency) (see Chapter 25)

Myocardial dysfunction
• Viral myocarditis (see Chapter 19)
• Kawasaki disease with myocardial ischemia or infarction (see Chapter 27)
• Dilated cardiomyopathy (see Chapter 19)
• Restrictive cardiomyopathy (see Chapter 19)
• Endocardial fibroelastosis (see Glossary)
• Anomalous origin of left coronary artery from the pulmonary trunk (see Chapter 13)
• Transient myocardial ischemia of the newborn
• Metabolic abnormalities
• Carnitine deficiency
• Mitochondrial disorders
• Muscular dystrophy
• Friedreich's ataxia
• Hypocalcemia

Miscellaneous causes
• Incessant supraventricular tachycardia (see Chapter 24)
• Neonatal complete heart block (see Chapter 23)
• Severe anemia
• Acute hypertension
• Acute cor pulmonale
• Cardiac arrest with successful resuscitation

Management

Diuretics
Diuretics are the mainstay of treatment for chronic heart failure and are usually used in combination.

Spironolactone is combined with furosemide or chlorthiazide. Chlorthiazide is weaker and longer acting than furosemide. The major complications are dehydration and hypovolemia together with electrolyte loss in the urine. Spironolactone is unique in not only in having a potassium-sparing effect but also in its influence on myocardial remodeling due to aldosterone antagonism and a direct myocardial effect.

ACE inhibitors

Used in combination with diuretics, the ACE inhibitors prescribed most frequently in pediatric practice are captopril, enalapril, and lisinopril. The latter carries the advantage of a single daily dose but is currently not used in infancy. By reducing systemic vascular resistance and blood pressure, their effect is to reduce the amount of left-to-right shunting or the severity of mitral or aortic insufficiency. By reducing left ventricular pressure loading, patients with heart muscle disease will also benefit. Because these drugs are poorly tolerated by some, a small test dose should be given prior to the introduction of a conventional dose regimen. ACE inhibitors should not be used in the presence of left heart obstruction. Complications include dizziness, hyperkalemia, skin rashes, and an irritable dry cough. Because of the risk of potassium retention, they should be used in combination with spironolactone with care and monitoring of serum electrolytes is advisable.

Beta-blockers

Carvedilol or metoprolol can benefit patients with heart muscle disorders, particularly those with a relative resting tachycardia. By reducing heart rate and increasing the time for ventricular filling, cardiac output and symptoms can improve. Patients whose cardiac output is heart rate dependent or those in whom beta-blockade further depresses ventricular function may manifest sudden deterioration. These drugs should therefore be used with care, beginning with small doses, and should not be instigated as the first line of treatment. It does appear, however, that some patients with poor ventricular function manifest significant symptomatic improvement when a combination of ACE inhibitor, spironolactone, and carvedilol are prescribed.

Oxygen

For infants with a left-to-right shunt or other cause of increased pulmonary blood flow who are admitted to hospital and found to have a slightly depressed systemic arterial oxygen saturation, almost certainly due to some degree of pulmonary edema, the temptation to give supplemental oxygen should be avoided. The consequences of an increased inspired oxygen concentration are a drop in pulmonary vascular resistance and a marked increase in pulmonary blood flow, causing congestive cardiac failure to become more severe.

Other treatments

There is little evidence of any benefit from the use of digoxin or sodium restriction. Fluid restriction used in combination with diuretics in a patient whose fluid intake is already reduced because of breathlessness is potentially dangerous and likely to lead to dehydration with subsequent risk of acute deterioration. In general, heart failure combined with dehydration and hypovolemia is potentially lethal.

Oral enoximone has been used to benefit patients with heart muscle disease but its exact role is not yet fully established.

Nutrition

Infants and children with chronic heart failure frequently manifest varying degrees of failure to thrive and even malnutrition. There is established evidence of malabsorption in these patients so that an increase in calorie intake with or without nasogastric, nasojejunal or even temporary parenteral feeding may be of help.

Cyanosis in the newborn (see Chapter 41)

For central cyanosis to be present, at least 5 g/dL of reduced hemoglobin must be present in the blood reaching the buccal mucosa and skin. For cyanosis to be evident on physical examination, the arterial oxygen saturation has to be below 85–89%. Neonatal hypoxia can be cardiovascular or pulmonary in origin. A high inspired fraction of oxygen leading to an increase in measured arterial oxygen saturation above 95% is likely to indicate a pulmonary cause for cyanosis. However, the site of measured desaturation is important because right-to-left shunting across the arterial duct will cause a lower saturation in the descending aorta or legs than in the upper body, regardless of the cause or inspired oxygen fraction. Elegant studies have demonstrated potential direct communications between the pulmonary arteries and veins which bypass lung parenchyma. Consequently in infants with lung disease, or in those receiving pulmonary vasodilators, such as prostacycline or prostaglandin E1 or

E2, there is the potential for ventilation–perfusion mismatch with intrapulmonary right-to-left shunting.

Duct-dependent pulmonary blood flow

The newborn infant with cyanotic congenital heart disease associated with severe pulmonary stenosis or pulmonary atresia depends upon patency of the arterial duct to maintain pulmonary blood flow from the aorta. Spontaneous closure of the duct, usually in the first few days after birth, will result in severe hypoxia and acidosis leading to inevitable death. The continuous intravenous infusion of prostaglandin E, by dilating the duct, causes pulmonary blood flow to increase, reduces the severity of hypoxia, and prevents or reverses acidosis. The infusion can be continued for several days, allowing elective surgery or cardiac catheter intervention to be performed. When an antenatal diagnosis of cyanotic heart disease has been made, prostaglandin E can be commenced at birth.

Complications of prostaglandins

- Systemic arterial vasodilatation and hypotension
- Pulmonary arterial dilatation
- Apnea
- Pyrexia
- Jitteriness
- Seizures
- Diarrhea
- Thrombocytopenia

Complete transposition of the great arteries (see Chapter 14)

There is an additional situation where prostaglandins are useful in the newborn with severe hypoxia. For complete transposition with intact ventricular septum, continued patency of the arterial duct may allow bidirectional shunting, which causes mixing of systemic and pulmonary venous return. More frequently however, the fall in pulmonary vascular resistance results in shunting from the aorta to the pulmonary artery, thus increasing pulmonary venous return to the left atrium. There is then improved mixing at atrial level because the raised left atrial pressure increases the left-to-right shunt across the patent foramen ovale. It is important to be aware that the raised left atrial pressure may result in pulmonary venous congestion and tachypnea.

Left heart obstruction in the newborn (see Chapters 11, 12, and 16)

Most cases of severe left heart obstruction are examples of so-called "duct-dependent systemic blood flow." Particularly in the newborn with coarctation, arch interruption or hypoplastic left heart, incipient closure of the duct soon after birth causes impaired lower body aortic blood flow with acidosis, renal failure, rapid deterioration, and death. An intravenous infusion of prostaglandin E usually will cause the duct to dilate, allowing shunting from the pulmonary trunk to the descending aorta, and preventing or reversing any metabolic acidosis and renal failure.

Potential causes of duct-dependent systemic blood flow

- Absent left atrioventricular connection and mitral atresia (see Chapter 16)
- Severe mitral stenosis (see Chapter 11)
- Hypoplastic left heart variants (see Chapter 16)
- Critical aortic stenosis (see Chapter 11)
- Coarctation of the aorta (see Chapter 12)
- Interruption of the aortic arch (see Chapter 12)

The mechanisms of acute deterioration in this group are varied and complex and depend not only on the interruption of systemic blood flow via the arterial duct but also on the primary etiology. These mechanisms include left ventricular dysfunction, an elevated left atrial and/or pulmonary venous pressure, raised pulmonary artery pressure and pulmonary vascular resistance, and right ventricular dysfunction. Right heart failure with hepatic congestion occurs in the majority and the emergency management is similar involving rapid sequence intubation, intravenous administration of prostaglandin E, fluid resuscitation followed by diuretic treatment, and inotropic support (see management of acute heart failure above).

Fluid balance and nutrition

Postoperative low cardiac output with variable degrees of capillary leak syndrome due to tissue reperfusion injury and the inflammatory response to cardiopulmonary bypass is common in infants. The early introduction of diuretics, peritoneal dialysis or hemofiltration is often needed because of renal dysfunction. The restriction of crystalloid fluid intake in the first 48 hours is part of successful postoperative management. Synthetic colloid replacement solutions carry less risk of infection and the molecular size of its particles is less likely to allow leakage into the extravascular space. Interference with hemostasis or renal function can be expected when large volumes are infused. Cautious use of inodilators (see above) or inotropes with peripheral vasoconstricting properties (norepinephrine [noradrenaline]) to maintain systemic blood pressure reduces the need for colloid administration.

Early enteral or parenteral nutrition is essential for full recovery. Enteral nutrition may be limited by reduced gut motility and absorption. Preoperative malnutrition, gastroesophageal reflux, and risk of necrotizing enterocolitis favor the early introduction of parenteral nutrition despite the restrictions dictated by reduced daily fluid allowance. Nutritional support in patients with chronic heart failure leads to improved outcome. Temporary fluid restriction should be supervised with care and is not compatible with adequate nutrition beyond a few days. Nasogastric or nasojejunal tube feeding using smaller volumes in short intervals or continuous regimens such as overnight feeding in older children usually overcomes difficulties with oral intake (nausea, poor appetite) caused by complications related to venous congestion in abdominal organs. The desired caloric intake (170 kcal/kg/day in infants, 70 kcal/kg/day in older children) should be reached gradually. Fluid balance, weight changes, and sodium intake should be monitored carefully (see also management of chronic heart failure above).

Further reading

Deakin CD, Knight H, Edwards JC, et al. Induced hypothermia in the postoperative management of refractory cardiac failure following paediatric cardiac surgery. *Anaesthesia* 1988;53:848–853.

Duggal B, Pratap U, Slavik Z, et al. Milrinone and low cardiac output following cardiac surgery in infants: is there a direct myocardial effect? *Pediatr Cardiol* 2005;26:642–645.

Hoffman TM, Wernovsky G, Atz AM, et al. Efficacy and safety of milrinone in preventing low cardiac output syndrome in infants and children after corrective surgery for congenital heart disease. *Circulation* 2003;107:996–1002.

Levin DL, Mills LJ, Parkey M. Morphologic development of the pulmonary vascular bed in experimental coarctation of the aorta. *Circulation* 1979;60:349–354.

Lister G, Hellebrand WF, Kleinman CS, et al. Physiologic effects of increasing hemoglobin concentration in left-to-right shunting in infants with ventricular septal defect. *N Engl J Med* 1982;306:502–506.

Miller SP, McQuillen PS, Vigneron DB, et al. Preoperative brain injury in newborns with transposition of the great arteries. *Ann Thorac Surg* 2004;77:1698–1706.

Monagle P, Chan A, Massicotte P, et al. Antithrombotic therapy in children: the Seventh ACCP Conference on Antithrombotic and Thrombolytic Therapy. *Chest* 2004;126 (Suppl 3):645S–687S.

Mori Y, Nakazawa M, Tomimatsu H, et al. (Long-term effect of angiotensin-converting enzyme inhibition on volume overloaded heart during growth. *J Am Coll Cardiol* 2000;36:270–275.

Stiller B, Weng Y, Hubler M, et al. Pneumatic pulsatile ventricular assist devices in children under 1 year of age. *Eur J Cardiothorac Surg* 2005;28:234–239.

Streif W, Mitchel LG, Andrew M, et al. (Antithrombotic therapy in children. *Curr Opin Pediatr* 1999;11:31–32.

33 Catheter intervention

Alan W. Nugent[1,2]

[1]University of Texas Southwestern Medical Center, Dallas, TX, USA
[2]Children's Medical Center, Dallas, TX, USA

Interventional catheterization continues to be an exciting, rapidly changing, and expanding field that has revolutionized the treatment of congenital heart disease. This chapter attempts to give an overview of interventions for congenital heart disease.

All interventional procedures carry additional risk for adverse events compared to hemodynamic cases, require additional specialized training, and should be performed in institutions with full anesthesia, critical care, and surgical support.

Cardiac catheterization interventions for congenital heart disease

- Valvuloplasty:
  - Pulmonary valve
  - Aortic valve
  - Mitral valve
- Balloon angioplasty/stent:
  - Aortic coarctation
  - Pulmonary artery
  - Right ventricle-to-pulmonary artery conduit
  - Systemic vein
  - Stenting of arterial duct
- Defect closure:
  - Atrial septal defect (ASD)
  - Patent foramen ovale (PFO)
  - Patent arterial duct (PDA)
  - Ventricular septal defect (VSD)
  - Fontan fenestration
  - Collaterals, fistulae, surgical shunt
- Defect creation:
  - Balloon atrial septostomy
  - Blade atrial septostomy
  - Balloon atrial dilatation
  - Fenestration creation

Planning for interventional catheterization

Patients scheduled for a catheterization require a complete history, physical examination, and laboratory testing. Informed consent is obtained after discussion of the risks/benefits, including the risks specific to a planned intervention, and available alternatives. The EKG, CXR, echocardiogram and prior catheterizations must be reviewed and a plan for the catheterization formulated.

Pre-catheterization plan

- Sedation/anesthesia: Patient factors, anticipated procedure
- Vascular access site: Anatomy, prior procedures, occluded vessels
- Hemodynamic/angiography: Necessary data/images to be obtained
- Intervention: Equipment, sheath size required
- Post-catheterization care: Outpatient, ward/intensive care admission

---

Valvuloplasty

Pulmonary valve stenosis

Balloon **pulmonary valvuloplasty** is a safe and highly effective procedure when performed with a balloon-to-annulus size ratio of 1.2–1.4:1. A peak gradient of greater than 50 mmHg was initially the threshold for catheter-based intervention. Lower profile balloons associated with lower procedural risks have not only liberalized the indication, but also allowed it to be routinely performed in newborn patients with critical pulmonary valve stenosis and membranous pulmonary atresia following perforation of the valve.

Pediatric Heart Disease: A Practical Guide, First Edition. Piers E. F. Daubeney, Michael L. Rigby, Koichiro Niwa, and Michael A. Gatzoulis.
© 2012 Blackwell Publishing Ltd. Published 2012 by Blackwell Publishing Ltd.

Aortic valve stenosis

Aortic stenosis is a more formidable problem but balloon **aortic valvuloplasty** provides results similar to surgery with low mortality and effective gradient relief with tolerable increases in aortic regurgitation. The usual indication remains a peak gradient of ≥50 mmHg with no more than mild regurgitation, and it can be performed in the newborn period. The initial balloon-to-annulus ratio should be no more than 0.9:1 with either antegrade (via femoral vein) or retrograde (via femoral artery) access. After each dilatation and before proceeding, there needs to be a reassessment of the gradient and degree of aortic regurgitation. Progression in this step-wise manner ensures that adequate gradient relief is achieved while minimizing regurgitation. This procedure is more challenging than pulmonary valvuloplasty, associated with increased morbidity, and should be viewed as palliative. It is now considered the primary therapy for most cases of significant aortic stenosis at any age.

Mitral valve stenosis

Balloon **mitral valvuloplasty**, initially described to treat rheumatic mitral stenosis, can also be performed for congenital mitral stenosis. This lesion has proven recalcitrant but balloon dilatation can ameliorate the condition, thereby potentially avoiding or delaying the need for surgery/prosthetic valve replacement in growing children.

Tricuspid valve stenosis

Of the four heart valves, there is least experience with the tricuspid valve, with few reports in patients with tricuspid stenosis.

Balloon angioplasty

Once the reason for success of balloon angioplasty in coronary arteries was shown to be due to a tear in the media, its potential in congenital heart disease was realized. However, it is not straightforward to achieve a controlled tear in a vessel wall that then needs to heal, particularly when the wall thickness and compliance of the lesion are unknown.

Primary coarctation of the aorta

Management of **native coarctation of the aorta** is controversial except early in life when the vast majority of physicians agree surgery remains the best option. The major problems with angioplasty in smaller patients are the high recurrence rate and incidence of arterial damage at the access site, although with technologic improvements the required sheath size is now smaller and angioplasty is possible even in premature infants. Native coarctation treated surgically has excellent long-term outcomes and balloon dilatation should therefore be offered to older children and adults; and only in younger patients who are a high surgical risk. Generally, the first balloon chosen is two to three times the narrowest diameter, but not more than the diameter of the aorta above or below the coarctation.

Recoarctation of the aorta

Recurrent coarctation of the aorta after prior surgery is a more complicated surgical procedure; therefore, balloon dilatation of recurrent coarctation has widespread acceptance and is the treatment of choice.

Pulmonary arterial stenosis

Branch pulmonary artery stenosis can be either proximal or multilevel into the peripheries; the latter is very challenging and has considerable morbidity and even mortality. Generally, balloons at least three times the size of the lesion are required for a therapeutic tear. Recently, cutting balloons have been utilized for lesions that are resistant to high-pressure angioplasty.

Dilatation of the main pulmonary artery is not rewarding in congenital supravalvar stenosis, but may be successful in an acquired postoperative lesion. Stenotic **right ventricle-to-pulmonary artery homografts/conduits** occur with patient growth, compression, calcification, and constriction. The decision to dilate a conduit needs to take into account the degree of regurgitation and right ventricular size and function. The procedure is palliative, but may delay time to surgical replacement of the stenotic homograft.

Systemic venous stenosis

Balloon dilatation of **systemic veins or atrial baffles after Mustard/Senning surgery** is often unrewarding and stent placement (see below) has dramatically improved the chances of a good outcome.

Pulmonary vein stenosis

Infants and children with discrete pulmonary vein stenosis can sometimes be managed successfully with balloon or cutting balloon angioplasty. Several repeat procedures are almost always required if a satisfactory outcome is to be achieved. However, when diffuse disease with vessel hypoplasia is present essentially all interventions are unsuccessful.

Other conditions

Palliative dilatation of the ductus arteriosus in newborns, or shunts and arterial collaterals later in life, to improve systemic saturation is less frequently performed. Aortopulmonary collaterals are often resistant even to high-pressure dilatation.

Stents

Following static balloon dilatation, there is immediate vessel recoil and varying rates of longer-term restenosis (due to intimal hyperplasia). This led to the development of stents (tubular metal mesh). Once inserted recoil is avoided, positive remodeling occurs, and restenosis rates are reduced. Stents have not only revolutionized coronary interventions, but also those for congenital heart disease, especially for vessels that are compliant, compressed, or kinked. The vast majority that are used are balloon expandable stainless steel stents. In a child, the obvious

disadvantage is somatic growth; however, stents can be later further dilated to adult size. Premounted stents are now available, enabling insertion through smaller sheaths, as well as improved deliverability.

Indications for stent insertion

Common indications

• Branch pulmonary artery stenosis
• Aortic coarctation (Figure 33.1)
• Right ventricle-to-pulmonary artery conduits
• Systemic venous pathway stenosis

Less frequent indications

• Arterial duct to maintain pulmonary blood flow
• Arterial duct to maintain systemic blood flow
• Stenosed systemic to pulmonary artery shunts
• Pulmonary vein stenosis

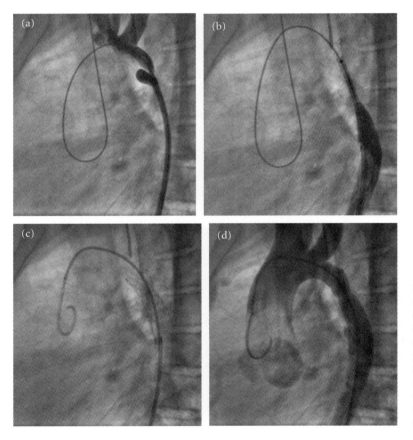

Figure 33.1 Stenting of coarctation. (a) Angiogram shows a juxtaductal coarctation. A guidewire has been passed across the coarctation site. Note the ductal diverticulum. (b) The stent is positioned over the wire across the coarctation site. (c) The stent has been expanded by balloon dilatation. (d) Ascending aortogram shows no residual coarctation. The ductal diverticulum has also been occluded.

Covered stents can manage emergent vessel rupture and severe arch obstruction, and cover aneurysms/shunts. Restenosis post coronary artery stent procedures has been significantly reduced with the use of drug-eluting stents specifically targeting intimal hyperplasia. While this technology is very appealing, at present the largest stent available is 3.5 mm in diameter and therefore too small to impact therapy significantly for congenital heart disease.

In addition to standard balloon angioplasty risks, stent implantation can also be complicated by malposition and embolization. In the long-term, stent fractures are well-recognized, particularly in right ventricle-to-pulmonary artery conduits. It is important to note that most stents utilized for congenital heart disease are designed for other purposes and are routinely inflated to diameters larger than manufacturers' recommendations.

Percutaneous valve replacement

The biggest advance in the last 10 years has been the development of percutaneous valves enabling valve replacement to be achieved without surgery. The first use was in congenital heart disease for pulmonary valve replacement in a surgically placed right ventricle-to-pulmonary artery conduit. Not surprisingly, following the success of the percutaneous pulmonary valve implantation, there has been an explosion of transcatheter aortic valve replacement, and also multiple devices designed for mitral valve intervention, in elderly patients.

Defect closure

Transcatheter devices to close defects have been used for a quarter of a century, but in the last decade there has been an explosion of experience.

Secundum atrial septal defect

Device closure of a secundum ASD is now routinely offered and can be performed with imaging by transesophageal or intracardiac echocardiography with or without fluoroscopy. Operators will familiarize themselves with a preferred method and most utilize a combination of imaging techniques. Currently, the Amplatzer septal occluder is the most frequently used device in most countries and presently has Food and Drug Administration (FDA) approval in the United States. It is constructed of a nitinol mesh woven into two discs with a connecting waist and has the advantages of being delivered through a relatively small delivery

sheath, and the capability to close large defects. Should malposition occur, both discs can be retracted and the device repositioned. Closure rates and safety are excellent and similar to those with surgery.

The Helex system is a spiral device applicable to small or fenestrated defects and when fully deployed consists of two circular discs. The patch material is expanded polytetrafluorethylene (ePTFE) attached to nitinol wire. A good feature of the device is a security cord, which enables retrieval if there is malposition after device release.

Many other devices have been trialled in the past and are no longer available, such as the CardioSEAL, STARFlex and BioSTAR family of devices.

It is important to be aware that superior or inferior sinus venosus defects, primum defects, and coronary sinus defects are all unsuitable for device closure.

Patent foramen ovale

PFO has been implicated in stroke due to paradoxical embolism, and also in migraine. Umbrella devices have been commonly used for closure, but devices have also been developed specifically for PFO closure and this trend will continue. The Amplatzer PFO occluder differs from the ASD device with a larger right atrial disc and a smaller connecting waist. Trials comparing the incidence of recurrent stroke with anticoagulation versus device closure have shown no benefit.

Patent ductus arteriosus

Various devices can close the persistently patent ductus arteriosus (PDA) (Figure 33.2). Coil occlusion remains a very effective and efficient way of closing restrictive PDAs outside the newborn period. If the minimum diameter is 2.5 mm or smaller, then a single coil will almost always be all that is required. A coil twice the size of the minimal diameter, with sufficient length to form four or five loops, is used. It is advisable to use at least 0.038-inch coils. The Amplatzer ductal occluder is FDA approved and able to close even very large defects. It is recommended for patients weighing more than 6 kg, although the small delivery system certainly means it can be used in smaller patients.

Ventricular septal defect

Device closure of VSDs is an extremely challenging procedure. Those VSDs that are difficult to visualize surgically in the apical or anterior portion of the septum are often best closed via catheterization with an Amplatzer muscular VSD device. Until recently, muscular position, surgical patch margin, or post-myocardial infarction defects were the common indications. Currently, the Amplatzer

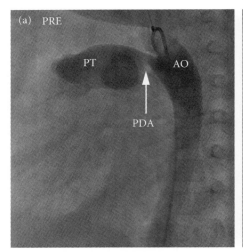 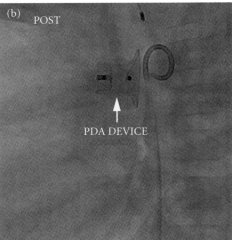

Figure 33.2 Device occlusion of a patent arterial duct (PDA). (a) Aortogram visualizes the arterial duct (arrow) and opacifies the pulmonary arteries. (b) An Amplatzer ductal occluder has been placed and released into the arterial duct, successfully occluding it. AO, aorta; PT, pulmonary trunk.

perimembranous VSD device is being tested in perimembranous inlet defects in children over the age of 2 years. Extensive experience has been gained in Europe and Asia. However, because the outcome of surgical closure of perimembranous defects is so good, only excellent procedural and follow-up results for closure devices will lead to their widespread acceptance. Initial concerns include damage to the conduction system and aortic valve leaflets.

Other uses of closure devices

Devices and coils can also close arterial/venous collateral vessels, fistulae (e.g. coronary arterial), surgical shunts, and perivalvar leaks. A small ASD device is ideal for closing a fenestration in the Fontan pathway.

Defect creation

Balloon atrial septostomy

The technique of balloon atrial septostomy is essentially performed in the same way today as initially described by Rashkind over 40 years ago. It is usually undertaken to improve preoperative mixing of blood in newborns with transposition of the great vessels. Access can be via the femoral or umbilical vein with fluoroscopic or echocardiographic guidance.

Additional indications for balloon atrial septostomy include:
• Tricuspid atresia;
• Absent left atrioventricular connection;
• Double inlet ventricle with stenotic atrioventricular valve;
• Pulmonary atresia with intact ventricular septum;
• Double outlet right ventricle with restrictive VSD.

Blade or balloon atrial septectomy

After the newborn period, a defect can be created with a blade atrial septostomy or a trans-septal Brockenbrough puncture, followed by static balloon atrial septal dilatation. This is sometimes performed in mitral atresia with a restrictive atrial septum, despite a hypoplastic left atrium. ASD creation may also be useful in advanced pulmonary hypertension with syncope or prior to pulmonary artery dilatation with right ventricular hypertension.

In the immediate postoperative period following a fenestrated Fontan procedure, spontaneous fenestration occlusion may result in a sudden increase in systemic saturation that may be accompanied by low cardiac output and acidosis. Usually the fenestration can be located and crossed without a trans-septal needle, and then reopened with a balloon ± stent.

The future

In the last few years, several innovative procedures have been introduced that may prove to have an impact on the care of patients with congenital heart disease. These include pulmonary valve replacement, hybrid procedures jointly performed by surgeons and interventionalists, and Fontan completion with covered stents.

With each new invention, there is always high initial enthusiasm, but the reality is that only a minority of devices will ultimately be accepted. It is imperative for those working in the field to perform careful long-term follow-up studies to rule out unforeseen long-term complications with each new procedure/device. The reports of late erosions with Amplatzer ASD devices serve as an important reminder of this. The Bjork–Shiley heart valve prosthesis enjoyed widespread use and was implanted for over a decade before problems were first noted. Despite the significant reoperation risk in this group of patients, some advocated prophylactic removal. Let us hope history does not repeat itself.

Key clinical points

- Many interventional procedures and devices have been introduced and modified over the last two decades with widespread acceptance.
- Equipment used is often not specifically designed for congenital heart disease.
- Experts in the field have a duty to monitor long-term outcomes of all new interventions/ devices.

Further reading

Lock JE, Keane JF, Perry SB. *Diagnosis and Interventional Catheterization in Congenital Heart Disease*, 2nd edn. Amsterdam: Kluwer Academic Publishers, 2000.

Mullins CE. *Cardiac Catheterization in Congenital Heart Disease: Pediatric and Adult*. Oxford: Blackwell Publishing, 2006.

34 Principles of surgical management

Hideki Uemura

Royal Brompton Hospital, London, UK

Cardiac surgery is performed with or without cardiopulmonary bypass, depending largely on the operation being undertaken.

> **Non-bypass procedures (often performed via lateral thoracotomy)**
> - Ligation of arterial duct
> - Repair of aortic coarctation
> - Banding of the pulmonary trunk
> - Modified Blalock–Taussig shunt
> - Other systemic artery-to-pulmonary shunts
> - Division of vascular ring

The classical or bidirectional Glenn operation (cavopulmonary anastomosis), completion of extracardiac total cavopulmonary connection and occasionally atrial septectomy can be performed without bypass. Other operations, the majority of which provide definitive repair, are always performed with the assistance of cardiopulmonary bypass.

Rationale for definitive repair

In congenital heart disease with intra- or extra-cardiac shunting, the principal purpose of definitive repair is to:
- Separate the pulmonary and systemic circulations;
- Eliminate arterial hypoxia;
- Avoid volume overloading;
- Avoid the development of pulmonary vascular disease.

When the ventricular–arterial connection is discordant or there is a double outlet right ventricle with a subpulmonary ventricular septal defect (VSD), establishing a circulation in series and normalizing oxygenation will usually require an arterial switch procedure, whereas an atrial switch (Mustard or Senning) was performed in a previous era. The relief of obstructive lesions will prevent ventricular or atrial pressure overloading and hypertrophy, and promote normal cardiac output. Lastly, for patients with complex "single" ventricle physiology, the emphasis is placed on optimizing the pulmonary blood flow and in time achieving the "Fontan circulation."

Biventricular repair

Biventricular repair is possible mainly in patients with biventricular atrioventricular connection (each atrium connected to a separate ventricle; see Chapter 3). When repair is established using the morphologically right ventricle for the pulmonary circulation and the morphologically left ventricle for the systemic circulation (**"anatomic repair"**), ventricles are expected to function well in the short- and long-term.

Conventional repair for congenitally corrected transposition (see Chapter 14) or intra-atrial redirection of blood for complete transposition also involves complete separation of the pulmonary and systemic circulations (see Chapter 14), but the morphologically right ventricle supports the systemic circulation (**"functional repair"**). There are legitimate concerns as to whether the morphologically right ventricle, designed for the low-pressure and compliant pulmonary vascular bed, can adequately support the systemic circulation for life. At present, anatomic repair (**arterial switch operation**) is regarded as the treatment of choice for infants with complete trans-

Pediatric Heart Disease: A Practical Guide, First Edition. Piers E. F. Daubeney, Michael L. Rigby, Koichiro Niwa, and Michael A. Gatzoulis.
© 2012 Blackwell Publishing Ltd. Published 2012 by Blackwell Publishing Ltd.

position of the great arteries (see Chapter 14). More extensive surgery is increasingly employed in patients with congenitally corrected transposition or discordant atrioventricular connection (**double switch procedure**), although it remains to be seen if the systemic left ventricle will function normally in this situation.

Univentricular repair (Fontan-type procedure)

When the atrioventricular connection is grossly abnormal, biventricular repair is usually not possible because ventricular inlet malformations frequently coexist with severe abnormalities in the ventricular architecture. For example, in classical tricuspid atresia, the morphologically right ventricle possessing no inlet valve is usually markedly hypoplastic (see Chapter 15). This is also the case in double inlet left or right ventricle (see Chapter

16). In visceral heterotaxy or isomerism (see Chapter 17), a common valve is frequently found opening to the ventricles in an unbalanced fashion. When the atrioventricular connection is mainly, or exclusively, to one dominant ventricle (univentricular atrioventricular connection), it is impossible to separate the pulmonary and systemic circulations in the normal way. The **"Fontan circulation"** refers to the systemic venous return being anastomosed to the pulmonary arteries, either directly, or via the right atrium (Figure 34.1). Exceptionally, in double inlet left ventricle, ventricular septation can provide a biventricular circulation.

Since the Fontan circulation has no ejecting chamber for the pulmonary circulation, blood flows passively and in a non-pulsatile fashion to the lungs, and depends on a static pressure difference between the systemic and pulmonary veins. Inevitably, therefore, the pressure in the superior and inferior caval veins is higher than normal so that venous congestion and inadequate perfusion of the

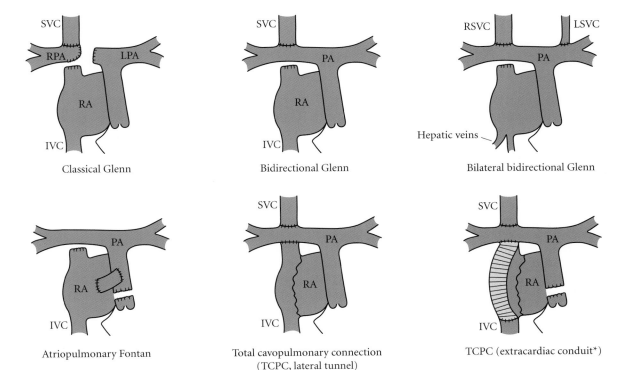

Figure 34.1 Types of venous anastomoses and Fontan operations. IVC, inferior caval vein; LPA, left pulmonary artery; LSVC, left superior vena cava; PA, pulmonary artery; RA, right atrium; RPA, right pulmonary artery; SVC, superior caval vein; RSVC, right superior vena cava; *, conduit or prosthetic tube. (Adapted from Gatzoulis MA, Swan L, Therrien J, Pantely GA, eds. *Adult Congenital Heart Disease, A Practical Guide*, 2005, with permission from Blackwell Publishing Ltd.)

body organs may lead to complications, such as hepatic cirrhosis, low cardiac output, and protein-losing enteropathy. The liver, in particular, is susceptible to elevated systemic venous pressure as up to 90% of its total perfusion is via the low pressure portal system.

The postoperative systemic venous pressure is dependent upon pulmonary vascular resistance and ventricular systolic and diastolic function. Atrioventricular valve regurgitation leading to pulmonary venous hypertension may also increase the pulmonary artery pressure.

The Fontan procedure was first reported by Fontan and colleagues in 1971, followed by Kreutzer and colleagues in 1973. Later, de Leval and colleagues proposed an alternative approach, the **total cavopulmonary connection (TCPC)** (see Figure 34.1), which had already been shown to be effective in patients with the hypoplastic left heart syndrome. The recommendation was based on studies of fluid kinetics and reducing energy loss at the connection between the systemic caval vein and the pulmonary artery. The superior caval vein was attached directly to the central pulmonary artery in an end-to-side (bidirectional) fashion, while the inferior caval vein was rerouted within the atrium (**"lateral tunnel"**) to the central pulmonary artery using a tube graft or baffle (see Figure 34.1). With this maneuver, the majority of the contractile atrial wall was excluded from the systemic venous pathway, and the pulmonary artery obtained was non-pulsatile and flow was laminar.

Numerous modifications have been proposed to the original Fontan procedure and TCPC. Direct anastomosis between the pulmonary trunk and the inferior caval vein has been attempted in selected patients. The channel for the inferior caval vein can be constructed outside of the atrium using a prosthetic tube graft or autologous pericardial roll – **"extracardiac Fontan"** (see Figure 34.1). This can be constructed without use of cardiopulmonary bypass (so-called off-pump Fontan). Such an approach can also be used in hearts with a biventricular atrioventricular connection for which intracardiac repair is inadvisable or impossible.

With increasing experience of the long-term outcome of the two main types of Fontan (atriopulmonary and TCPC; see Figure 34.1), most centers now show preference for the TCPC and would consider converting to a TCPC when there is a failing atriopulmonary Fontan. Marked right atrial dilatation, thrombosis, and intractable arrhythmia are considered by some as good indications for conversion, although patient selection and timing remain unclear. Arrhythmia prevention and preservation of ventricular function may be helped if the

---

Preoperative criteria identifying individuals who do well after the Fontan/TCPC

- Mean pulmonary artery pressure $\leq 15\,mmHg$
- Pulmonary vascular resistance ≤ 4 units/m^2
- Ratio of pulmonary artery-to-aorta diameter ≥ 0.75 without distortion or narrowing of the pulmonary arteries
- Systemic ventricular ejection fraction $\geq 60\%$
- Ventricular end-diastolic pressure $\leq 12\,mmHg$
- Systemic valve regurgitation not greater than mild

---

sinus node and cardiac veins (coronary sinus) remain outside the pulmonary venous atrium.

Fenestrated Fontan procedure

In individuals judged at higher surgical risk, a fenestration is added. The creation of a window or the insertion of a short prosthetic tube between the systemic venous channel and the functional left atrium ("fenestration") allows a right-to-left shunt, which secures a greater preload to the systemic ventricle, increasing cardiac output, albeit at the expense of cyanosis. A fenestration can improve the early postoperative course of the Fontan procedure; the fenestration (4–6 mm in size), may close spontaneously or can be closed with a transcatheter approach when no longer required.

Superior cavopulmonary anastomosis (partial right heart bypass or Glenn anastomosis)

The Glenn procedure reduces ventricular volume loading and usually improves arterial oxygen saturation (see Figure 34.1). The superior caval venous drainage is directly to the pulmonary artery without passing through the ventricles. The inferior caval and hepatic venous drainage mixes with pulmonary venous return and flows to the systemic circulation.

In the classical Glenn procedure, the right pulmonary artery was divided and connected to the superior caval vein (see Figure 34.1); the pulmonary arteries inevitably became non-confluent, producing unbalanced right and left lung perfusion. Furthermore, pulmonary arteriovenous fistulae frequently developed in the ipsilateral lung, making cyanosis worse. These issues were partly addressed with the introduction of the bidirectional Glenn anastomosis, in which the superior caval vein is transected and anastomosed to the central pulmonary artery in an end-to-side fashion.

Such partial right heart bypass can be considered as a semi-definitive repair in patients who are not suitable for the complete (non-fenestrated) Fontan operation, but usually it is the first step in the staged Fontan approach. It reduces the risk of a sudden decrease in ventricular volume and the consequential increase in wall thickness causing ventricular dysfunction, sometimes seen after the one-stage Fontan procedure. Furthermore, overall surgical risks may be reduced with a staged approach.

There is still some controversy about preserving additional forward flow from the ventricle to the pulmonary arteries (so-called competitive flow). Patients with the bidirectional Glenn anastomosis alone without competitive flow may remain more cyanosed and pulmonary artery growth may be suboptimal.

One-and-a-half ventricle repair

The term refers to the use of a Glenn anastomosis combined with relief of pulmonary stenosis or atresia in patients with moderate hypoplasia of the tricuspid valve and right ventricle and intact ventricular septum (see Chapter 15). Thus, there are two sources of pulmonary blood supply, from the right ventricle and from the superior caval vein. The indications and rationale for one-and-a-half ventricle repair remain contentious. The author employs a one-and-a-half ventricular repair when right ventricular end-diastolic volumes are 25–50% of normal or when the diameter of the tricuspid valve orifice is 50–70% of normal.

Palliative procedures

Palliative procedures when performed well enable early survival and preparation for later definitive surgical repair They are designed to decrease or increase pulmonary blood flow or, less frequently, to increase systemic flow in cases with aortic obstruction.

Blalock–Taussig shunt

The Blalock–Taussig (BT) shunt involves an anastomosis between the subclavian and pulmonary arteries, usually in severely cyanosed small infants, to increase pulmonary blood and reduce hypoxia. The original operation was a direct anastomosis, but now a prosthetic tube is interposed between the subclavian and pulmonary arteries. The amount of blood flow across the shunt is determined not only by the size but also by the diameter of the proximal artery and by pulmonary resistance. Excellent palliation can be achieved even with very small pulmonary arteries.

Central shunt

When the brachiocephalic artery or aorta is chosen as the proximal anastomotic site for the source of a shunt, or a short prosthetic tube is used to connect the ascending aorta to the proximal pulmonary arteries, the shunt is described as "central." Central shunts carry the risk of inconsistent and variable control of pulmonary blood flow.

Palliative reconstruction of the right ventricular outflow tract

In the neonate with tetralogy of Fallot and severe pulmonary stenosis or atresia, when there is extreme hypoplasia of the pulmonary arteries, establishing a direct connection from the right ventricle to the central pulmonary arteries is an alternative to a systemic artery-to-pulmonary artery shunt, but requires the use of cardiopulmonary bypass.

Pulmonary artery banding

Pulmonary artery banding is employed to reduce pulmonary blood flow in early infancy. Its major indications include hearts with absent atrioventricular connection or double inlet ventricle without pulmonary stenosis, and cases with multiple VSDs. Banding is often performed at the time of coarctation repair when there is a large VSD, including in cases with complete transposition or double outlet right ventricle. Banding of the pulmonary trunk and a concomitant BT shunt are employed in some patients with transposition of the great arteries when an early arterial switch operation is considered inadvisable (see Chapter 14).

Promotion of an adequate aortic pathway

Much more complex palliative procedures include the Norwood operation (see Chapter 16) in which the entire aortic arch is reconstructed and connected to the pulmonary trunk; pulmonary blood flow to the disconnected pulmonary arteries being supplied via a BT shunt or a conduit from the right ventricle. The Damus–Kaye–Stansel anastomosis or additional aortopulmonary anastomosis can also be performed to provide an unobstructed systemic ventricular outflow tract using the proximal pulmonary trunk in selected cases with severe subaortic stenosis and VSD, including those with a univentricular atrioventricular connection.

Atrial septectomy

If the interatrial communication is restrictive, systemic or pulmonary venous return can be congested (as in tricuspid or mitral atresia respectively). Balloon or blade atrial septostomy/septectomy (see Chapter 33) is the treatment of choice, although occasionally the surgical creation of an atrial septal defect may be required.

Further reading

Choussat A, Fontan F, Besse P, Vallot F, Chauve A, Bricand H. Selection criteria for Fontan's procedure. In: Anderson RH, Shinebourne EA, eds. *Pediatric Cardiology*. Edinburgh: Churchill Livingstone, 1978, pp. 559–566.

de Leval MR, Kilner P, Gewillig M, Bull C. Total cavopulmonary connection: a logical alternative to atriopulmonary connection for complex Fontan operations: experimental studies and early clinical experience. *J Thorac Cardiovasc Surg* 1988;96:682–695.

Fontan F, Baudet E. Surgical repair of tricuspid atresia. *Thorax* 1971;26:240–248.

Jonas RA. The importance of pulsatile flow when systemic venous return is connected directly to the pulmonary arteries. *J Thorac Cardiovasc Surg* 1993;105:173–175.

Kawashima Y, Kitamura S, Matsuda H, Shimazaki Y, Nakano S, Hirose H. Total cavopulmonary shunt operation in complex cardiac anomalies. *J Thorac Cardiovasc Surg* 1984;87:74–81.

Kirklin JK, Blackstone EH, Kirklin JW, Pacifico AD, Bargeron LM. The Fontan operation: ventricular hypertrophy, age, and date of operation as risk factors. *J Thorac Cardiovasc Surg* 1986;92:1049–1064.

Marcelletti C, Corno A, Giannico S, Marino B. Inferior vena cava-pulmonary artery extracardiac conduit. *J Thorac Cardiovasc Surg* 1990;100:228–232.

Mavroudis C, Backer CL, Deal BJ, Johnsrude CL. Fontan conversion to cavopulmonary connection and arrhythmia circuit cryoablation. *J Thorac Cardiovasc Surg* 1998;115:547–556.

Mendelsohn AM, Bove EL, Lupinetti FM, Crowley DC, Lloyd TR, Beekman RH. Central pulmonary artery growth patterns after the bidirectional Glenn procedure. *J Thorac Cardiovasc Surg* 1994;107:1284–1290.

Numata S, Uemura H, Yagihara T, Kagisaki K, Takahashi M, Ohuchi H. Long-term functional results of the one and one half ventricular repair for the spectrum of patients with pulmonary atresia/stenosis with intact ventricular septum. *Eur J Cardio-thorac Surg* 2003;24:516–520.

Uemura H, Anderson RH, Yagihara T. Surgical implications in hearts with isomeric atrial appendages. In: Karp RB, Laks H, Wechsler AS, eds. *Advances in Cardiac Surgery*, volume 7. St Louis: Mosby-Year Book, Inc., 1996:101–135.

Uemura H, Yagihara H, Yamashita K, Ishizaka T, Yoshizumi K, Kawahira Y. Establishment of total cavopulmonary connection without use of cardiopulmonary bypass. *Eur J Cardio-Thorac Surg* 1998;13:504–508.

Wilcox BR, Anderson RH. Valvar morphology. In: Wilcox BR, Anderson RH, eds. *Surgical Anatomy of the Heart*, 2nd edn. London: Gower Medical Publishing, 1992, pp. 6.7–6.8.

35 Heart, lung, and heart–lung transplantation

Steven A. Webber[1,2]

[1]University of Pittsburgh School of Medicine, Pittsburgh, PA, USA
[2]Children's Hospital of Pittsburgh of UPMC, Pittsburgh, PA, USA

Transplantation offers the only hope for survival and improved quality of life for selected children with end-stage heart and lung disease due to:
- Cardiomyopathy;
- Congenital defects;
- Idiopathic pulmonary arterial hypertension;
- Parenchymal lung disease.

The first pediatric thoracic transplant was performed by Kantrowitz in 1967, only a few days after Dr Christian Barnard's pioneering operation in an adult. Interest in heart transplantation declined throughout the 1970s, due to the high mortality from lack of effective immunosuppression. There was a resurgence in the early 1980s with the introduction of cyclosporine, the first oral immunosuppressive agent with relative specificity for inhibition of T lymphocytes, the primary mediators of allograft rejection. This resulted in dramatic improvements in survival of all transplanted organs. There have been significant improvements over the last two to three decades in perioperative care and first year survival after all forms of thoracic transplantation in children, but the procedure remains palliative. This is due to our poor understanding of, and lack of treatments for, chronic allograft rejection, the main cause of late mortality after heart and lung transplantation.

Heart transplantation

Indications and contraindications

A consensus group of the American Heart Association recently addressed the indications for heart transplantation in children. Heart transplantation is generally considered to be indicated when expected survival is less than 2 years, and/or when there is unacceptable quality of life. Cardiomyopathy (predominantly dilated forms) and complex congenital heart defects remain the primary indications, and together account for approximately 90% of transplantations undertaken in children. Diagnoses leading to transplantation are age dependent, with congenital heart disease accounting for two-thirds of transplants in infancy, and cardiomyopathy a similar proportion among adolescents. For neonates with hypoplastic left heart syndrome there has been a move away from transplantation, and towards staged reconstruction in most centers. This reflects donor shortage, high pre-transplant mortality, and improving (though imperfect) results of staged reconstruction (Norwood procedure and subsequent palliations).

Relative and/or absolute contraindications include:
- Chronic infection with either hepatitis B or C, or human immunodeficiency virus;
- Prior non-adherence with medical therapy;
- Recent treatment of malignancy with inadequate follow-up to ensure likely cure;
- Active acute viral, fungal or bacterial infections;
- Excessive and fixed pulmonary vascular resistance (above 10 IU);
- Inadequate intraparenchymal pulmonary vascular bed;
- Diffuse pulmonary vein stenosis;
- Major extracardiac disease considered to preclude good quality of life and long-term survival.

Candidate evaluation

The evaluation includes the assessment of expected survival without transplantation, the patient's current quality of life, the potential for alternate surgical or medical therapies, as well as the inherent risks of the transplant surgery itself. The evaluation includes careful assessment of anatomic and hemodynamic findings, including pulmonary vascular resistance. Excessive fixed resistance will result in acute donor right ventricular failure and an inability to wean the patient from cardiopulmonary bypass. Each candidate is evaluated by a multidisciplinary team. Evaluation of past history of non-adherence to medical therapy is critical.

Typical evaluation protocol for candidates for heart transplantation

- History and physical examination
- Required consultations:
  - Pediatric cardiologist
  - Congenital cardiovascular surgeon
  - Cardiac anesthesiologist
  - Infectious disease specialist
  - Psychiatrist or psychologist
  - Transplant coordinator
  - Social worker
- Cardiac diagnostic studies:
  - CXR
  - EKG
  - Echocardiogram
  - Cardiac catheterization
  - In selected patients: Exercise test, ventilation–perfusion scan, chest CT or MRI, pulmonary function tests
- Laboratory tests:
  - Blood type (ABO)
  - Anti-HLA antibody screen
  - Complete blood count and white cell differential
  - Platelet count
  - Coagulation screen
  - Blood urea nitrogen
  - Serum creatinine, glucose, calcium, magnesium, liver function tests, lipid profile, brain natriuretic peptide
  - Serologic screening for antibodies to cytomegalovirus (CMV), Epstein–Barr (EBV), herpes simplex, human immunodeficiency, varicella, hepatitis A, B, C, D, and measles; antibodies to *Toxoplasma gondii*
- PPD/ Mantoux placement
- Update immunizations including hepatitis B, pneumococcal, and influenza (in season)

Donor evaluation

Evaluation of the donor heart begins with a careful review of the history. This includes:

- Donor age and gender;
- Body size;
- Cause of death;
- Presence of any chest trauma;
- Need for cardiopulmonary resuscitation. A history of cardiopulmonary resuscitation is not, in itself, a contraindication to cardiac donation for pediatric recipients;
- Length of resuscitation;
- Evaluation of the hemodynamic status of the donor (including blood pressure, heart rate, and central venous pressure if available). The amount of inotropic support, and trends in usage over time, are noted.

To rule out structural abnormalities and to evaluate cardiac function, a complete echocardiogram should be performed. Most centers avoid the use of donor hearts whose systolic function is more than mildly impaired after treatment with inotropic agents or thyroid hormone. A 12-lead EKG should be performed. Mild, non-specific ST and T wave changes are commonly present, and usually reflect central nervous system effects, electrolyte disturbances, or hypothermia. These do not contraindicate organ donation. Use of older donors (e.g. above 35 years of age) for pediatric recipients is associated with high risk of post-transplant coronary disease and poor long-term survival. Such donors are generally avoided.

Size matching is a critical issue in the selection of potential donors. Most centers avoid undersizing the donor below 75–80% of recipient weight. Below this, cardiac output of the donor may be insufficient to meet the needs of the recipient. Use of oversized donors is common in pediatric transplantation.

All donors should be screened for evidence of infection. Evidence of donor retroviral infection (HIV or HTLV) is considered an absolute contraindication to heart transplantation. The presence of donor hepatitis B surface antigen is also usually considered an absolute contraindication to heart donation.

Evaluation of the cardiac donor

- History:
  - Donor age, height, weight, and gender
  - Cause of brain death
  - History of cardiac arrest and length of resuscitation
  - Evidence of chest trauma
  - History of intravenous drug usage
  - Past history of cardiovascular disease
  - Distance from transplant center
  - History of malignancy

- Cardiovascular status:
  - Heart rate, blood pressure, central venous pressure
  - Fluid balance
  - Blood gas
  - Types and doses of intravenous inotropes
- Cardiovascular testing:
  - EKG
  - CXR
  - Echocardiogram
  - Cardiac enzymes
- Infection screening:
  - CMV, EBV, *T. gondii*, HIV-1, HIV-2, HTLV-1, HTLV-2, RPR (for syphilis), hepatitis B and C
  - All culture results since admission to intensive care unit

Surgical techniques of graft implantation

Detailed review of surgical techniques is beyond the scope of this text and has recently been reviewed (see Further reading). In 1960, Lower and Shumway enumerated the basic surgical principles of orthotopic (i.e. into the same site as the original organ that failed) heart transplantation, initially in dogs, and several years later in humans. The pioneering efforts led to the adoption of the **biatrial anastomoses** for cardiac transplantation. This technique has been applied to thousands of patients, of all ages, with excellent results. Many centers now perform **bicaval anastomoses** in children of all ages undergoing orthotopic heart transplantation. It is believed by some that this may result in less sinus node dysfunction and less tricuspid regurgitation. Some specific forms of congenital heart disease lend themselves particularly well to the bicaval technique, e.g. patients who have previously undergone Mustard or Senning operations, and those with a Glenn anastomosis. The bicaval technique may be associated with superior caval vein stenosis, especially in infants.

Transplantation for congenital heart disease is often performed after multiple palliative procedures, and may present formidable surgical challenges. The anatomic substrate can be broadly classified as abnormalities of the systemic venous return, abnormalities of the pulmonary venous return, and abnormalities of the great vessels, including hypoplastic left heart syndrome. Surgical modifications of the two basic techniques, atrial and bicaval anastomoses, are required for transplantation of these anatomic variants.

Postoperative management and early complications
Cardiovascular considerations

Abnormalities in cardiac function are inevitable due to the obligatory hypoxic/ischemic insult that the donor heart endures. Recovery of systolic function is usually rapid. Abnormalities in diastolic function, however, may persist for many weeks. Most heart transplant recipients will benefit from low-dose inotropic support in the immediate postoperative period. Occasionally, and particularly in infants with markedly oversized donors, the simplest way to improve cardiac function is to leave the chest open at the end of the transplant procedure.

The term **primary graft failure** is often reserved for the finding of acute left ventricular or biventricular failure not due to high pulmonary vascular resistance, resulting in failure to wean from cardiopulmonary bypass or need for mechanical circulatory support within the first 48 hours after transplantation. Poor donor selection, very prolonged ischemic time, poor preservation technique, and hyperacute rejection (due to preformed donor-specific anti-HLA antibodies) should all be considered. When primary graft failure occurs, recovery is frequently possible if the circulation can be supported. This is usually achieved with extracorporeal membrane oxygenation (ECMO). Retransplantation for early graft failure is generally associated with very poor outcomes, and many consider this a contraindication to retransplantation.

When there is acute failure of the right ventricle, the usual cause is excessive **pulmonary vascular resistance**. Inadequate repair of stenotic pulmonary arteries must also be ruled out. For excessive pulmonary arteriolar resistance, nitric oxide (up to 80 ppm) is commenced in the operating room. Hypercarbia is avoided, sedation provided, and there is no attempt at early weaning from artificial ventilation. The right heart may require significant inotropic support. Mechanical assistance can be provided, but if acute donor right heart failure reflects poor candidate selection (e.g. indexed pulmonary resistance greater than 10 IU), then recovery of right heart function is unlikely.

Postoperative **tachy- and brady-arrhythmias** have been observed in children following heart transplantation. The commonest rhythm abnormality is sinus node dysfunction leading to sinus bradycardia, with or without an atrial or junctional escape rhythm. The denervated sinus node responds appropriately to exogenous chronotropic agents and isoproterenol (isoprenaline) is useful in this respect. A simpler approach is atrial pacing, and all transplant recipients should have temporary pacing wires placed in the operating room. Sinus node dysfunction reflects ischemic and/or traumatic injury, but usually recovers in a few days. Ventricular ectopy and non-sustained ventricular tachycardia are also quite common in the first week or two after transplantation, but rarely require treatment.

Systemic hypertension is also common early after heart transplantation. Many factors contribute, including vigorous function of an oversized donor organ and use of high-dose corticosteroids.

Renal dysfunction

The combination of chronic heart failure, cardiopulmonary bypass, and use of cyclosporine or tacrolimus all contribute to postoperative renal dysfunction. This is exacerbated if there is a low cardiac output state postoperatively. Oliguria is common. Fortunately, acute renal failure is rare in children and dialysis is seldom required. When urine output remains low, it may be necessary to delay the introduction of calcineurin inhibitor immunosuppressant medication (tacrolimus or cyclosporine) for a few days. This can be facilitated by the use of intravenous induction agents as part of the early immunosuppressive regimen (see below).

Infectious complications and their prevention

Infections are a leading cause of death and morbidity in the first year following heart transplantation. Most severe infections occur during the initial hospitalization. During the first week after transplantation, invasive lines and drains are removed as soon as possible. A short course of antibiotics is given as prophylaxis against mediastinal wound infection. Usually a first-generation cephalosporin will suffice. Broader staphylococcal coverage (i.e. vancomycin) is given if the patient has had a prolonged ICU stay, long-standing lines are in place, or the recipient is colonized with methicillin-resistant *Staphylococcus aureus* (MRSA). Oral nystatin is started in the ICU, along with ganciclovir, if the recipient or donor is seropositive for CMV. Patients at high risk for yeast infections (e.g. patients on pre- or post-transplant ECMO) are frequently given prophylaxis with fluconazole. It should be noted that all "azole" antifungals have a profound effect on calcineurin inhibitor metabolism (via the cytochrome P450 system) and a marked reduction in tacrolimus or cyclosporine dosing is required during concomitant use of an azole antifungal agent. Initiation of prophylaxis against *Pneumocystis jiroveci* (formerly *Pneumo-*

cystis carinii) can follow nearer to the time of hospital discharge.

Initial immunosuppression and early acute rejection

High-dose intravenous methylprednisolone (e.g. 15–20 mg/kg) is given in the operating room. A tapering course of corticosteroids is often given over the next 1–2 weeks. Historically, the majority of centers discharged patients on maintenance corticosteroid therapy. However, there is increasing use of steroid-free immunosuppressive regimens in pediatric practice. Cyclosporine or tacrolimus is commenced generally within 24–48 hours of surgery once good urine output has been established. Both agents can be given intravenously or enterally, though the latter is the preferred route of administration. Approximately half of centers use "induction therapy," either with anti-T cell agents that deplete T cells (most commonly polyclonal rabbit antithymocyte globulin) or less often with an interleukin-2 receptor.

There are many strategies for **maintenance immunosuppression** (Table 35.1). All centers currently use a calcineurin inhibitor as the primary immunosuppressive agent and there is approximately equal use of tacrolimus and cyclosporine at this time. Most centers also use a second, adjunctive, antimetabolite or antiproliferative agent. There is highly variable use of long-term corticosteroids. In general, agents of similar classes are not given together as this tends to enhance toxicities. Combination therapies use two or three agents of different classes with different mechanisms of action.

Acute cellular rejection is primarily associated with infiltration of T cells (CD4 and CD8) into the graft (Figure 35.1a). Infants and young children experience less acute rejection than adolescents. Pallor, increasing tachycardia, abdominal pain, gallop rhythm, and oliguria are all suggestive of severe rejection. Ideally, rejection is identified by echocardiography and/or surveillance biopsy before such signs develop. The EKG may show reduced precordial voltages. The tempo of rejection can be quite abrupt in the early post-transplant period and any deterioration in the patient's condition after initial recovery from surgery must be taken very seriously. If there is unequivocal evidence of new graft dysfunction, empiric treatment (usually consisting of bolus intravenous corticosteroids) or immediate endomyocardial biopsy should be performed. Biopsy generally shows lymphocytic infiltrates (predominantly T cells) with varying degrees of edema and myocyte damage. Endomyocardial biopsies are graded according to an internationally agreed classi-

Table 35.1 Potential combinations of maintenance immunosuppressive drugs used in pediatric heart transplantation. All maintenance regimens may be used with or without induction therapy with T-cell depleting antibody preparations or with interleukin-2 receptor antagonists

Number of agents	Potential combinations	Comments
Monotherapy	Tacrolimus or cyclosporine	Monotherapy rarely used with cyclosporine
Dual therapy	Tacrolimus or cyclosporine with	Little experience with the mTOR (target of rapamycin) inhibitors sirolimus and everolimus in children
	Azathioprine or mycophenolate mofetil or sirolimus/everolimus or corticosteroids	Steroid avoidance increasingly common in pediatric heart transplantation
Triple therapy	Tacrolimus or cyclosporine with	Mycophenolate mofetil is being used with increasing frequency *in lieu* of azathioprine
	Corticosteroids with	
	Azathioprine or mycophenolate mofetil or sirolimus/ everolimus	

(a)   (b)

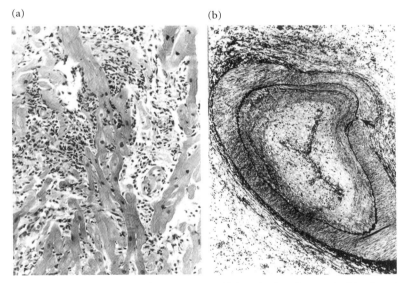

Figure 35.1 Cardiac allograft rejection. (a) Moderately severe acute cellular rejection characterized by dense lymphocytic infiltrates, edema, and myocyte necrosis. (b) Chronic rejection characterized by diffuse graft coronary arterial vasculopathy, with severe myointimal proliferation leading to luminal occlusion.

fication system developed by the International Society for Heart and Lung Transplantation.

Medium-term and late complications

A detailed discussion of all complications of heart transplantation is beyond the scope of this text and readers are referred to other reviews (see Further reading). Immunologic complications of transplantation fall into two main groups:

• Allograft rejection with or without graft dysfunction (both acute and chronic), reflecting inadequate or ineffective immunosuppression;
• Manifestations of non-specific immunosuppression, including infections and malignancy.

Non-immune side effects of immunosuppressive therapy (i.e. tissue and organ toxicities) are also an important cause of morbidity and, occasionally, mortality.

Acute rejection

Early acute rejection is described above. Patients remain at risk for acute rejection indefinitely. There is no evidence that heart transplant recipients become truly tolerant to their allograft. Acute rejection is the commonest cause of death between 30 days and 3 years after heart transplantation, accounting for almost 30% of all deaths. The peak hazard, or instantaneous risk, for first rejection is between 1 and 2 months after transplantation. Onset to first rejection is generally delayed by the use of induction therapy. By 1 year after transplantation, only 40–60% of pediatric heart recipients are free of acute rejection.

Late acute rejection episodes (occurring beyond the first year after transplantation) appear to carry a particularly poor long-term prognosis, especially if associated with graft dysfunction. When there is any degree of systolic dysfunction with acute rejection, rapid deterioration is common. Treatment for acute rejection is generally with intravenous methylprednisolone 10–15 mg/kg (maximum 1 g) daily for 3 days. In less severe cases, a course of high-dose oral prednisolone (e.g. 2 mg/kg for 5 days) may be used, with or without a subsequent taper.

Acute rejection with hemodynamic compromise can rapidly lead to graft failure. Unless there are specific contraindications, such patients should receive full hemodynamic support, including mechanical support, since the condition is generally reversible in nature.

The presence of donor-specific anti-HLA antibodies may lead to **antibody-mediated rejection**, with complement activation, graft endothelial cell damage, and severe graft dysfunction. This type of rejection can be difficult to treat, though often responds to high-dose steroids and plasmapheresis.

Chronic rejection or post-transplantation coronary arterial disease

The terms chronic rejection and post-transplant coronary arterial disease are generally used synonymously. Coronary disease subsequent to transplantation is an accelerated vasculopathy and is the leading cause of death among late survivors of pediatric heart transplantation. It accounts for approximately 40% of deaths in the period 3–5 years after transplantation. The pathology differs somewhat from that of ischemic heart disease in the normal adult population. Typical allograft coronary arterial disease consists of myointimal proliferation that is generally concentric and involves the entire length of the vessel, including intramyocardial branches. Eventually, luminal occlusion occurs (Figure 35.1b). There is often associated inflammation. Both immune

and non-immune mechanisms likely contribute to the development of graft vasculopathy, though immune mechanisms are probably of central importance in children. Use of older donors, late acute rejection episodes, older recipient age, CMV infection, and antibody-mediated rejection are all risk factors for the development of post-transplant coronary arterial disease.

Symptoms of angina are often absent, though some children will experience episodes of abdominal pain and/or chest pain, despite operative denervation of the heart. Syncope and sudden death are also common presentations of graft coronary arterial disease. The diagnosis is most often made during surveillance selective coronary angiography. Intravascular ultrasound has much greater sensitivity for this diagnosis, though experience in children is much more limited than that in adults.

Unfortunately, no curative treatment exists for established coronary arterial disease. Retransplantation is the primary therapeutic option for advanced coronary arterial disease at this time. Results of late retransplantation (beyond 1 year) are similar to those for primary transplantation.

Infections

An increased prevalence of all forms of infection is seen compared to the general population. Most infections are caused by pathogens that also cause infection in the non-immunocompromised host. Common examples include respiratory viruses, *Streptococcus pneumoniae*, and varicella virus. All infections that occur in non-immunocompromised patients can cause greater disease severity in the transplant recipient. Of particular note in this respect are infections due to CMV and EBV, which only rarely cause severe disease in the immunocompetent host. More rarely, opportunistic infections are seen, e.g. *Pneumocystis jiroveci* (formerly *Pneumocystis carinii*).

Primary CMV infection is less problematic in heart transplant patients than in lung recipients. Nonetheless, pneumonitis, gastroenteritis, hepatitis, and bone marrow suppression may all be observed. Diagnosis is facilitated by evaluation of peripheral blood by PCR or antigenemia (pp65) testing. Diagnosis of CMV disease remains a tissue diagnosis. When the diagnosis is made early, treatment with intravenous ganciclovir and/or oral valganciclovir is usually very effective.

EBV infection in the immunocompromised host can be asymptomatic, or may cause a non-specific viral syndrome, mononucleosis, fulminant "viral sepsis" or a **post-transplant lymphoproliferative disorder (PTLD)**. The strongest risk factor for the development of PTLD is the development of primary EBV infection post-transplantation. PTLD occurs in 5–10% of pediatric heart transplant recipients. Although it frequently resolves with reduced immunosuppression, overall morbidity and mortality remain significant, including graft loss due to reduced immunosuppression. Second-line therapies include anti-CD20 monoclonal antibodies (which eliminate B cells), chemotherapy, and rarely, cellular (adoptive) immunotherapy.

Non-immune complications

In addition to the consequences of over- or under-immunosuppression, transplant recipients experience a wide array of non-immune toxicities of immunosuppressive therapies. These include systemic hypertension, hyperlipidemia, diabetes mellitus, decreased bone mineral density, and bone marrow suppression, among others. One complication worthy of particular attention is that of **progressive renal dysfunction** due to calcineurin inhibitor renal toxicity. This is becoming increasingly problematic as larger numbers of children survive long-term after heart transplantation. Up to 5% of long-term survivors develop end-stage renal failure requiring renal transplantation.

Survival after listing for transplantation and after transplantation

Data from the United States Scientific Registry of Transplant Recipients reveal that children in all age groups have substantially shorter waiting times for heart transplants than do adults, but they have a greater risk of **pretransplant mortality**. The highest death rate is among infant candidates. It is hoped that improved mechanical circulatory support systems (e.g. ventricular assist devices specifically designed for infants and children) may decrease this high wait-list mortality in the future.

Early **post-transplant survival** has improved in recent years; the improved survival is most evident in the infant age group and in smaller volume centers. Most of the improvement appears to be due to reduction in perioperative mortality. One-year survival is now approximately 90%. There is slightly higher early mortality for infant recipients, but interestingly, these youngest recipients have the greatest conditional graft half-life based on analysis of 1-year survivors. It is likely that this reflects a lower incidence of post-transplant coronary arterial disease in these very young recipients and a degree of immune privilege. The results of transplantation for congenital heart disease still lag slightly behind those of transplantation for cardiomyopathy; this difference is due to slightly

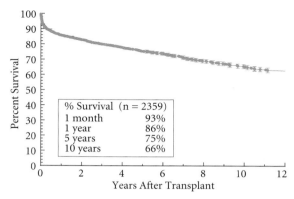

Figure 35.2 Survival after pediatric heart transplantation. (Data from the Pediatric Heart Transplant Study, 1993–2007.)

higher perioperative mortality. Importantly, there is evidence of significantly reduced survival among black pediatric recipients compared to other racial groups, though the reasons for this are not entirely clear. For all recipients, it is evident that heart transplantation is palliative and not curative, and that current immunosuppressive regimens are associated with significant drug-related toxicities. Graft coronary arterial disease remains the primary barrier to very long-term survival. Five- and 10-year patient survival rates are approximately 75% and 65% respectively (Figure 35.2).

Lung and heart–lung transplantation

A detailed discussion of lung and heart–lung transplantation is outside the scope of this book. However, it is important for the pediatric cardiologist to understand the indications and outcomes of these procedures in order to determine when referral is appropriate, and to help counsel patients and families about the outcomes following transplantation.

Indications

The primary indications for lung or heart–lung transplantation for cardiovascular disorders are the presence of irreversible pulmonary hypertension, inadequately developed central pulmonary arteries, or the presence of pulmonary venous obstructive disease. Pulmonary hypertension may be idiopathic, secondary to long-standing left-to-right shunts (Eisenmenger complex), or due to long-standing pulmonary venous hypertension (e.g. due to Shone complex or restrictive cardiomyopathy).

Double-lung transplantation (performed as separate, sequential single-lung transplants) is indicated for most cases of idiopathic pulmonary hypertension and for rare cases of congenital heart disease where there is a simple lesion amenable to repair at the time of lung transplantation (e.g. patent ductus arteriosus or atrial septal defect). Heart–lung transplantation is performed for pulmonary vascular disease associated with more complex congenital heart disease, or with long-standing cardiomyopathy.

Candidate evaluation

The principles of candidate selection are similar to those for heart transplantation, i.e. alternative therapies have been exhausted, life expectancy is considered to be very limited, and/or quality of life is extremely poor. Enthusiasm for referral for lung transplantation is significantly dampened compared to heart transplantation due to the poorer long-term outcomes, and the ethical dilemmas of performing these complex palliative procedures, particularly in young candidates who cannot participate in the consent process.

Complications

The complications of heart–lung and lung transplantation are similar, and are driven primarily by the lung allograft. The heart of the heart–lung allograft appears relatively protected from acute rejection, and the lung bears the brunt of the host immune response. Compared to isolated heart transplantation, there is an increased prevalence of severe infection due to the externalized nature of the allograft and the greater levels of immunosuppression required to control allograft rejection compared to the isolated heart transplant. Chronic rejection takes the form of a progressive obliterative bronchiolitis,

which eventually leads to respiratory failure. Approximately 50% of heart–lung and lung recipients have some evidence of this complication by 2–3 years after transplantation.

Survival after heart–lung and lung transplantation is similar and currently disappointing. One-year survival has improved and is currently approximately 85%. However, 5- and 10-year survival is only approximately 50% and 30% respectively. These poor late results largely reflect the development of obliterative bronchiolitis and its complications.

Further reading

Webber SA, McCurry K, Zeevi A. Seminar: Heart and lung transplantation in children. *Lancet* 2006;368:53–69.
Canter CE, Shaddy RE, Bernstein D, *et al*. Indications for heart transplantation in pediatric heart disease: A scientific statement from the American Heart Association. *Circulation* 2007;115:658–676.
Kirk R, Edwards LB, Aurora P, *et al*. Registry of the International Society for Heart and Lung Transplantation: Eleventh official pediatric heart transplantation report – 2008. *J Heart Lung Transplant* 2008;27:970–977.
Pigula FA, Webber SA. Donor evaluation, surgical technique and perioperative management. In: Fine R, Webber SA, Harmon W, Olthoff K, Kelly D, eds. *Pediatric Solid Organ Transplantation*. Oxford: Blackwell Publishing, 2007, Chapter 33.
Stewart S, Winters GL, Fishbein MC, *et al*. Revision of the 1990 working formulation for the standardization of nomenclature in the diagnosis of heart rejection. *J Heart Lung Transplant* 2005;24:1710–1720.
Chin C, Naftel D, Pahl E, *et al*. Cardiac retransplantation in pediatrics: A Multi-institutional study. *J Heart Lung Transplant* 2006;25:1420–1424.
English RF, Pophal SA, Bacanu S, *et al*. Long-term comparison of tacrolimus and cyclosporine induced nephrotoxicity in pediatric heart transplant recipients. *Am J Transplant* 2002;2:769–773.

36 Murmurs in asymptomatic patients

William H. Neches[1] and Gregory H. Tatum[2]

[1]Children's Hospital of Pittsburgh of UPMC, Pittsburgh, PA, USA
[2]Duke University Medical Center, Durham, NC, USA

Murmurs represent the most common reason for referral to a pediatric cardiologist. More than 90% of children will have a murmur during their first 5 years of life, but most of these murmurs are benign physiologic phenomena.

History

Patients with innocent murmurs will be asymptomatic, while pathologic murmurs may be present prior to the onset of any cardiac symptoms. Several historical features can help guide the practitioner to the correct diagnosis. It is important to know when the murmur was first noted and whether it was found by a new physician, or by the physician who has seen the patient on a number of previous occasions. Is the murmur always present, or does it come and go? While cyanosis is important to note at any age and poor weight gain can always be a sign of heart failure, other symptoms will vary with age.

> **Important symptoms to ascertain**
>
> **In infants**
> - Rapid breathing
> - Diaphoresis (sweatiness)
> - Feeding difficulties
>
> **In older children**
> - Exercise intolerance
> - Shortness of breath
> - Fatigue
> - Palpitations
> - Lightheadedness
> - Syncope

It is important to ask about any family members with congenital heart defects or syndromes.

Physical examination

A complete physical examination should be performed, including assessment for cyanosis and any dysmorphic features. A rapid respiratory rate, hyperinflation or rales on pulmonary examination may be due to congestive heart failure and would suggest a pathologic murmur. A complete cardiac examination should be performed as detailed in Chapter 4. A normal precordial impulse and normal heart sounds will be present in patients with innocent heart murmurs. Any abnormalities in these findings would argue for a pathologic murmur. In particular, innocent murmurs are never associated with a palpable thrill. The murmur should be characterized in terms of timing, duration, intensity, pitch, location, and radiation. The abdomen should be assessed for enlargement of the liver or spleen. The peripheral perfusion and strength of pulses in all four extremities (especially the femoral pulses) should be determined.

Differential diagnosis

Still's murmur

- The classic innocent murmur; most common in early school-age children, but can present in infancy.
- Vibratory or musical systolic murmur usually best heard along the mid or upper left sternal border. Sometimes heard best between the left sternal border and apex.

Pediatric Heart Disease: A Practical Guide, First Edition. Piers E. F. Daubeney, Michael L. Rigby, Koichiro Niwa, and Michael A. Gatzoulis.
© 2012 Blackwell Publishing Ltd. Published 2012 by Blackwell Publishing Ltd.

• Usually grade 1 or 2/6 in intensity, but may be as loud as grade 3/6; loudest with the patient in a supine position.
• Often becomes more pronounced with increased cardiac output such as during febrile illnesses or after exercise.
• Heart sounds are normal and there is no ejection sound.

Venous hum
• Another common innocent murmur in the early school-age child.
• Low-pitched continuous murmur heard in the supra-clavicular or infraclavicular area.
• Diminishes significantly, or disappears, with lying down, turning the head, or external compression of the jugular vein.
• Can occur on either side, but is more common on the right.

Neonatal peripheral pulmonary stenosis
• Common innocent murmur found in infants
• Particularly common in preterm and small-for-dates infants.
• Soft, medium-pitched systolic ejection murmur that is loudest at the left upper sternal border.
• Pattern of radiation is distinctive with the murmur being audible in either, or both, axillae and often over the back as well.
• Arises from a relative size discrepancy between the main pulmonary artery and branch pulmonary arteries due to differential blood flow during fetal circulation, when the majority of pulmonary blood flow goes through the ductus arteriosus into the systemic circulation.
• Normally resolves by 6 months of age.

Innocent aortic or pulmonic systolic murmurs
• Occur in children and adolescents.
• Systolic ejection murmurs localized to the right upper sternal border and left upper sternal border respectively.
• Medium pitched and not as harsh as the pathologic murmurs from aortic or pulmonary stenosis.
• No associated ejection sound.
• Tend to occur during times of illness, fever, excitement or exercise.
• Common during pregnancy and anemia.

Murmur from a closing patent arterial duct
• Occasionally heard in neonates.
• Crescendo systolic murmur in the left infraclavicular area, which normally disappears within 24–48 hours after birth.

• Can be difficult to distinguish from a large patent ductus arteriosus (PDA) at onset, but the murmur from a pathologic PDA will persist and often is accompanied by bounding pulses.

Systolic murmur along the left lower sternal border
• May be heard in neonates due to transient tricuspid regurgitation.
• Can sound very similar to a ventricular septal defect.
• Most commonly associated with transient myocardial ischemia and resolves as myocardial function improves.

Murmur over the cranium
• Rarely, may be heard in children younger than 4 years of age, especially with fever.
• Low intensity continuous murmur.
• Mechanism for this innocent murmur is unknown.
• Differential diagnosis includes cranial arteriovenous malformations.

Mammary soufflé murmur
• Occurs in pregnant and early postpartum women.
• Loudest in systole and can be limited to systole.
• Distinct delay from S1 to the onset of the murmur.
• Audible anywhere along the breast.
• Can be differentiated from an arteriovenous malformation or PDA in that it can be eliminated with compression or sometimes with standing, and it will disappear after breast feeding is discontinued.

Many patients with cardiac disorders, both congenital and acquired, may have murmurs and yet remain asymptomatic. These include septal defects, valvar stenosis or regurgitation, cardiomyopathies, coarctation of the aorta, and rheumatic heart disease, just to name a few.

Investigation and referral

The majority of murmurs in pediatric patients are innocent and no diagnostic testing is required. The classic innocent murmurs frequently can be distinguished from pathologic murmurs by physical examination. Patients should be referred to a cardiologist if they have any cardiovascular symptoms, other abnormal physical findings, or if the diagnosis is in doubt. When the murmur is not classical for an innocent murmur, several tests can be useful.
• **EKG:** Look for any signs of chamber enlargement, ventricular hypertrophy, or conduction abnormalities

- **CXR:** Useful for assessing the heart size, as well as the pulmonary vascular markings
- **Echocardiogram:** May be needed to assess for any underlying structural heart disease if the latter cannot be definitively excluded on clinical examination, but is not indicated when the diagnosis of an innocent murmur is certain

---

Key clinical points

- Asymptomatic murmur is the commonest reason for referral to a pediatric cardiologist
- Most children will exhibit an innocent murmur at some point in childhood
- Nature of the murmur is age dependent:
  - "Peripheral pulmonary stenosis" is the most common innocent murmur in newborns
  - "Still's type" murmur is the most common innocent murmur in toddlers and young school-age children
- Most innocent murmurs can be accurately diagnosed by clinical examination
- Echocardiography is indicated if doubt exists after evaluation by a cardiologist

---

Further reading

Danford DA, Martin AB, Fletcher SE, Gumbiner CH. Echocardiographic yield in children when innocent murmur seems likely but doubts linger. *Pediatr Cardiol* 2002; 23:410–414.

Pelech AN. Evaluation of the pediatric patient with a cardiac murmur. *Pediatr Clin North Am* 1999;46:167–188.

Rosenthal A. How to distinguish between innocent and pathologic murmurs in childhood. *Pediatr Clin North Am* 1984;31:1229–1240.

37 Syncope and presyncope

William H. Neches[1] and Gregory H. Tatum[2]

[1]Children's Hospital of Pittsburgh of UPMC, Pittsburgh, PA, USA
[2]Duke University Medical Center, Durham, NC, USA

Syncope and presyncope are common in the pediatric population. While most cases will be benign, syncope or presyncope can be indicative of potentially life-threatening illnesses.

History

Prodromal symptoms are commonly reported:
- Weakness;
- Nausea;
- Blurred vision;
- Diaphoresis;
- Lightheadedness;
- Dizziness;
- Palpitations;
- Tachycardia.

The setting in which the syncope occurred and its frequency are important. Precipitating factors, duration of loss of consciousness, how the patient appears during the event, the patient's state during the recovery period, and whether these events always follow the same pattern should be recorded. It is important to know of any underlying medical conditions. Family history may reveal relatives with arrhythmias, sudden cardiac death or history of fainting. Patients should also be asked about their dietary habits with particular attention paid to their total fluid and salt intake. Any medications or dietary supplements that the patient is using should be documented. All patients should be asked about any recreational drug use. In young children, the family should be asked about any medications or drugs that are in the household.

Physical examination

Even though in most patients the physical examination will be normal, all patients should have a thorough and complete examination with particular attention paid to the cardiac and neurologic systems. Patients should be assessed for orthostatic hypertension by obtaining the pulse rate and blood pressure when supine and then after 5–10 min of standing. A drop in blood pressure by more than 10 mmHg is abnormal. During the eye examination, one should assess for papilledema. Any abnormalities on cardiac or neurologic examination warrant referral to the appropriate specialist.

Differential diagnosis

Vasovagal syncope

The most common form of syncope or presyncope in the pediatric population is **vasovagal syncope**. This disorder is known by many names including neutrally-mediated syncope, neurocardiogenic syncope, vasodepressor syncope, positional orthostatic tachycardia syndrome, orthostatic hypotension, or common faint.

The history is usually diagnostic with symptoms occurring during postural changes due to altered sympathetic tone. With standing, blood pools in the lower extremities, resulting in decreased venous return to the heart. This causes a decreased cardiac output, leading to cerebral blood flow that is inadequate to maintain consciousness. Vasovagal syncope can occur after prolonged standing (such as in church) and during times of emotional distress (such as at the sight of blood). Syncope after taking a hot shower, after combing hair, or after voiding or defecating are all classic variants of vasovagal syncope. This form of syncope is most common in adolescents but can be seen in younger children. Most patients will have resolution of the symptoms during late adolescence or early adulthood.

Testing for orthostatic hypotension during the physical examination is a useful screening tool for this disorder

Pediatric Heart Disease: A Practical Guide, First Edition. Piers E. F. Daubeney, Michael L. Rigby, Koichiro Niwa, and Michael A. Gatzoulis.
© 2012 Blackwell Publishing Ltd. Published 2012 by Blackwell Publishing Ltd.

but has low sensitivity. Most patients respond to increased daily fluid and salt intake, but some may need medical treatment.

Treatment of vasovagal syncope

- Reassurance
- Avoidance of precipitating factors, e.g. waiting in line
- Recognition of warning symptoms
- Once symptoms experienced:
  - Sitting on floor or lying down
  - Isometric maneuvers, e.g. Jendrassik or
  - Vigorous movement of lower limbs
- Increase fluid intake and add salt to diet
- Medication: fludrocortisone, midrodine
- Dual chamber pacemaker rarely required

Neurologic cause

Neurologic causes of syncope and presyncope are significantly less common than vasovagal syncope. These include seizure disorders, migraines, intracranial tumors, and transient ischemic attacks. While not diagnostic, a history of seizure-like movements, posturing, loss of bowel or bladder function, or a postictal state are all concerning for a neurologic etiology.

Cardiac causes

Patients with cardiac causes of syncope or presyncope are at greatest risk of sudden death. Symptoms that occur with exercise are more worrisome for a cardiac etiology.

Arrhythmias are the most common cardiac causes of syncope or presyncope (see Chapters 23 and 24). Especially serious are arrhythmias associated with long QT syndrome, Wolff–Parkinson–White syndrome, Brugada syndrome, or arrhythmogenic right ventricular dysplasia. These arrhythmias include ventricular tachycardia, ventricular fibrillation, sick sinus syndrome, and complete heart block. Patients will most commonly report palpitations, but may have syncope without warning.

Acquired heart disease, such as myocarditis or cardiomyopathies may present with syncope or presyncope due to arrhythmias, but usually is associated with other symptoms such as fatigue, exercise intolerance, or shortness of breath.

In the rare circumstance when patients with congenital heart diseases such as aortic stenosis or congenital coronary abnormalities have syncope, it is typically associated with exercise. Patients with single ventricle physiology are at risk for developing arrhythmias that may lead to syncope.

Pulmonary hypertension is a final cardiac cause of syncope and presyncope. Often a loud P2 will be the only abnormality on physical examination, and a high index of suspicion may be needed to make the diagnosis. The EKG commonly shows a right axis deviation with right ventricular hypertrophy and perhaps secondary T-wave abnormalities.

Other causes

Other non-cardiac causes include electrolyte abnormalities due to any cause, such as eating disorders, or hypoglycemic spells. Drug intoxications are an important part of the differential diagnosis. Finally, psychiatric disorders may produce syncope or presyncope symptoms.

Investigation and referral

The majority of patients will not require an extensive work-up or cardiology consultation. Patients with vasovagal syncope do not require further testing, although an EKG may be considered. Tilt table testing may be useful to help confirm the diagnosis of vasovagal syncope in cases where the etiology is not certain, or when the patient does not respond to initial therapy. However, this test has a relatively low sensitivity and specificity and is not recommended routinely.

Patients who do not clearly have vasovagal syncope should receive a screening EKG. A cardiologist should always be consulted if:

- Syncope occurred with exercise;
- Family history of sudden death, cardiomyopathy or other cardiac disease;
- Abnormal findings on cardiac examination;
- Abnormal EKG.

The cardiologist may choose to perform an echocardiogram to evaluate for structural heart disease, or use a Holter or event monitor to evaluate for arrhythmias. An exercise test may be useful if the symptoms occur with exercise. Occasionally, the patient may be referred for an electrophysiologic study to elicit arrhythmias, or for a cardiac CT, MRI or cardiac catheterization to assess for coronary abnormalities, or arrhythmogenic right ventricular dysplasia.

Further reading

Driscoll DJ, Jacobsen SJ, Porter CJ, Wollan PC. Syncope in children and adolescents. *J Am Coll Cardiol* 1997;29:1039–1045.

Johnsrude C. Current approach to pediatric syncope. *Pediatr Cardiol* 2000;21:522–531.

Sapin SO. Autonomic syncope in pediatrics: a practice-oriented approach to classification, pathophysiology, diagnosis, and management. *Clin Pediatr* 2004;43:17–23.

38   Chest pain

William H. Neches[1] and Gregory H. Tatum[2]

[1]Children's Hospital of Pittsburgh of UPMC, Pittsburgh, PA, USA
[2]Duke University Medical Center, Durham, NC, USA

Chest pain is a common complaint in pediatric patients of all ages and is one of the most common reasons for a pediatric cardiology office consultation.

History

A thorough history of the pain is essential, including the localization, nature, intensity, duration, and radiation, as well as any associated symptoms, alleviating or aggravating factors, and the frequency of episodes. The setting in which the pain occurs is important. Exercise-induced pain is more worrisome for a cardiac etiology. A history of participation in sports, or trauma and/or pain that is positional or varies with respiration, suggest a musculoskeletal origin. Family history may reveal relatives with sudden death, early myocardial infarction, familial hypercholesterolemia, arrhythmias, or congenital heart defects. Social history should include information regarding the use of alcohol, tobacco, recreational drugs, and any significant psychologic stressors.

The most frequently encountered type of chest pain typically occurs at rest and is located centrally or slightly to the left of the midline, in children from 11 to 16 years during periods of growth. The pain may be continuous or wax and wane, lasting anything from a few minutes up to 2 hours and is sometimes particularly severe. Bouts of pain can be grouped together over several days or weeks with pain free periods of several weeks or months in between. Intermittent bouts of pain may occur for 2–3 years. This is one of the most common symptoms encountered in a pediatric cardiac clinic and is probably more common in those who have had a previous median sternotomy although certainly not confined to patients who have undergone cardiac surgery. The exact cause is unknown and such pain is often described as "idiopathic" or "nonspecific." The term "growing pains" may well be correct. The condition is benign, probably musculoskeletal in origin but not associated with local tenderness.

Physical examination

Vital signs, the patient's general state, and all organ systems should be assessed. The quality and timing of the heart sounds, any murmur, rub or gallop, the femoral pulses, and distal perfusion should be noted. In addition to palpation of the precordial area, the entire chest wall should be palpated vigorously in an attempt to reproduce the pain, both with and without deep inspiration.

Differential diagnosis

Causes of chest pain in childhood

- **Idiopathic chest pain** is the most common type in the pediatric population. The pain may persist for years, but is benign.
- **Musculoskeletal chest pain,** such as costochondritis or trauma, is the next most common type. The physical examination is diagnostic, with palpation of the affected muscle group or joint reproducing the pain. Treatment is supportive and should include a period of avoiding strenuous activity.
- **Respiratory causes** account for 12–21% of chest pain and include asthma, pneumonia, pleural effusion, pneumothorax, and pulmonary embolism.

Pediatric Heart Disease: A Practical Guide, First Edition. Piers E. F. Daubeney, Michael L. Rigby, Koichiro Niwa, and Michael A. Gatzoulis.
© 2012 Blackwell Publishing Ltd. Published 2012 by Blackwell Publishing Ltd.

- **Gastrointestinal causes** occur at a frequency similar to cardiac causes. Patients typically describe a burning pain localized to the mid or lower chest that is temporally related to eating. These disorders include esophagitis, gastritis, gastroesophageal reflux, peptic ulcers, cholecystitis, pancreatitis, hiatal hernia, foreign bodies, and esophageal rupture.
- **Cardiac problems** are among the least common causes of pediatric chest pain (see below).
- **Psychiatric causes** for chest pain occur in 5–17% of cases and are more common in adolescents.
- There are numerous other rare causes of chest pain.

Cardiac causes

Cardiac causes of chest pain can be divided into arrhythmias, acquired heart diseases, and underlying congenital defects.

- Children with **arrhythmias** commonly present with chest pain, but normally have tachycardia or an irregular heart beat on history and/or physical examination.
- Acquired lesions can also produce chest pain:
  ○ **Pericarditis**, which frequently presents with chest pain, is most often non-specific but can follow a viral illness or be a part of rheumatic fever
  ○ **Endocarditis, cardiomyopathies, myocarditis, and rheumatic fever** are more likely to present with other classic symptoms, such as fevers or exercise intolerance, but also can be associated with chest pain
  ○ **Acquired coronary artery lesions** due to Kawasaki disease, accelerated atherosclerotic coronary artery disease, or cocaine use produce chest pain.
- **Pulmonary hypertension** is a rare cause of chest pain, but these patients normally have fatigue, exercise intolerance, palpitations, and/or syncope.
- The vast majority of structural cardiac abnormalities are not associated with chest pain.

- Patients who have undergone **heart surgery** in the past month may have postpericardiotomy syndrome.
- Lesions such as aortic stenosis, which can lead to decreased myocardial perfusion and ischemia, may cause chest pain, which almost always occurs with exercise.
- Other less common cardiac problems associated with chest pain include aortic aneurysm with dissection (as can be seen in Marfan syndrome or coarctation of the aorta), mitral valve prolapse, and congenital coronary artery abnormalities.

Investigation and referral

In the vast majority of cases no further evaluation will be required. Patients should be referred to a cardiologist if there are:
- Other cardiac symptoms;
- An abnormal cardiac examination; or
- Chest pain is exercise-induced without associated asthma.

Most cardiac causes of chest pain can be assessed with EKG and echocardiography. Holter monitoring can be useful to assess for possible arrhythmias. When the chest pain is exercise-induced, exercise testing can be useful. Other studies, such as CT, MRI or cardiac catheterization, may be required.

Further reading

Cava JR, Sayger PL. Chest pain in children and adolescents. *Pediatr Clin North Am* 2004;51:1553–1568.

Ives A, Daubeney PEF, Balfour-Lynn IM. Recurrent chest pain in the well child. *Arch Dis Child* 2010;95:649–654.

Talner NS, Carboni MP. Chest pain in the adolescent and young adult. *Card Rev* 2000;8:49–56.

39 Palpitations

William H. Neches[1] and Gregory H. Tatum[2]

[1]Children's Hospital of Pittsburgh of UPMC, Pittsburgh, PA, USA
[2]Duke University Medical Center, Durham, NC, USA

Palpitations are a perception of an unusually strong or abnormal heart beat. This is a common complaint in the general pediatric population. Although normally benign in nature, palpitations can be indicative of serious underlying heart disease.

History

The history is the most important element in differentiating benign causes of palpitations from potentially life-threatening causes. Some patients will describe palpitations as the sensation of a single heart beat, while others use it to describe a fast heart rate. Any precipitating factors, duration of the palpitations, and any associated symptoms should be described, as well as the frequency of palpitations. The setting in which the palpitations occurred is also important – Did they occur at rest or with exercise? It is important to know of any underlying medical conditions. Inquiry should be made into any family history of palpitations, arrhythmias, congenital heart disease, or sudden death. Any medications or dietary supplements that the patient is using should be documented. All patients should be asked about any recreational drug use. It is also important to document the amount of caffeine intake, as caffeine use often is associated with isolated premature beats.

Physical examination

In most patients with palpitations, the physical examination will be normal. All patients should have a thorough and complete examination, including a complete cardiac examination. Patients with premature atrial or ventricular beats sometimes have premature beats audible during auscultation. Any abnormalities on cardiac examination, other than isolated premature beats, warrant referral to the cardiologist.

Differential diagnosis

The majority of patients with palpitations are not at risk of serious problems. The most common causes of palpitations are isolated premature atrial or ventricular beats, and generally these are benign. These are particularly common in patients who consume large amounts of caffeine, and symptoms may resolve with discontinuation of caffeine use. In addition to isolated premature beats, isolated ventricular bigeminy and trigeminy also generally are benign. On the other hand, four or more premature ventricular beats in a row is considered **ventricular tachycardia** and warrants further evaluation.

Another common cause for palpitations is the sensation of **sinus tachycardia**. In patients with sinus tachycardia, the symptoms normally occur at times when the heart rate would be expected to be increased, such as with emotional stress, illness or exercise; alternatively they may occur as a response to postural hypotension. If the patient describes palpitations with exercise, he or she can be asked to perform brief exercise in the office. If the symptoms are reproduced and the patient is found to be in sinus tachycardia, then he or she can be given appropriate reassurance.

Palpitations may be the presenting symptom of any arrhythmia (see Chapters 23, 24, and 37) either as an isolated abnormality or in conjunction with underlying structural heart disease. If the palpitations occur with exercise, it is more concerning for a cardiac etiology;

Pediatric Heart Disease: A Practical Guide, First Edition. Piers E. F. Daubeney, Michael L. Rigby, Koichiro Niwa, and Michael A. Gatzoulis.
© 2012 Blackwell Publishing Ltd. Published 2012 by Blackwell Publishing Ltd.

although palpitations due to cardiac disorders most certainly also do occur at rest.

Causes of palpitations in children with a structurally normal heart

- Isolated premature atrial or ventricular beats (benign)
- Isolated non-conducted P waves with forceful next beat (benign)
- Isolated atrial or ventricular bigeminy and trigeminy (generally benign)
- Atrial of ventricular couplets and triplets (generally benign)
- Sensation of sinus tachycardia (benign):
  - Emotional stress, dehydration, illness or exercise
  - Secondary to postural hypotension
- Supraventricular tachycardia: four or more premature atrial beats in a row (warrants further evaluation)
- Ventricular tachycardia: four or more premature ventricular beats in a row (warrants further evaluation)
- Other arrhythmia

Investigation and referral

The majority of patients will not require an extensive work-up, or a cardiology consultation. It is reasonable to obtain a CXR to look for signs of underlying cardiac disease. Additionally, all patients should have an EKG to investigate for evidence of pre-excitation, arrhythmias, premature beats, or conduction abnormalities.

Patients who are suspected of having a rhythm disorder, or underlying structural heart disease, should be referred to a pediatric cardiologist. Further testing will depend on the suspected abnormality and may include echocardiography, exercise testing, cardiac CT or MRI, cardiac catheterization, and/or electrophysiologic studies.

Further reading

Nehgme R. Recent developments in the etiology, evaluation, and management of the child with palpitations. *Curr Opin Pediatri* 1998;10:470–475.

40 Stridor

William H. Neches[1] and Gregory H. Tatum[2]

[1]Children's Hospital of Pittsburgh of UPMC, Pittsburgh, PA, USA
[2]Duke University Medical Center, Durham, NC, USA

The majority of patients with stridor do not have any cardiac disease, and thus routine referral of patients with stridor is not common.

History

Historical findings may help in the differential diagnosis of stridor, including the age of onset, changes with position or time of day, or if the stridor is persistent or intermittent. Respiratory symptoms should be noted. Fever, rhinorrhea or rash suggests an infectious cause. Swallowing difficulties and stridor may be indicative of a tracheoesophageal fistula. Cardiovascular symptoms are not common even with cardiac causes. A detailed past medical, surgical, family, and social history, including any prior intubation, should be obtained.

Physical examination

Any dysmorphic features should be noted. Nasal congestion or cervical lymphadenopathy suggests an infectious cause. The effect of positional changes on the degree of stridor should be assessed by evaluating the patient in the prone and supine positions, and with the neck flexed and extended. Any signs of respiratory distress should be noted. Cardiovascular signs that may be present include a pulsatile mass in the neck, or diminished pulses in the extremities. Any murmurs should be noted as they may indicate underlying congenital heart disease.

Differential diagnosis

Respiratory causes

The most common causes of stridor are respiratory diseases. With either an infectious or anatomic etiology, the pathology results in a significantly narrowed airway diameter.

The most common infectious cause of stridor is **viral croup**. These patients normally have other signs and symptoms of infection. They typically have worsening of the stridor at night and often improvement with exposure to cold or humidified air.

Patients with **epiglottitis** also may present with stridor. These patients usually appear toxic and obtaining a secure airway is an emergency. Bacterial tracheitis may have a similar, less severe presentation.

Numerous anatomic abnormalities may result in stridor, with **tracheomalacia** and **laryngomalacia** being the most common. These patients normally present in infancy and may worsen significantly before improving over time. Symptoms often improve in the prone position and may worsen with inhaled beta-agonists.

Foreign body aspiration is a common cause of acute onset of stridor during the early childhood years.

Other respiratory causes include choanal atresia, laryngeal webs or cysts, vocal cord paralysis, subglottic stenosis, and vocal cord papillomas. Patients with macroglossia (as in Down syndrome) or micrognathia (as in Pierre–Robin syndrome) may have stridor. Another frequent cause of stridor is spasmodic croup, which is a recurrent sudden-onset stridor that typically occurs at night. Unlike viral croup, it is not preceded by an upper respiratory tract infection.

Cardiac causes

Cardiac causes of stridor are extremely rare and typically present with very severe stridor in early infancy. These include any form of a **vascular ring**, such as aortic arch and pulmonary artery anomalies, which can cause extrinsic compression of the airway. The majority of these patients never experience stridor, and the disorder is

Pediatric Heart Disease: A Practical Guide, First Edition. Piers E. F. Daubeney, Michael L. Rigby, Koichiro Niwa, and Michael A. Gatzoulis.
© 2012 Blackwell Publishing Ltd. Published 2012 by Blackwell Publishing Ltd.

diagnosed as an incidental finding. Referral to a cardiologist is usually made after a pulsatile mass is seen to compress the airway during laryngoscopy or bronchoscopy.

Cardiac causes of stridor (see Chapter 12)

- Pulmonary artery sling
- Double aortic arch
- Right aortic arch with aberrant left subclavian artery and left-sided ligamentum arteriosum
- Right aortic arch with mirror-image branching and retroesophageal ligamentum arteriosum from diverticulum of Kommerell (rare)
- Left aortic arch with aberrant right subclavian artery and right-sided ligamentum arteriosum (rare)
- Left aortic arch with retroesophageal right descending aorta, aberrant right subclavian artery, and right ligamentum arteriosum (rare)
- Right aortic arch with aberrant left innominate artery and left-sided ligamentum arteriosum (very rare)
- Cervical aortic arch with aberrant subclavian artery and ipsilateral ligamentum arteriosum

---

These lesions can occur as isolated anomalies, but are more commonly associated with other structural heart disease.

Investigation and referral

Patients with stridor who have any findings suggestive of cardiac disease should be referred to a cardiologist. In addition, clinicians should have a higher suspicion for a cardiac etiology in patients who have very severe stridor early in life. When severe stridor is present, a CXR should be obtained to evaluate for any signs of underlying heart disease. If this is normal, then evaluation by an otolaryngologist or pulmonologist should occur. If any extrinsic compression of the airway is seen, then further cardiac evaluation is appropriate. The cardiologist usually will obtain an echocardiogram to assess the anatomy, but also may obtain a cardiac CT, MRI, or catheterization if further imaging is needed.

Further reading

Kussman BD, Geva T, McGowan FX. Cardiovascular causes of airway compression. *Paediatr Anaes* 2004:14:60–74.

Maiya S, Ho Y, Daubeney PEF. Vascular rings, pulmonary slings and other abnormalities. In: Gatzoulis MA, Webb GD, Daubeney PEF, eds. *Diagnosis and Management of Adult Congenital Heart Disease*, 2nd edn. Elsevier, 2010, pp. 277–287.

41 Cyanosis and cyanotic spells

William H. Neches,[1] Gregory H. Tatum,[2] and Michael L. Rigby[3]

[1]Children's Hospital of Pittsburgh of UPMC, Pittsburgh, PA, USA
[2]Duke University Medical Center, Durham, NC, USA
[3]Royal Brompton Hospital, London, UK

Cyanosis is a blue/gray color to the skin or mucous membranes resulting from an increased concentration of reduced hemoglobin; 5 g/100 mL of reduced hemoglobin in the cutaneous blood vessels is needed for the clinical recognition of cyanosis. It may result from the desaturation of arterial blood ("central cyanosis") or an increased extraction of oxygen by peripheral tissues in the presence of normal systemic arterial oxygen saturation ("peripheral cyanosis"). Normal transient physiologic peripheral cyanosis, particularly around the lips and extremities of the arms and legs, is extremely common and may be brought on by exposure to cold water or cool air. Any type of cyanosis is much more obvious in patients with polycythemia and less so with anemia.

History

It is important to document in what setting the cyanosis occurred, how frequently, and over what time period.
• Was the cyanosis limited to the hands and feet?
• Was it noted around the mouth, or does it involve the mucous membranes?
• Was the cyanosis associated with rapid or deep breathing, or any respiratory distress?
• Has a murmur been noted previously, or is there a diagnosis of congenital heart disease?

Any respiratory or infectious symptoms should be detailed. A complete review of systems, and past medical, family, and social history should be obtained.

Physical examination

The presence of any dysmorphic features should be noted. Differentiating tachypnea from respiratory distress is an important part of the physical examination. Patients with respiratory distress should have significant retractions and may have nasal flaring with grunting.

The cardiac examination should include assessment of precordial activity, heart sounds, as well as any extra heart sounds such as murmurs or clicks. It is important to remember that no murmur may be present during a hypoxemic spell in a patient with congenital heart disease.

A complete assessment of all other organ systems should be performed as well. **Clubbing**, although sometimes associated with chronic lung disease, is almost always present in cyanotic heart disease in patients older than 6–8 months of age. Patients with arterial hypoxemia will demonstrate central cyanosis best detected in the oral mucosa. Perioral and peripheral cyanosis, or acrocyanosis, do not reflect a hypoxemic state unless accompanied by central cyanosis. Acrocyanosis is due to vasoconstriction. This finding in a newborn or a small infant is a normal physiologic phenomenon.

Breath-holding spells are another common cause of reported cyanotic episodes. In these patients, the history of a fright, or serious crying episodes, followed by breath holding, cyanosis, and often transient loss of consciousness, is quiet characteristic.

Pediatric Heart Disease: A Practical Guide, First Edition. Piers E. F. Daubeney, Michael L. Rigby, Koichiro Niwa, and Michael A. Gatzoulis.
© 2012 Blackwell Publishing Ltd. Published 2012 by Blackwell Publishing Ltd.

Classification and causes

> **Peripheral cyanosis**
> - Normal intermittent "physiological" cyanosis
> - Congestive heart failure
> - Low cardiac output
> - Circulatory shock
> - Acrocyanosis of the newborn
> - Polycythemia
>
> **Abnormal hemoglobin**
> - Methemoglobinemia
> - Carbon monoxide poisoning
> - Sulfhemoglobinemia
>
> **Central cyanosis**
> - Cyanotic heart disease:
>   ◦ Intracardiac right-to-left shunts
>   ◦ Common mixing situations
> - Intrapulmonary shunting:
>   ◦ Pulmonary arteriovenous fistula
>   ◦ Chronic liver disease with multiple arteriovenous fistulae
> - Pulmonary hypertension and Eisenmenger syndrome
> - Inadequate alveolar ventilation:
>   ◦ Weakness of respiratory muscles
>   ◦ Parenchymal lung disease
>   ◦ Airway obstruction (congenital or acquired)
>   ◦ Obesity and "Pickwickian" syndrome
>   ◦ Asthma
>   ◦ Central nervous system depression
>   ◦ Seizures

Peripheral cyanosis

One of the most frequent reasons for referral to a pediatric cardiologist before the age of 3 years is a history of intermittent blue coloration of the lips and around the mouth in an infant or toddler who is well and symptom-free even during episodes of appearing cyanosed. This is best described as "normal intermittent peripheral cyanosis." There will be a normal systemic arterial saturation, normal physical examination, and absence of finger clubbing, together with a normal EKG, CXR, and echocardiogram (if performed). Peripheral cyanosis is a common finding after variants of the Fontan operation, and is frequently observed in patients with other low cardiac output situations, including tachyarrhythmia, congestive heart failure, and circulatory shock.

Central cyanosis

Cyanotic congenital heart disease includes common mixing situations, right-to-left intracardiac shunts, and complete transposition.

> **Common mixing** (see Chapter 16)
> - Common atrium
> - Total anomalous pulmonary venous connection
> - Tricuspid atresia
> - Mitral atresia and other variants of absent left atrioventricular connection
> - Double inlet ventricles (variants of "single ventricle")
> - Truncus arteriosus ("common arterial trunk")
>
> **Right-to-left shunts** (see Chapters 10, 15, and 21)
> - Ebstein malformation with oval fossa atrial septal defect
> - Tetralogy of Fallot with pulmonary stenosis or atresia
> - All variants of pulmonary atresia with ventricular septal defect (VSD)
> - Severe pulmonary stenosis
> - Pulmonary atresia with intact ventricular septum
> - Pulmonary hypertension (pulmonary vascular disease)

The classical form of intrapulmonary shunting is due to focal or multiple pulmonary arteriovenous fistulae. These may be congenital or related to the "Fontan" operation or liver disease. So-called intrapulmonary shunting encountered in parenchymal lung disease (pneumonia, respiratory distress syndrome, cystic fibrosis, and fibrosing alveolitis), pulmonary edema, and others is a form of ventilation–perfusion mismatch of some lung segments. Other reasons for inadequate alveolar ventilation include CNS depression caused by opiates and other respiratory depressants, obesity, airway obstruction and respiratory muscle weakness caused by myopathy, muscular dystrophy, peripheral neuropathy, and other neurologic problems.

Hyperoxia test (nitrogen washout test)

The hypoxia test is used with decreasing frequency, but is still of use when it is difficult to distinguish parenchymal lung disease or persistent pulmonary hypertension from cyanotic heart disease.

Infants are placed in 90–100% oxygen for 10 min via a head box or mask. With a right radial artery blood gas the following is a useful guide:
- $pO_2 > 33$ kPa (>250 mmHg): Excludes cyanotic heart disease;
- $pO_2 > 26$ kPa (>200 mmHg): Cyanotic heart disease very unlikely;
- $pO_2 < 13$ kPa (<100 mmHg): Cyanotic heart disease extremely likely.

> **Consequences of central cyanosis**
> - Polycythemia
> - Clubbing of fingers and toes
> - Hypercyanotic spells (*vide infra*)
> - Squatting
> - CNS complications:
>   - Brain abscess
>   - Cerebrovascular accident
>   - Hemiplegia

Hypercyanotic ("hypoxic") spells (see also Chapter 15 and Appendix A)

The mechanism of hypercyanotic or "hypoxic" spells in congenital heart disease is not completely understood. Predisposing conditions include not only tetralogy of Fallot with pulmonary stenosis but also any form of pulmonary atresia with VSD, "classical" tricuspid atresia, or the much rarer Holmes heart (double inlet left ventricle), each with concordant ventricular–arterial connection, restrictive VSD, and pulmonary stenosis. Approximately 40% of infants with tetralogy will develop increasingly severe hypercyanotic spells during the first year of life. Other heart malformations are implicated much less frequently.

Mild at first but becoming progressively more severe, hypercyanotic spells are very variable in duration and last anything from 5 to 20 min. They are characterized by paroxysms of rapid and often deep breathing, variable irritability with whining rather than crying loudly, and a shorter murmur of pulmonary stenosis which may disappear completely. A severe spell may lead to limpness, convulsions, stroke or even death.

There is no relationship between the degree of resting cyanosis and the likelihood of a spell. Although infundibular spasm might be the cause in tetralogy, any event that suddenly lowers systemic vascular resistance and causes an increased right-to-left ventricular shunt may precipitate a spell. Examples are defecation, crying, or induction

of anesthesia. The resulting fall in systemic arterial PO_2, along with the increase in PCO_2 and fall in pH, stimulates the respiratory center and produces hyperpnea. This in turn increases the impact of the negative intrathoracic pressure, increasing systemic venous return. In the presence of fixed pulmonary stenosis or pulmonary atresia with systemic pulmonary collaterals or a small systemic artery-to-pulmonary artery shunt, the increased systemic venous return to the ventricles must go to the aorta, further decreasing the arterial oxygen saturation. Thus the vicious spiral of a hypoxic spell is established. The same mechanism can be responsible for paroxysms of severe cyanosis when pulmonary vascular disease is associated with a large VSD. It is important to be aware that seizures in infancy and reflex anoxic seizures in older children may cause severe arterial desaturation and can masquerade as cyanotic spells similar to those encountered in tetralogy.

Treatment
The principles of treatment are aimed at breaking the spiral of events described above by the use of the following maneuvers:
- The knee–chest position trapping venous blood in the legs and reducing systemic venous return;
- Intravenous morphine to suppress the respiratory center and abolish hyperpnea;
- Sodium bicarbonate by intravenous infusion to correct acidosis;
- Nasal oxygen to increase arterial oxygen saturation (minimally);
- Intravenous vasoconstrictors such as phenylephrine to increase systemic resistance;
- Intravenous propranolol to relieve infundibular spasm.

Familial types
- **Erythrocyte reductase deficiency** (autosomal recessive): Bluish coloration of skin in a patient likely to be otherwise well.
- **Generalized reductase deficiency** (autosomal dominant): Causes developmental delay, failure to thrive, mental retardation, seizures, and premature death.
- **Hemoglobin M disease** (autosomal dominant defect of the hemoglobin molecule): Bluish coloration of skin in a patient who is likely to be otherwise well.

Abnormal hemoglobin
Acquired methemoglobinemia
Cyanosis may result from the build-up of methemoglobin (MHb) in the blood. Acquired methemoglobine-

mia, which is more common that familial types of cyanosis, arises from exposure to certain drugs and chemicals:
- Benzocaine and xylocaine;
- Benzene;
- Antimicrobials (dapsone and chloroquine);
- Nitrites and nitrates.

Blue coloration of the skin, headache, fatigue, lack of energy, and breathlessness on exertion or even at rest are characteristic symptoms.

Diagnosis
- Arterial blood gas analysis and pulsed oximetry will be normal
- Blood sampling detects abnormal hemoglobin
- Family history may be important

Treatment
- Methylene blue, but avoid in glucose-6-phospate dehydrogenase (G6PD) deficiency or if family history (hemolysis has been reported even in patients without G6PD deficiency).
- Ascorbic acid may reduce methemoglobin levels.
- Hyperbaric oxygen or exchange transfusion in severe cases.
- Identify and avoid responsible drug or chemical in acquired type.

Sulfhemoglobinemia
Sulfhemoglobinemia is a rare disorder of hemoglobin characterized by severe cyanosis without congenital heart disease in which there is excess sulfhemoglobin (SHb) in the blood. The pigment is a greenish derivative of hemoglobin which cannot be converted back to normal, functional hemoglobin. It causes intense cyanosis even at very low blood levels. Automated blood gas analysis using spectrophotometry does not distinguish between SHb and MetHb. Another confusing aspect is that some agents known to cause methemoglobinemia also cause sulfhemoglobinemia.

It is usually drug induced:
- Acetanilid;
- Phenacetin;
- Nitrates;
- Trinitrotoluene;
- Sulfur compounds (mainly sulfonamides, sulfasalazine);
- Occupational exposure to sulfur compounds;
- Phenazopyridine.

Chronic constipation may also be a cause.

There are few adverse clinical consequences because cyanosis is so apparent at low concentrations of SHb.

Treatment
Careful observation until the SHb gradually disappears with the normal physiologic turnover of red cells is usually adequate.

Summary

There are many causes of cyanosis and it is important to be aware of those conditions that can masquerade as cyanotic heart disease or hypoxic spells. In general, a good history and examination coupled with an EKG and CXR will provide a short differential diagnosis. Cross-sectional echocardiography will not always be required to provide a definitive diagnosis but should be performed if an underlying congenital heart malformation is possible.

Further reading

Hutter D, Redington AN. The principles of management, and outcomes for, patients with functionally univentricular hearts. In: Anderson RH, Baker EJ, Penny D, Redington AN, Rigby ML, Wernovsky G (eds) *Paediatric Cardiology*. Philadelphia: Churchill Livingstone/Elsevier, 2010, pp. 687–696.

42 Activity restriction

William H. Neches[1] and Gregory H. Tatum[2]

[1]Children's Hospital of Pittsburgh of UPMC, Pittsburgh, PA, USA
[2]Duke University Medical Center, Durham, NC, USA

Determining which patients are at risk for sudden cardiac death is a daunting task. While some patients with underlying heart disease obviously warrant restrictions being placed on their activity, the more difficult task is detecting those previously healthy patients who are at risk for sudden death. Any patient who has had cardiovascular symptoms, such as chest pain with exercise, palpitations, racing heart rate, lightheadedness, or syncope, should be referred for further evaluation. Likewise, any patient with an abnormal cardiac examination should also be referred. The recommended screening of athletes varies from region to region; therefore, any further screening should be in accordance with regional guidelines.

It is important to consider both the type of activity and the setting in which the patient would be participating when determining if a patient with known heart disease should have restrictions placed on his or her activities. The key element in determining whether a patient can participate in any activity is their being able to stop immediately upon feeling any chest pain or lightheadedness, without affecting the outcome of a play. Invariably, this is impossible in organized, competitive, varsity level athletics. Thus, when counseling families, it is important to differentiate between competitive athletics and unorganized sports activities played with friends.

The majority of patients with underlying congenital heart disease will be able to participate in some form of sports activity. As a general rule, patients who never required repair, either because of spontaneous closure of a defect, or because their defect was trivial, can participate fully in sports programs. Patients who have undergone complete repair and have no residual problems may be able to participate in sports activities, while others may require significant limitations to their activity. There are extensive guidelines for the assessment of patients with congenital heart disease and for the restrictions on their participation in competitive sports activities. At a minimum, patients with a history of congenital heart disease will need an extensive physical examination to be cleared for sports participation. Further testing may be warranted based on the patient's condition. This testing may include an EKG, exercise testing, and echocardiography, or other modalities.

Recommendations for exercise proscription for patients with congenital heart disease

- No restriction on physical activity:
  - Patients with left-to-right shunting lesions with normal pulmonary pressure and no cardiomegaly
  - Patients with mild right- or left-sided obstructive lesions (mild pulmonary stenosis, mild aortic stenosis, and mild coarctation of the aorta)
- Restricted physical activity to class IA type activities (low static and low dynamic impact):
  - Patients with left-to-right shunting lesions and some degree of pulmonary hypertension or Cardiomegaly
  - Patients with moderate-to-severe obstructive lesions
  - Patients with clinically stable repaired tetralogy of Fallot, Mustard, arterial switch, Ebstein, and the Fontan procedure
- Contraindication to physical activity:
  - Patients with severe pulmonary hypertension
  - Patients with severe cardiomegaly
  - Patients with life-threatening arrhythmias
  - Patients with class IV symptoms

Pediatric Heart Disease: A Practical Guide, First Edition. Piers E. F. Daubeney, Michael L. Rigby, Koichiro Niwa, and Michael A. Gatzoulis.
© 2012 Blackwell Publishing Ltd. Published 2012 by Blackwell Publishing Ltd.

As for patients with congenital heart disease, there are published guidelines for screening patients with acquired heart disease for sports participation. Many patients with acquired diseases, such as myocarditis and rheumatic fever, will have sufficient recovery that may allow full participation. However, patients who have significant valvar damage, from either rheumatic fever or endocarditis, or those with hypertrophic cardiomyopathy, should be restricted from some activities. Athletes often will have enlarged hearts which can make differentiating a healthy athlete from a patient with hypertrophic cardiomyopathy challenging. Patients who had Kawasaki disease with evidence of coronary artery disease may need to be restricted in their activities. Patients who are known to have Marfan syndrome are at risk for developing aortic dissection, and should not participate in strenuous, organized sports activities, especially if there is a possibility of a blow to the chest. In addition, in these patients, as well as those with aortic valve regurgitation, isometric activities such as wrestling and weight lifting are to be discouraged since the increased blood pressure from these activities may contribute to progressive aortic root dilation.

Patients who have arrhythmias, with or without underlying structural heart disease, may be at risk for sudden death. Patients who are noted to have isolated asymptomatic premature beats (without a prolonged QT interval) should have an EKG to confirm the diagnosis, but usually require no further testing. Patients with any other form of arrhythmia should be evaluated by a cardiologist to determine their need for activity restrictions. Some of the arrhythmias associated with sudden death include arrhythmogenic right ventricular dysplasia, long QT syndrome, Brugada syndrome, and catecholaminergic polymorphic ventricular tachycardia. Any patient who requires an implantable automated cardioverter–defibrillator should be restricted from competitive athletics.

Clearance for airline travel

During air travel the plane is pressurized at an altitude of 5000 feet and therefore the oxygen content in the plane may be below 21%. For most cardiac patients this will not cause any problems. However, the FiO_2 is an important determinant of pulmonary vasodilation and any decrease in the oxygen content may result in some degree of pulmonary vasoconstriction. In patients with a single ventricle physiology, or with pulmonary hypertension, this may result in adverse sequelae. These patients should discuss their travel plans with a cardiologist before flying.

Further readings

Maron BJ. Sudden death in young athletes. *N Engl J Med* 2003;24:845–899.

Maron BJ, Chaitman BR, Ackerman MJ, *et al.*; Working Groups of the American Heart Association Committee on Exercise, Cardiac Rehabilitation, and Prevention. Councils on Clinical Cardiology and Cardiovascular Disease in the Young. Recommendations for physical activity and recreational sports participation for young patients with genetic cardiovascular diseases. *Circulation* 2004:109:2807–2816.

Appendix A
Resuscitation algorithms

Margarita Burmester

Royal Brompton Hospital, London, UK

Bradycardia algorithm (with a pulse and poor perfusion)

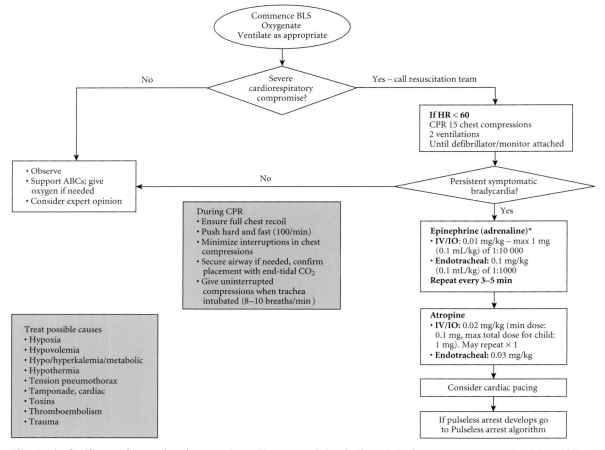

Commence BLS
Oxygenate
Ventilate as appropriate

Severe cardiorespiratory compromise?

No → • Observe
• Support ABCs; give oxygen if needed
• Consider expert opinion

Yes – call resuscitation team

If **HR < 60**
CPR 15 chest compressions
2 ventilations
Until defibrillator/monitor attached

Persistent symptomatic bradycardia?

No → (to Observe box)

Yes →

Epinephrine (adrenaline)*
• **IV/IO:** 0.01 mg/kg – max 1 mg (0.1 mL/kg) of 1:10 000
• **Endotracheal:** 0.1 mg/kg (0.1 mL/kg) of 1:1000
Repeat every 3–5 min

Atropine
• **IV/IO:** 0.02 mg/kg (min dose: 0.1 mg, max total dose for child: 1 mg). May repeat × 1
• **Endotracheal:** 0.03 mg/kg

Consider cardiac pacing

If pulseless arrest develops go to Pulseless arrest algorithm

During CPR
• Ensure full chest recoil
• Push hard and fast (100/min)
• Minimize interruptions in chest compressions
• Secure airway if needed, confirm placement with end-tidal CO_2
• Give uninterrupted compressions when trachea intubated (8–10 breaths/min)

Treat possible causes
• Hypoxia
• Hypovolemia
• Hypo/hyperkalemia/metabolic
• Hypothermia
• Tension pneumothorax
• Tamponade, cardiac
• Toxins
• Thromboembolism
• Trauma

*Give atropine first if suspected increased vagal tone or primary AV block.
ABCs, airway, breathing, circulation; BLS, basic life support; CPR, cardiopulmonary resuscitation; HR, heart rate.

(Adapted with permission from 2010 American Heart Association guidelines. 2010 International Consensus on Cardiopulmonary Resuscitation and Emergency Cardiovascular Care Science with Treatment Recommendations (COSTR).)

Pediatric Heart Disease: A Practical Guide, First Edition. Piers E. F. Daubeney, Michael L. Rigby, Koichiro Niwa, and Michael A. Gatzoulis.
© 2012 Blackwell Publishing Ltd. Published 2012 by Blackwell Publishing Ltd.

Narrow complex tachycardia algorithm (with poor perfusion)

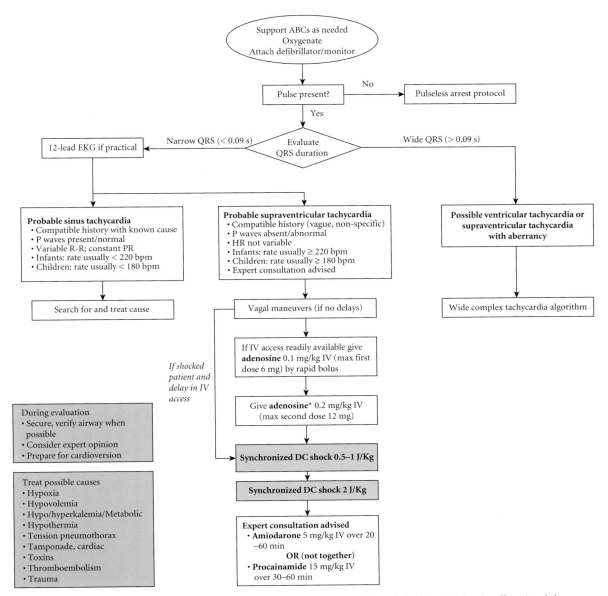

Support ABCs as needed
Oxygenate
Attach defibrillator/monitor

Pulse present? → No → Pulseless arrest protocol

Yes

Evaluate QRS duration

Narrow QRS (< 0.09 s) → 12-lead EKG if practical

Wide QRS (> 0.09 s)

Probable sinus tachycardia
- Compatible history with known cause
- P waves present/normal
- Variable R-R; constant PR
- Infants: rate usually < 220 bpm
- Children: rate usually < 180 bpm

Probable supraventricular tachycardia
- Compatible history (vague, non-specific)
- P waves absent/abnormal
- HR not variable
- Infants: rate usually ≥ 220 bpm
- Children: rate usually ≥ 180 bpm
- Expert consultation advised

Possible ventricular tachycardia or supraventricular tachycardia with aberrancy

Search for and treat cause

Vagal maneuvers (if no delays)

Wide complex tachycardia algorithm

If IV access readily available give **adenosine** 0.1 mg/kg IV (max first dose 6 mg) by rapid bolus

If shocked patient and delay in IV access

Give **adenosine*** 0.2 mg/kg IV (max second dose 12 mg)

During evaluation
- Secure, verify airway when possible
- Consider expert opinion
- Prepare for cardioversion

Synchronized DC shock 0.5–1 J/Kg

Synchronized DC shock 2 J/Kg

Treat possible causes
- Hypoxia
- Hypovolemia
- Hypo/hyperkalemia/Metabolic
- Hypothermia
- Tension pneumothorax
- Tamponade, cardiac
- Toxins
- Thromboembolism
- Trauma

Expert consultation advised
- **Amiodarone** 5 mg/kg IV over 20 –60 min
OR (not together)
- **Procainamide** 15 mg/kg IV over 30–60 min

*European Resuscitation Council (ERC) 2010 Guidelines recommend a **further third** adenosine dose at 0.3 mg/kg followed by a **fourth** adenosine dose at 0.4–0.5 mg/kg (max 12 mg) prior to cardioversion.
ABCs, airway, breathing, circulation; HR, heart rate.

(Adapted with permission from 2010 American Heart Association guidelines. 2010 International Consensus on Cardiopulmonary Resuscitation and Emergency Cardiovascular Care Science with Treatment Recommendations (COSTR).)

Wide complex tachycardia algorithm

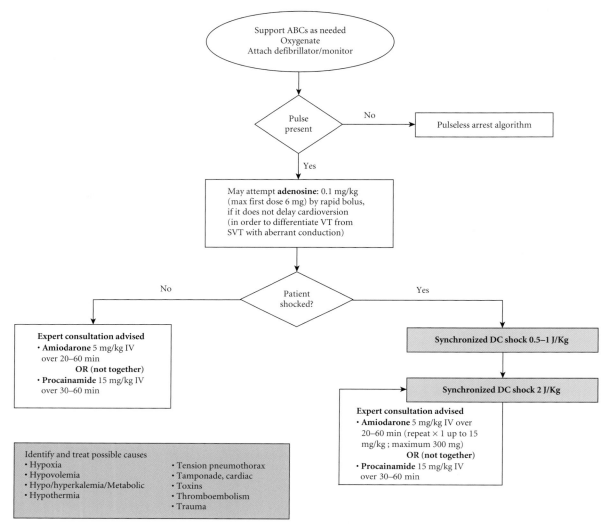

ABC, airway, breathing, circulation; SVT, supraventricular tachycardia; VT, ventricular tachycardia.

(Adapted with permission from 2010 American Heart Association guidelines. 2010 International Consensus on Cardiopulmonary Resuscitation and Emergency Cardiovascular Care Science with Treatment Recommendations (COSTR).)

Pulseless arrest algorithm

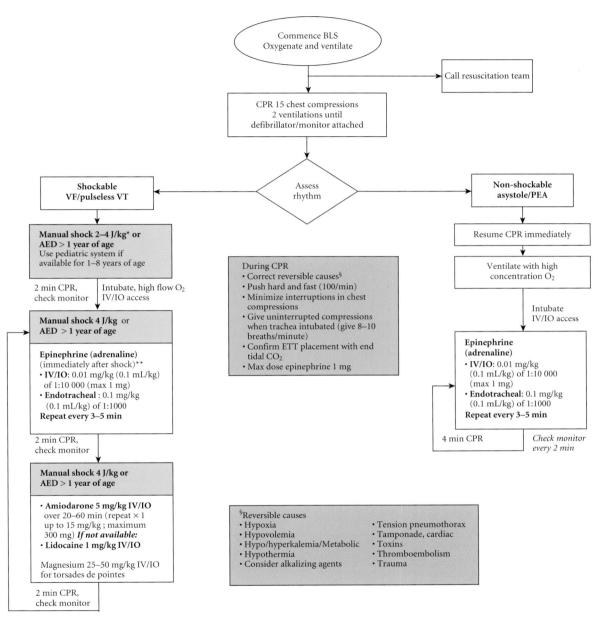

*European Resuscitation Council (ERC) 2010 Guidelines recommend first shock to be **4 J/kg**.

ERC 2010 Guidelines recommend adrenaline immediately after **third shock.

AED, automated external defibrillator; BLS, basic life support; CPR, cardiopulmonary resuscitation; PEA,

pulseless electrical activity; VF, ventricular fibrillation; VT, ventricular tachycardia.

(Adapted with permission from 2010 American Heart Association guidelines. 2010 International Consensus on Cardiopulmonary Resuscitation and Emergency Cardiovascular Care Science with Treatment Recommendations (COSTR).)

Hypercyanotic spell algorithm

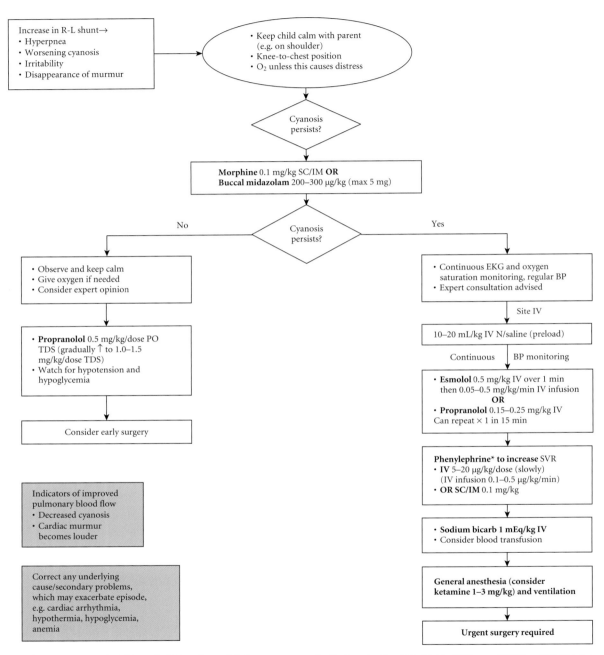

*In UK may use metaraminol 0.01 mg/kg IV (continuous infusion at 0.1–1 µg/kg/min).

BP, blood pressure; SVR, supraventricular rhythm.

(Based on information from Park MK, *The Pediatric Cardiology Handbook*, 3rd edn. Philadelphia: Mosby, 2003; Chang AC *et al. Pediatric Cardiac Intensive Care*. Philadelphia: Williams and Wilkins, 1998; Lieh-Lai M *et al. Pediatric Acute Care*, 2nd edn. Philadelphia: Williams and Wilkins, 2001.)

Appendix B
Glossary of terms commonly used in pediatric cardiac disease

Nick Hayes

Royal Brompton Hospital, London, UK

aberrant subclavian artery – anomalous origin of either subclavian artery. Most commonly the right in the context of a left aortic arch; it arises from the arch distal to the left subclavian and passes posterior to the esophagus. This generally does not produce a vascular ring, unlike a right aortic arch with aberrant left subclavian which can produce a ring if there is a left-sided duct.

absent pulmonary valve syndrome – virtual absence of pulmonary valvar tissue, resulting in free pulmonary regurgitation. Markedly dilated central pulmonary arteries cause bronchial compression, bronchomalacia, and obstructive emphysema. Found in about 2% of patients with tetralogy of Fallot, rarely associated with tricuspid atresia, ventricular septal defect, double outlet right ventricle, or an otherwise normal heart. Most cases do not have an arterial duct and the morphogenesis has been attributed to its congenital absence or premature closure.

aneurysm – discrete area of blood vessel dilatation, which may be fusiform or saccular.

angioplasty – dilatation of blood vessel with balloon catheter to alleviate area of stenosis.

annuloplasty – repair of a valve annulus using plication and/or a synthetic ring to reshape or resize valve area.

anomalous left pulmonary artery (pulmonary artery sling) – left pulmonary artery arises from the right pulmonary artery instead of the pulmonary trunk, passing behind the distal trachea, often resulting in airway compression ("stove pipe" trachea). Associated congenital heart defects occur in 50%.

anomalous origin of left coronary artery from pulmonary artery (ALCAPA) – the left coronary artery arises from the pulmonary artery instead of the aortic root. Once pulmonary vascular resistance falls, flow reversal occurs in the left coronary artery with progressive myocardial ischemia and infarction.

anomalous pulmonary venous connection – either some (partial/PAPVC) or all four (total/TAPVC) pulmonary veins fail to connect with the left atrium. Can be:
    supracardiac – drainage to innominate vein/superior vena cava/azygos vein
    cardiac – drainage to coronary sinus or occasionally directly to the right atrium
    infracardiac – drainage below diaphragm, frequently to portal veins
    mixed – drainage to more than one of the above.

aortic override – shift in the aortic root location, so that it is positioned (to a varying degree) above the interventricular septum, with connections to both the right and left ventricles.

aortopulmonary collateral – abnormal vessel connecting the systemic arterial and pulmonary arterial circulations.

Pediatric Heart Disease: A Practical Guide, First Edition. Piers E. F. Daubeney, Michael L. Rigby, Koichiro Niwa, and Michael A. Gatzoulis.
© 2012 Blackwell Publishing Ltd. Published 2012 by Blackwell Publishing Ltd.

Frequently associated with pulmonary atresia and ventricular septal defect.

aortopulmonary window – defect between the aorta and pulmonary artery, resulting from failure of complete septation of the embryonic truncus. May be in continuity with the semilunar valves, and often displays similar hemodynamics to common arterial trunk.

arrhythmogenic right ventricular dysplasia (ARVD) – there is progressive replacement of the myocardium (predominantly, but not exclusively the right ventricle) with fibro-fatty tissue; results in an increasingly dilated and poorly functioning right ventricle, which is prone to ventricular arrhythmias.

arterial switch procedure (Jatene operation) – surgical procedure used in transposition repair, involving transection and translocation of the great vessels to re-establish ventricular–arterial concordance, along with coronary artery transfer.

arteriovenous fistula/malformation – abnormal vessel between the arterial and venous circulations, which bypasses the capillary bed. If systemic, can result in progressive heart failure; if pulmonary, then cyanosis.

asplenia – anatomic or functional absence of splenic tissue. Often found in association with right atrial isomerism (heterotaxy).

atresia/atretic – imperforate or congenital absence of.

atrial isomerism – group of conditions characterized by the presence of two morphologically identical atria; either right (also termed asplenia/Ivemark syndrome) or left (also termed polysplenia syndrome). There is frequently mirror imaging of bronchial and lobar pattern, visceral heterotaxy, and associated complex congenital cardiac defects.

atrial redirection/switch procedure – procedure involving baffling of the systemic and pulmonary venous pathways, so the blood is redirected from the atrium into which it drains, to the opposite atrioventricular valve. Palliation used in previous eras in patients with transposition prior to the arterial switch and still used when performing a double switch in congenitally corrected transposition.

atrial septal defect (ASD) – defect in the interatrial septum allowing communication between both atria. Strictly speaking, the only true atrial septal defect is the oval fossa (or secundum) defect, as the primum defect is really part of the atrioventricular septal defect (AVSD) spectrum and other communications, such as sinus venosus or coronary sinus defects are not a result of deficiency in the true interatrial septum and are best termed "interatrial communications".

atrial tachycardia – tachyarrhythmia with the focus or re-entrant circuit located entirely within the atria (e.g. atrial flutter, multifocal ectopic atrial tachycardia).

atrioventricular (AV) connection – describes the relationship of the connection between the atria and ventricles. May be univentricular or biventricular, and concordant (left atrium to left ventricle, right atrium to right ventricle), discordant (left atrium to right ventricle, right atrium to left ventricle) or ambiguous (in the setting of right atrial isomerism – right-sided right atrium to right ventricle, left-sided right atrium to left ventricle; or left atrial isomerism – right-sided left atrium to right ventricle, left-sided left atrium to left ventricle). Importantly, the AV valve morphology is independent of the junctional connections.

atrioventricular re-entry tachycardia (AVRT) – commonest tachyarrhythmia in pediatric setting. An accessory pathway connects the atria and ventricular myocardium, producing a circuit with the AV node with the potential for rapid perpetual conduction. Pathway is termed "concealed" if no pre-excitation present on resting EKG.

atrioventricular nodal re-entry tachycardia (AVNRT) – as with AVRT, but the re-entry circuit is located within the AV node.

atrioventricular septal defect (AVSD) (also termed endocardial cushion defect) – congenital defect characterized by deficiency of the atrioventricular septum and a common AV junction. There is a common AV valve typically consisting of five leaflets (including superior and inferior bridging leaflets) and associated defects in either the atrial and/or ventricular septum. Often subclassified into:

    partial AVSD/primum atrial septal defect – isolated atrial component, with no ventricular defect

intermediate AVSD – atrial component with only small ventricular defect

complete AVSD – both atrial and ventricular defects. The term "unbalanced AVSD" refers to ventricular disproportion, which can be marked.

autologous – denotes re-implantation of tissue or organ within an individual person ("autograft"), as opposed to between different individuals of the same species ("allograft" or "homograft"), and between different species ("xenograft" or "heterograft").

baffle – surgically created structure used to divert blood.

balloon atrial septostomy (BAS) – palliative procedure employed to improve atrial mixing of blood. First described by Rashkind in 1966. The atrial communication is enlarged by pulling an inflated balloon from the left atrium, through the patent foramen ovale to the right atrium.

Barth syndrome (Type II 3-methylglutaconic aciduria) – X-linked neurometabolic syndrome with variable penetrance characterized by cyclical neutropenia, skeletal myopathy, dilated cardiomyopathy, and 3-methylglutaconic aciduria.

bicuspid aortic valve – the aortic valve consists of two, rather than the usual three, leaflets. Sometimes this is "functionally bicuspid," where there is a rudimentary third leaflet fused to another. There may be associated aortic stenosis and/or regurgitation. Present in approximately 2% of the population, although seen in up to 75% of patients with coarctation.

bidirectional superior cavopulmonary anastomosis/ bidirectional Glenn (BDG)/hemi-Fontan – procedure involving anastomosis of the superior caval vein to the pulmonary artery in patients undergoing univentricular palliation. Superior systemic venous return fills the pulmonary circulation passively, which offloads the ventricle compared to a systemic–pulmonary shunt. The original description by Glenn involved end-to-end anastomosis of the distal superior caval vein to the disconnected right pulmonary artery, but patients often remained significantly cyanosed. The procedure has been subsequently modified to end-to-side anastomosis of the distal superior caval vein to a right pulmonary artery still confluent

with the left pulmonary artery (hence the term "bidirectional Glenn").

bilateral bidirectional cavopulmonary anastomosis – as with bidirectional cavopulmonary anastomosis, but performed when there are bilateral superior caval veins without a bridging vein, with both being anastomosed to the pulmonary arteries.

biventricular atrioventricular connection – morphologic description of the AV connection when both atria are connected to their own ventricle. Also see atrioventricular connections.

blade atrial septostomy – as with balloon atrial septostomy, but the defect in the atrial septum is created using a wire blade passed through a long venous sheath.

Blalock–Hanlon atrial septectomy – palliative procedure involving partial resection of atrial septum from a right thoracotomy to improve mixing across the atrial septum.

Blalock–Taussig (BT) shunt – palliative shunt procedure employed to either supply or increase pulmonary blood flow. An anastomosis is created between the subclavian artery and the pulmonary artery, either by transection and anastomosis of the subclavian artery (classic BT shunt) or, now more commonly, by using an interposition tube graft between both arteries (modified BT shunt).

bridging leaflets – the superior and inferior leaflets of a common atrioventricular valve, so termed as they "bridge" the interventricular septum.

Bruce protocol – a standardized exercise stress test protocol on a treadmill that increases in both slope and speed over time.

cardiac catheterization – use of catheters for either cardiac diagnostic purposes (e.g. angiography, direct pressure measurements, and hemodynamic calculations) or interventional cardiac procedures (e.g. angioplasty, stenting, and device closure of defects).

cardiac tamponade – accumulation of fluid in pericardial cavity causing cardiac compression and consequent hemodynamic compromise.

cardiomegaly – cardiac enlargement, typically defined on anteroposterior chest radiography as a cardiothoracic ratio > 50%.

cardiomyopathy – pathologic process affecting the myocardium, resulting in impaired systolic and/or diastolic ventricular function. Traditionally classified into three types: hypertrophic, dilated, and restrictive, with distinct etiologic factors and pathophysiologic features.

cardioversion – use of DC electrical shock to terminate cardiac arrhythmia.

Carpentier procedure – a technique for repairing Ebstein anomaly, where the tricuspid valve annulus and atrialized portion of the right ventricle are plicated, and the atrial septal defect closed.

CATCH 22 – an acronym encompassing the associated features observed in patients with a microdeletion at chromosome 22q11, also known as DiGeorge and velocardiofacial syndromes: **C**ardiac defects (typically conotruncal abnormalities), **A**bnormal facies, **T**hymic hypoplasia, **C**left palate, and **H**ypocalcemia (secondary to parathyroid abnormalities).

cervical aortic arch – an elongated, usually right-sided, aortic arch extending into the neck above the clavicle and producing a pulsating mass palpable in the right supraclavicular fossa.

Chagas disease – an important cause of dilated cardiomyopathy in Central and South America. Due to the protozoan parasite *Trypanosoma cruzi*.

CHARGE association – group of associated defects including: **C**oloboma, **H**eart defects (commonly conotruncal and arch abnormalities), choanal **A**tresia, growth and mental **R**etardation, **G**enitourinary abnormalities, and **E**ar abnormalities (including deafness).

"cleft" left atrioventricular valve – description of the abnormal trileaflet left atrioventricular valve found in partial atrioventricular septal defects, formed by the commissure between the superior and inferior bridging leaflets, and therefore not strictly a "cleft".

coarctation of the aorta – discrete narrowing of the aortic arch, usually around the point of ductal insertion (isthmus). Obstruction to systemic outflow occurs once the patent ductus arteriosus has closed which, depending on the severity of coarctation, can present with neonatal collapse or adult hypertension.

commissurotomy – surgical relief of valve leaflet fusion to increase the effective orifice size and reduce obstruction.

common atrium (also termed single atrium) – condition where the atrial septum is completely absent. Seen in Ellis–van Creveld syndrome and atrial isomerism.

common arterial trunk (also termed truncus arteriosus) – a single great vessel arises from the ventricles, which subsequently branches to give rise to both the aorta and pulmonary arteries. The aortic arch is right sided in around 30% and interrupted in around 10% of patients. Up to one-third of patients also have 22q11 deletion.

concordant atrioventricular connection – see atrioventricular connection.

concordant ventricular–arterial connection – see ventricular–arterial connection.

conduit – surgically inserted tube, connecting adjacent parts of the cardiovascular system.

congenital complete heart block – complete heart block originating in fetal life as a result of damage to the atrioventricular conduction system. Frequently associated with maternal lupus (systemic lupus erythematosus) and Sjögren syndrome with anti-Ro and La antibodies.

congenitally corrected transposition of the great arteries (also termed l-transposition and double discordance) – there is atrioventricular and ventricular–arterial discordance, resulting in the right ventricle becoming the systemic ventricle. Often associated with ventricular septal defects and pulmonary stenosis.

conotruncal defect – encompasses a group of defects arising from abnormal septation of the aortic and pulmonary outflow tracts (including tetralogy of Fallot, common arterial trunk and interrupted aortic arch). Strong association with 22q11 deletion.

constrictive pericarditis – chronic inflammation results in pericardial fibrosis, causing compression of the myocardium and severe restriction in diastolic ventricular filling.

coronary fistula – abnormal communication between a coronary artery and cardiac chamber, great artery or vein. May be isolated or occur in the setting of pulmonary atresia with intact ventricular septum, with fistulae between the coronary artery and right ventricle, sometimes with associated coronary artery stenoses.

cor pulmonale – right-sided heart failure secondary to pulmonary hypertension resulting from pulmonary vascular or parenchymal lung disease.

cor triatriatum (sinister) (also known as divided left atrium) – condition where the left atrium is divided into two chambers (one receiving the pulmonary veins and the other adjoining the mitral valve) by a membrane. More rarely, this can occur in the right atrium by failure of regression of the right valve of the sinus venosus (cor triatriatum dexter; *also* known as divided right atrium).

criss-cross atrioventricular connection/criss-cross heart – rotation of the atrioventricular relationship results in an apparent crossing of the atrioventricular connections which can be either concordant or discordant. Frequently associated with other cardiac defects.

Dallas criteria – histopathologic criteria for the diagnosis of myocarditis from myocardial biopsy: inflammatory infiltrate and associated myocyte necrosis or damage.

Damus–Kaye–Stansel operation – procedure involving pulmonary artery transection and anastomosis of the proximal end to the ascending aorta, thereby committing both great arteries to the systemic circulation. Pulmonary blood flow supplied by either a Blalock–Taussig shunt (with subsequent cavopulmonary connection) or right ventricle-to-pulmonary artery conduit.

Danon disease – an X-linked condition characterized by mutation in the lysosomal-associated membrane protein 2 (LAMP2). Presents in teenage years with hypertrophic cardiomyopathy and impaired systolic function.

dextrocardia – the heart is abnormally located in the right hemithorax. This can be isolated or associated with situs inversus, atrioventricular discordance, isomerism, lung abnormality or scimitar syndrome.

diaphoresis – sweatiness.

diastolic dysfunction – impairment in myocardial relaxation, results in a reduction in ventricular compliance, and consequently abnormal and often reduced diastolic ventricular filling. The ventricular end-diastolic pressure is high.

DiGeorge syndrome – an association of abnormalities (see CATCH 22) resulting from abnormal development of the pharyngeal pouches. Over 80% of patients have a documented microdeletion at chromosome 22q11. Cardiac defects, which are predominantly conotruncal in origin, are observed in around 80%. There is marked cross-over with other reported 22q11 syndromes, although the hallmark of DiGeorge is thymic hypoplasia resulting in defective T-lymphocyte function.

discordant atrioventricular connection – see atrioventricular connection.

discordant ventricular–arterial connection – see ventricular–arterial connection.

double aortic arch – type of vascular ring, with persistence of both right and left aortic arches (which arise from the single ascending aorta and combine to form the single descending aorta). Encircles the trachea and esophagus, often producing secondary obstructive symptoms.

double chambered right ventricle – hypertrophy of muscle bundles within the right ventricle results in cavity obstruction, but at a point proximal to the pulmonary infundibulum. Often associated with a ventricular septal defect.

double discordance – atrioventricular and ventricular–arterial discordance. See congenitally corrected transposition of the great arteries.

double inlet ventricle – both atria connect predominantly to one ventricle either through two separate atrioventricular valves or less commonly through a common atrioventricular valve. Straddling or overriding of a valve may occur. Double inlet left ventricle is the most common (70%) while double inlet right ventricle or solitary indeterminate ventricle are more likely to be associated with a common valve.

double orifice mitral/left atrioventricular valve – a fibrous bridge of tissue connects the anterior and posterior leaflets of the mitral valve, creating two orifices (which may be stenotic), both connecting to the left ventricle. May be associated with coarctation and atrioventricular septal defect.

double outlet ventricle – both great arteries arise predominantly from one ventricle, which is far more commonly the right (DORV) than the left (DOLV). Ventricular septal defect location and commitment varies, as does the great artery relationship.

double switch procedure – combination of an atrial redirection and arterial switch operation for patients with congenitally corrected transposition. Also used to describe the reversal of a previous atrial switch procedure and then arterial switch operation for patients with transposition.

doubly-committed sub-arterial ventricular septal defect – see ventricular septal defect.

Down syndrome – chromosomal disorder, resulting from trisomy 21, with typical phenotypic features and associated abnormalities. Around 40% have a congenital cardiac lesion, most commonly atrioventricular septal defect (40%), atrial septal defect, ventricular septal defect, and tetralogy of Fallot.

Duckett Jones criteria – see Jones criteria.

Duke criteria – set of major and minor criteria used when establishing a diagnosis of infective endocarditis.

Ebstein anomaly – anomaly of the tricuspid valve, where the septal and inferoposterior leaflets are displaced into the right ventricular (RV) cavity, resulting in a portion of the RV becoming incorporated into the right atrium (i.e. "atrialized") and functional RV hypoplasia. There is frequently significant tricuspid regurgitation and 25% of patients have associated Wolff–Parkinson–White syndrome.

Edwards syndrome – almost invariably fatal chromosomal disorder, resulting from trisomy 18. Typical phenotypic features include overlapping fingers, rocker-bottom feet, micrognathia, low set ears, and associated cardiac defects (predominantly ventricular septal defect, atrial septal defect, patent arterial duct, and bicuspid aortic valve).

Ehlers–Danlos syndrome – group of heritable connective tissue disorders characterized by hyperextensibility of joints and hyperelasticity of skin. Associated with mitral and tricuspid valve prolapse and arteriopathy of the ascending aorta.

Eisenmenger syndrome – severe, irreversible pulmonary hypertension secondary to pulmonary vascular obstructive disease because of a pre-existing large systemic to pulmonary shunt. As pulmonary pressures become supra-systemic, the shunt reverses and cyanosis ensues.

endocardial cushion defect – see atrioventricular septal defect.

endocardial fibroelastosis – diffuse fibrosis of the endocardium (which may, but not always, appear highly echogenic) with associated myocardial dysfunction. May be primary or secondary when associated with congenital heart defects, notably hypoplastic left heart syndrome and critical aortic stenosis.

extracorporeal membranous oxygenation (ECMO) – use of cardiopulmonary bypass circuit to support either oxygenation (V-V ECMO) or both oxygenation and circulation (V-A ECMO) in intensive care unit patients with critical cardiopulmonary disease.

Fabry disease – X-linked recessive lysosomal storage disease, due to deficiency of alpha-galactosidase A. Associated with hypertrophic cardiomyopathy, abnormalities of the aortic and mitral valves, and a short PR interval.

fenestration – an opening or communication between two structures.

Fick principle – principle developed by Adolf Fick through which cardiac output and systemic-to-pulmonary shunting can be calculated on the basis of measured oxygen concentration and consumption.

Fontan procedure – palliative "univentricular" operation performed in patients in whom a biventricular repair is not feasible. Following previous superior cavopulmonary connection, the inferior systemic venous return is diverted to flow passively into the pulmonary arteries, committing the entire systemic venous return to the pulmonary circulation. Various modifications to the original procedure have now been adopted, and the term "total cavopulmonary circulation (TCPC)" tends to be used instead of "Fontan procedure" to reflect this.

> **classic Fontan** – direct connection between right atrium and pulmonary artery with a valved conduit
> **lateral tunnel** – inferior vena cava is baffled within the right atrium to the pulmonary arteries
> **extracardiac** – the inferior vena cava is disconnected from the right atrium and anastomosed to the pulmonary arteries via an extracardiac conduit.

fusion beat – EKG complex formed when a ventricular ectopic beat occurs so late in the cardiac cycle that a sinus impulse has already caused partial ventricular depolarization, resulting in a complex that is midway between a true ventricular ectopic and a normally conducted QRS complex.

Gerbode defect – rare defect in the atrioventricular septum, resulting in a shunt from the left ventricle to the right atrium.

Ghent criteria – set of clinical criteria used in establishing a diagnosis of Marfan syndrome.

Glenn shunt – see bidirectional superior cavopulmonary anastomosis.

"goose neck" deformity – description of the left ventricular outflow tract deformity resulting from unwedging of the aorta in an atrioventricular septal defect

hemi-Fontan – see bidirectional superior cavopulmonary anastomosis.

hepatopulmonary syndrome – development of pulmonary arteriovenous malformations in patients with chronic liver disease and cirrhosis, resulting in blood bypassing alveolar gas exchange with consequent cyanosis.

heterotaxy – abnormal "sidedness" of the abdominal and thoracic organs in contrast to situs solitus/inversus. Often associated with atrial isomerism.

Holt–Oram syndrome – autosomal dominant condition comprising of radial defects of the forearm and wrist, and associated with cardiac defects (typically atrial septal defect and ventricular septal defect).

Holter monitoring – 24-h ambulatory EKG monitoring.

homograft – transplanted tissue or organ from another individual of same species. Synonymous with "allograft".

hypercyanotic spell – episode of increased cyanosis in patients with tetralogy of Fallot related to acute spasm of the pulmonary infundibulum causing further reduction in the pulmonary blood flow and increase in the degree of right-to-left shunting. Often leads to attempts by the patient to increase systemic vascular resistance (e.g. by squatting). Now less common with the trend for earlier surgical repair.

hyperoxic test (also termed nitrogen wash-out test) – test aimed at establishing whether cyanosis is likely to be secondary to congenital heart disease (where arterial PaO_2 remains <14 kPa despite 100% O_2) or other pathology.

hypertrophic obstructive cardiomyopathy (HOCM) – type of cardiomyopathy characterized by inappropriate myocardial hypertrophy (typically asymmetrical hypertrophy of interventricular septum), which can result in progressive left ventricular outflow obstruction and be associated with sudden death (particularly on exertion).

hypoplastic left heart syndrome (HLHS) – congenital defect characterized by hypoplasia of the left ventricle and often encompassing a spectrum of hypoplasia and stenosis throughout the left heart (including mitral/aortic atresia, arch hypoplasia, and coarctation). Systemic circulation initially depends on right-to-left shunting through the duct and subsequent surgical palliation involves the Norwood procedure.

infundibulum – describes any funnel-shaped passage or structure, but in the context of cardiac morphology more specifically refers to the sleeve of myocardium connecting the right ventricle to the pulmonary artery. A subaortic infundibulum can also occur in certain congenital heart defects.

innocent murmur (also termed functional/physiologic/vibratory) – murmur in the absence of structural heart disease, which can occur in up to 25% of children and is of no significance. Subdivided into various types (e.g. Still's, pulmonary flow murmur, and venous hum) depending on character and location.

interrupted aortic arch – can be thought of as extreme form of coarctation, where complete discontinuity occurs between the ascending and descending aorta. Categorized according location of interruption:

Type A (30%) – distal to left subclavian artery

Type B (50%) – between left common carotid and left subclavian (aberrant right subclavian artery common)

Type C (20%) – between innominate (brachiocephalic) and left carotid arteries.

Frequently associated with a ventricular septal defect and bicuspid aortic valve; 22q11 deletion is found in around 15% of patients.

interrupted inferior vena cava (IVC) – the IVC is interrupted below the confluence with the hepatic veins and usually drains to the superior vena cava via the azygos system. Frequently seen in left atrial isomerism.

Ivemark syndrome – see atrial isomerism.

Jatene operation – see arterial switch procedure.

Jervell–Lange–Nielsen syndrome – autosomal recessive condition characterized by congenital deafness and prolonged QT interval (through mutations in *KCNE1* and *KCNQ1* genes).

Jones criteria (also termed Duckett Jones criteria) – consist of five major (arthritis, carditis, erythema marginatum, nodules, and chorea) and four minor manifestations that provide criteria for diagnosis of acute rheumatic fever (revised in 1993).

junctional rhythm – cardiac rhythm originating from the atrioventricular junction (either within or adjacent to the atrioventricular node), which can occur as an automatic tachycardia (JET) or as an escape mechanism in either heart block or marked sinus bradycardia.

juxtaposition of atrial appendages – rare anomaly seen in transposition and other complex congenital cardiac conditions where the atrial appendages are situated side by side.

Kartagener syndrome – autosomal recessive condition consisting of situs inversus, dextrocardia, and ciliary dysmotility (leading to chronic sinusitis and bronchiectasis).

Katz–Wachtel phenomenon – eponymous term for the presence of large equiphasic RS voltages in the mid-precordial EKG leads – implying biventricular hypertrophy.

Kawasaki disease (also termed mucocutaneous lymph node syndrome) – a multisystem vasculitis of unknown etiology characterized by pyrexia of 5 days or more and a number of clinical criteria, including rash, non-purulent conjunctivitis, mucositis, extremity changes, and cervical lymphadenopathy. There is frequently a pancarditis, but the main concern revolves around coronary arteritis, with a proportion suffering from coronary aneurysm formation.

Kommerell's diverticulum – enlarged proximal portion of an aberrant right subclavian artery at its origin from the descending part of a left aortic arch. Term also often used to describe a similar "aortic diverticulum" sometimes observed in the left subclavian artery when associated with a right aortic arch, although this did not form part of the original case report.

Konno procedure/aortoventriculoplasty – augmentation of the left ventricular outflow tract (LVOT) by creating and then patching a ventricular septal defect, enlargement of the aortic "annulus," and aortic valve replacement. Performed in patients with long segment subvalvar LVOT obstruction and also as part of the Ross procedure when the native pulmonary valve is significantly larger than the aortic annulus (Ross/Konno).

Lecompte maneuver – maneuver employed during arterial switch operation to bring the pulmonary artery anterior to the aorta.

left superior vena cava (SVC) – may be isolated, but usually persists in the presence of a right SVC (where there may or may not be a connecting bridging vein). Usually drains via the coronary sinus to the right atrium, but can connect directly to the left atrium.

LEOPARD syndrome – genetic condition related to Noonan syndrome with mutation of the *PTPN11* gene. Acronym of **L**entigines, **E**lectrocardiographic conduction abnormalities (bundle branch block), **O**cular hypertelorism, **P**ulmonary stenosis, **A**bnormal genitalia, **R**etarded growth, and **D**eafness. Also aortic stenosis, mitral valve prolapse, and hypertrophic cardiomyopathy may occur.

levocardia – strictly refers to the situation where the heart is normally located in the left hemithorax, but there is visceral situs inversus. However, the term is commonly used to describe the usual situation of situs solitus with left-sided heart.

Lincoln–Danielson heart – form of double outlet right ventricle with subaortic ventricular septal defect, muscular subpulmonary stenosis and "L-malposition" or left-sided aortic valve.

long QT syndrome (LQTS) – condition characterized by an abnormal delay in ventricular repolarization, resulting in an increased risk of ventricular arrhythmias and sudden death (particularly on exertion). The majority of patients, but not all, demonstrate a prolonged QT interval at rest. Genetic LQTS results from a heterogeneous group of defects of myocardial ion channels, with over twelve distinct "channelopathies" now reported.

Lown–Ganong–Levine syndrome – condition characterized by short PR interval, but normal QRS duration (i.e. no pre-excitation). James fibers bypass the upper part of the atrioventricular node, but allow normal ventricular depolarization via the His–Purkinje system.

major aortopulmonary collateral artery (MAPCA) – abnormal arterial vessel originating from the aorta and connecting with the pulmonary arterial circulation. Principally found in complex congenital defects with severely reduced pulmonary blood (typically pulmonary atresia with ventricular septal defect). Collaterals originating from other arteries (e.g. subclavian) should strictly be termed systemic-pulmonary, as they do not originate from the aorta.

maladie de Roger – outdated term for a small restrictive ventricular septal defect, which is easily audible, but has no hemodynamic consequences.

Marfan syndrome – an autosomal dominant connective tissue disorder caused by a defective fibrillin gene on chromosome 15. Phenotypic features include dolichostenomelia, arachnodactyly, scoliosis, high palate, and ligamental laxity. Diagnosis is currently based on a set of clinical features (Ghent criteria). There is an increased incidence of mitral valve prolapse, valvar regurgitation, aortic root dilatation, and aortic dissection, and patients require regular cardiac screening to identify these.

Mee procedure – palliative procedure advocated in patients with pulmonary atresia, ventricular septal defect and severely hypoplastic pulmonary arteries. A direct end-to-side anastomosis is formed between the hypoplastic main pulmonary artery and the side of the ascending aorta.

mesocardia – the heart is abnormally located in the central thorax.

moderator band – broad muscular strap that crosses the right ventricular cavity and is useful in determining morphologic ventricular status.

mucocutaneous lymph node syndrome – see Kawasaki disease.

Mustard procedure – an atrial redirection procedure.

myocarditis – myocardial inflammation, usually secondary to a viral or autoimmune process, which can result in significantly impaired myocardial function.

Nikaidoh procedure – an alternative to the Rastelli procedure in transposition of the great arteries with ventricular septal defect and pulmonary stenosis. Surgical repair involves aortic translocation and reconstruction of the ventricular outflow tracts.

nodal rhythm – cardiac rhythm originating from the atrioventricular node. See junctional rhythm.

non-compaction – deep, fine trabecular clefts are present on the endocardial surface of the ventricular myocardium, giving a "spongy" appearance. Often associated with marked systolic and diastolic ventricular dysfunction.

Noonan syndrome – autosomal dominant condition, resulting from a defect on chromosome 12 and causing a mutation of the gene *PTPN11*. Overlap with LEOPARD syndrome and has similar phenotypic features to Turner syndrome. Frequently associated cardiac defects include pulmonary valve and artery stenosis, tetralogy of Fallot, and hypertrophic cardiomyopathy.

Norwood procedure – palliative procedure for hypoplastic left heart syndrome or other functionally univentricular hearts with marked aortic hypoplasia. The main pulmonary artery is disconnected and anastomosed to the augmented aorta, resulting in the right ventricle providing systemic output. The pulmonary arterial circulation is supplied by a modified Blalock–Taussig shunt (or with the Sano modification, a right ventricular to pulmonary artery conduit). Patients subsequently undergo a staged Fontan-type palliation.

one-and-half ventricle repair – palliative procedure, where a superior cavopulmonary anastomosis is created, but the native pulmonary tract remains patent with some degree of antegrade flow into the lungs. Performed in some cases of pulmonary atresia with intact ventricular septum where the right ventricular hypoplasia is moderate but not severe.

orthotopic – into the same site as the original organ that failed, as occurs in, for example, heart transplantation.

overriding valve – describes the situation when either an atrioventricular valve drains into both ventricles or a ventricular-arterial valve has origins from both ventricles. By convention, if the degree of override is > 50%, the valve is considered to be committed to the other ventricle.

oxygen consumption – metabolic rate of tissue as defined by the amount of oxygen used over a period of time.

parachute mitral valve – abnormality of the mitral valve, where the chordae from both leaflets attach to a single papillary muscle, which can often result in mitral stenosis.

partial anomalous pulmonary venous connection/ drainage (PAPVC/PAPVD) – see anomalous pulmonary venous connection.

Patau syndrome – almost invariably fatal chromosomal disorder, resulting from trisomy 13. Typical phenotypic features include holoprosencephaly, microphthalmia, cleft lip/palate, scalp defects, and polydactyly. Associated cardiac defects in 80% include ventricular septal defect, atrial septal defect, and patent arterial duct.

patent ductus arteriosus (PDA) (also patent arterial duct) – describes continued patency of the ductus, a common finding in the neonatal period, but term usually used in relation to abnormal persistence of the duct beyond the immediate perinatal period (i.e. persistent ductus arteriosus).

patent foramen oval (PFO) – lack of fusion of the secundum septum to the primum septum results in persistence of a communication between the atria. Usually there is no shunt as long as the left atrial pressure > right atrial pressure. Probe patency of the oval fossa is found in up to 25% of adults.

pentalogy of Cantrell – condition of associated midline thoracoabdominal defects, characterized by two major anomalies: ectopia cordis and abdominal wall defect (typically gastroschisis), and defects in the distal sternum, anterior diaphragm, and diaphragmatic pericardium.

pericardial defect – defect in the pericardium due to defective formation of the pleuropericardial membrane. Can lead to herniation of cardiac chambers depending on its location.

pericardiocentesis – needle perforation of pericardial sac to aspirate a pericardial effusion.

pericardotomy – surgical incision of the pericardial sac.

persistent pulmonary hypertension of the newborn (PPHN) – situation where the pulmonary vascular resistance remains markedly elevated for longer than anticipated in the neonatal period. Number of etiologies including meconium aspiration and perinatal hypoxia. Often mimics cyanotic congenital heart disease due to pulmonary V/Q mismatch and right-to-left shunting at ductal level, and can improve with prostaglandin infusion (which lowers pulmonary vascular resistance as well as maintaining ductal patency).

perimembranous ventricular septal defect – see ventricular septal defect.

polysplenia – presence of multiple areas of splenic tissue, frequently associated with left atrial isomerism.

Pompe disease (also known as glycogen storage disease type II or acid maltase deficiency) – an autosomal recessive metabolic storage disorder caused by deficiency of alpha-1,4 glucosidase, resulting in impaired breakdown of glycogen to glucose. Leads to hypertrophic cardiomegaly as well as myopathy, hepatomegaly, failure to thrive, and death.

Potts shunt – palliative procedure to increase pulmonary blood flow by formation of a direct anastomosis between the descending aorta and ipsilateral pulmonary artery (usually left). Technically difficult to control flow and with time patients frequently end up with excessive pulmonary circulation and secondary pulmonary hypertension.

pre-ductal saturations – oxygen saturations recorded from any part of the systemic circulation proximal to the ductus arteriosus, typically the right hand. Comparison with post-ductal saturations (e.g. foot) can demonstrate any right-to-left shunt at the ductal level.

pre-excitation – describes presence of a delta wave on resting EKG, indicating the existence of an accessory pathway, and hence Wolff–Parkinson–White syndrome.

protein-losing enteropathy (PLE) – complication of uncertain etiology occurring in patients following the Fontan procedure, where protein is lost in the gut, resulting in hypoalbuminemia with consequent ascites, edema, pleural effusions, and sometimes death.

pulmonary artery band – surgically created stenosis of main pulmonary artery using ligature to limit excessive pulmonary blood flow, thereby protecting the pulmonary vasculature when definitive correction of the congenital defect is not immediately advisable.

pulmonary artery sling – see anomalous left pulmonary artery.

pulmonary atresia – the right ventricular outflow tract is totally imperforate with no direct communication between the right ventricle and pulmonary artery. Pulmonary blood flow is therefore dependent on ductal shunt. The obstruction may be either membranous (i.e. valvar) or muscular. If the ventricular septum is intact, varying degrees of right ventricular hypoplasia are observed. When associated with a ventricular septal defect (essentially an extreme form of tetralogy of Fallot), the right ventricular cavity is usually of reasonable size, although the pulmonary arteries are frequently hypoplastic with associated multiple aortopulmonary collateral arteries (MAPCAs).

pulmonary hypertension – [also termed pulmonary arterial hypertension (PAH)]. The pulmonary arterial pressure is elevated above normal levels. May be primary (idiopathic) or secondary to a number of causes, including excessive volume and pressure load from an unrestrictive systemic-to-pulmonary shunt.

pulmonary vascular resistance (PVR) – the resistance that needs to be overcome (using pressure) to allow forward flow through the pulmonary circulation. Predominantly dictated by small arteriolar tone (i.e. diameter). From Ohm's law: Pressure (difference) = Flow × Resistance.

Rashkind procedure – see balloon atrial septostomy.

Rastelli classification of atrioventricular septal defect (AVSD) – subdivision of types of complete AVSD into A, B or C depending on morphology of the superior bridging leaflet and location of chordal attachments. In Type A, there are chordal attachments from the superior bridging leaflet to the crest of the ventricular septum; in Type B, to the papillary muscles of the right ventricle; and in Type C, the superior bridging leaflet is free standing without chordal attachments.

Rastelli procedure – surgical procedure involving use of an intraventricular baffle to connect the aorta to the left ventricle through the ventricular septal defect and insertion of a right ventricle-to-pulmonary artery conduit.

restrictive physiology – describes diastolic ventricular dysfunction resulting from impaired ventricular compliance. Commonly affects the right ventricle following tetralogy of Fallot repair, where characteristic antegrade flow is observed in the pulmonary artery during atrial systole.

REV procedure – similar to the Rastelli procedure, but the pulmonary artery is anastomosed directly to the right ventricle using a pericardial patch, avoiding the use of a right ventricleto-pulmonary artery conduit.

right aortic arch – the aortic arch passes to the right of the trachea, with the first head and neck vessel branching to the left. Often seen in association with tetralogy of Fallot, pulmonary atresia, and common arterial trunk. The left subclavian artery may in addition be aberrant.

Romano–Ward syndrome – autosomal dominant condition characterized by prolonged QT interval.

Ross procedure – aortic valve replacement using autologous pulmonary valve with coronary artery translocation and homograft replacement of pulmonary valve. Preferred technique in pediatric aortic valve replacement as somatic valvar growth can occur and the native pulmonary valve tends to perform better than a homograft in the aortic position.

scimitar syndrome – sequestered right lower (and occasionally middle) lobe, with systemic arterial supply from the descending aorta, and partial anomalous pulmonary venous drainage to the inferior vena cava resulting in a vertical radiographic shadow along lower right cardiac border resembling a "scimitar." Frequently associated with other cardiac defects and abnormalities of the bronchial tree.

Senning procedure – type of atrial redirection procedure.

septostomy – see balloon or blade atrial septostomy.

Shone complex – associated series of left heart obstructive lesions occurring at multiple levels, including mitral stenosis, left ventricular outflow tract obstruction, including sub-, valvar, supravalvar aortic stenosis, and coarctation.

Shprintzen syndrome – see velo-cardio-facial syndrome and CATCH 22.

shunt – surgically created connection between two circulations. Also used to indicate abnormal flow of blood from the right-to-left or left-to-right sides of the circulation.

single ventricle – strictly describes complete absence of a contralateral ventricle. Extremely rare in reality, as there is nearly always a second, albeit extremely hypoplastic, ventricle present.

single ventricle palliation – encompasses the surgical strategy employed in palliating all congenital heart defects not suitable for biventricular repair, which ultimately results in a Fontan-type circulation.

sinus venosus defect – inter-atrial communication with similar hemodynamic consequences to an atrial septal defect, but occurring as a result of abnormal development of the sinus venosus as opposed to the atrial septum. Located either posterosuperior to the oval fossa in association with the superior vena cava or, more rarely, posteroinferior in association with the inferior vena cava. Superior defects frequently associated with partial anomalous pulmonary venous connection (PAPVC) (typically right upper love pulmonary vein to superior vena cava).

situs – sidedness:
 situs solitus – usual visceral arrangement
 situs inversus – mirror image visceral arrangement
 situs ambiguous – visceral heterotaxy (isomerism).

Starnes' procedure – operation that may be required in the most severe cases of neonatal Ebstein. The tricuspid valve is sutured closed, atrial septal defect enlarged, and systemic-to-pulmonary artery shunt created, effectively creating tricuspid atresia and a single ventricle physiology.

stent – intravascular mesh prosthesis, which maintains shape once inflated to preserve vessel patency following balloon dilatation.

Still's murmur – see innocent murmur.

straddling – describes the situation where chordae from either atrioventricular valve straddle the septum and insert into both ventricles.

subaortic stenosis – obstruction to the left ventricular outflow tract just beneath the aortic valve. Usually caused by a discrete fibro-muscular ridge, although occasionally results from posterior deviation of the outlet septum.

supraventricular tachycardia (SVT) – abnormally rapid heart rate (typically >200 bpm) originating above the ventricular mass. May be focal (atrial/nodal) or re-entrant (atrial, AVRT, AVNRT) in mechanism.

Sydenham chorea – neuropsychiatric disorder, characterized by choreiform movements, occurring in approx. 20% of patients with acute rheumatic fever and forming one of the major revised Jones criteria.

syncope – transient loss of consciousness as a result of reduced oxygenated blood flow to brain.

Takeuchi repair – procedure involving formation of an intrapulmonary aortocoronary tunnel, for patients with ALCAPA in whom direct transfer of the left coronary artery is not feasible.

Taussig–Bing anomaly – type of double outlet right ventricle, with malposed great arteries and subpulmonary ventricular septal defect. Physiology similar to transposition of the great arteries with ventricular septal defect.

tetralogy of Fallot – commonest cyanotic congenital defect. There is anterocephalad deviation of the outlet septum, which fails to unite, resulting in a ventricular septal defect, right ventricular outflow tract obstruction, and aortic override. Right ventricular hypertrophy subsequently develops and is thought to be secondary to the pressure loaded ventricle. Frequently associated with pulmonary arterial stenoses, bicuspid pulmonary valve, and right aortic arch (25%). Occasionally, the pulmonary valvar tissue is absent (see absent pulmonary valve syndrome).

torsades de pointes – type of ventricular tachycardia, with characteristic "twisting" of ventricular complexes around the baseline (sinusoidal pattern). Typically occurs in patients with long QT syndrome.

total anomalous pulmonary venous connection/drainage (TAPVC/TAPVD) – see anomalous pulmonary venous connection.

total cavopulmonary circulation (TCPC) – see Fontan procedure.

transannular – crossing the valve annulus. A "transannular patch" may be required in repair of tetralogy of Fallot if the valve annulus is small.

transposition of the great arteries (TGA) (also termed d-transposition or ventricular-arterial discordance) – there is discordance of the ventricular–arterial connection, so that the pulmonary artery arises from the left ventricle and aorta from the right. Simple TGA refers to the absence of any other cardiac defects, whilst complex TGA implies the presence of other anomalies (most commonly a ventricular septal defect). Systemic oxygenation requires mixing of the circulations, which can occur at the atrial, ventricular or ductal level depending on communications.

tricuspid atresia – there is compete absence of the right atrioventricular connection, with no direct communication between the right atrium and ventricle. An obligate right-to-left shunt across the atrial septum results in systemic cyanosis. Hemodynamic consequences depend on the great artery relationship, degree of pulmonary stenosis, and size/location of ventricular septal defect.

trisomy – conditions where, in addition to the normal diploid set, an extra chromosome is present in all cell lines. Often occurs as a result of non-disjunction during meiosis.

truncus arteriosus – see common arterial trunk.

Turner syndrome – chromosomal disorder, resulting from monosomy of the X chromosome (45 XO). Typical phenotypic features include short stature, short webbed neck, and broad "shield" chest with wide-spaced nipples. Associated cardiac defects include bicuspid aortic valve (30%), coarctation of the aorta (10%), aortic stenosis, and mitral valve prolapse.

unifocalization – surgical technique involving anastomosis of multiple systemic-to-pulmonary artery collaterals to form a common vessel, which can then be connected back to the pulmonary artery. Technique utilized in repair of pulmonary atresia with ventricular septal defect and MAPCAs

univentricular atrioventricular connection – see atrioventricular connection.

unroofed coronary sinus – defect in septation of the coronary sinus (which runs in the atrioventricualr groove) and left atrium. Partial unroofing is associated with a "coronary sinus atrial septal defect". Complete unroofing causes a left superior vena cava to connect to the left atrium and may result in central cyanosis.

VACTERL association – describes sequence of associated defects: **V**ertebral anomalies, **A**nal anomalies, **C**ardiac anomalies, **T**racheo-Esophageal fistula, **R**enal anomalies, **L**imb anomalies.

valvotomy – surgical relief of valvar obstruction involving release of cusp fusion and dilatation.

valvuloplasty – cardiac catheter relief of valvar obstruction involving dilatation with balloon.

vascular ring – group of anomalies where abnormal or aberrant vascular structures completely encircle the trachea and esophagus, resulting in various degrees of compression. Commonest examples include double aortic arch, and right arch with aberrant left subclavian artery and left ligamentum arteriosum.

vascular sling – as with vascular ring, although trachea/esophagus not completely encircled. Examples include aberrant right subclavian artery and anomalous left pulmonary artery.

vasovagal syncope (also referred to as neurocardiogenic syncope) – commonest cause of syncope, where lack of neuroendocrine control of vascular tone and heart rate results in transient decrease in blood pressure and oxygenated blood flow to brain. Commonly termed a faint.

velo-cardio-facial syndrome (also termed Shprintzen syndrome) – an association of palatal abnormalities, congenital heart defects (typically conotruncal defects), and phenotypic facial features resulting from abnormal pharyngeal pouch development. Around 90% of patients have a documented microdeletion at chromosome 22q11 and there is frequently cross-over with other 22q11 deletion syndromes, with many other associated abnormalities (see CATCH 22).

venous hum – see innocent murmur.

ventricular assist device (VAD) – a mechanical pump that aids or replaces a failing heart. Termed an RVAD where the right heart is supported, LVAD where the left heart is stopped, and BiVAD where both are supported. Usually a "bridge" to transplantation.

ventricular imbalance – disproportion between left and right ventricular cavity size.

ventricular septal defect (VSD) – defect in interventricular septum allowing communication between left and right ventricles, which can occur in a number of locations and may be multiple. Symptoms and hemodynamic consequences depend on the direction and degree of shunt, which is determined by the VSD size, vascular resistance, and existence of other cardiac defects.

Location:
   muscular – all borders of the defect are muscular, and may be further described as inlet, trabecular/apical or outlet, depending on the location of the defect with respect to the right ventricular aspect of the interventricular septum. Defects extending into more than one area can be described as confluent.
   perimembranous – part of the border is formed by the membranous septum and hence located just beneath the aortic valve and in continuity with the tricuspid valve. May well extend into the inlet or outlet portions of the right ventricle.
   doubly-committed subarterial – rare defect, resulting in absence of the outlet septum and hence fibrous continuity of the aortic and pulmonary valves.

Hemodynamics:
   restrictive – implies a small left-to-right shunt with minimal symptoms of cardiac failure and protected pulmonary vasculature.
   unrestrictive – implies large left-to-right shunt with significant symptoms, cardiac failure, and elevated right-sided pressures.

ventricular tachycardia (VT) – defined as a series of three or more beats, which are typically broad complex, originating from the ventricular mass at a rate of >100 bpm. Can be polymorphic/monomorphic and sustained/non-sustained (<30 s), and results from a range of etiologies.

ventricular–arterial (VA) connection – describes the relationship between the ventricles and great arteries. Can be concordant (left ventricle to aorta, right ventricle to pulmonary artery), discordant (left ventricle to pulmonary artery, right ventricle to aorta), single or double outlet.

Waterston shunt – palliative procedure to increase pulmonary blood flow by formation of a direct anastomosis between the ascending aorta and right pulmonary artery. Technically difficult to control flow and with time patients frequently end up with excessive pulmonary circulation and secondary pulmonary hypertension.

Williams syndrome – autosomal dominant condition resulting from deletion of the *elastin* allele in chromosome 7q11. Phenotypic features include "elfin" facies, stellate pattern iris, developmental delay, "cocktail party" speech, and hypercalcemia. Frequently associated with supravalvar aortic stenosis, peripheral pulmonary artery stenosis, ventricular septal defect, and atrial septal defect. May have a generalized arteriopathy.

Wolff–Parkinson–White syndrome (WPW) – an additional abnormal connection (accessory pathway) between the atria and ventricles allows early activation of the ventricular myocardium. This results in a typical resting EKG pattern (short PR interval and delta wave) and acts as a substrate for re-entry tachyarrhythmias.

Wood unit – a unit measure of vascular resistance, typically calculated when assessing PVR (1 Wood unit = $80\,dyn{\cdot}cm{\cdot}s^{-5}$). Usually normalized for body size in pediatrics – Wood unit $\times\,m^2$.

Appendix C
Pediatric cardiac drugs and dosages

Sian Bentley
Royal Brompton Hospital, London, UK

This is the drug glossary in use at the Royal Brompton Hospital. Recommended drug doses vary around the world and from institution to institution. Clinicians should seek local advice before prescribing from these recommendations.

Pediatric Heart Disease: A Practical Guide, First Edition. Piers E. F. Daubeney, Michael L. Rigby, Koichiro Niwa, and Michael A. Gatzoulis.
© 2012 Blackwell Publishing Ltd. Published 2012 by Blackwell Publishing Ltd.

Drug	Indication	Route	Dose			Comments
			Neonates <1 month	Child 1 month – 12 years	Child >12 years	
Adenosine	Supraventricular arrhythmias	IV	Initial dose: 100 µg/kg (max 3 mg) Increase by 100 µg/kg every 1–2 min until tachycardia terminated or until maximum dose of 300 µg/kg if <1-month old or 500 µg/kg if >1-month old (max 12 mg) reached		<50 kg: see <12 years >50 kg: initial dose 3–6 mg, increased to 12 mg after 1–2 min if necessary	Rapid IV bolus over 1–2 s, flushing after each dose with 0.9% sodium chloride. Preferably via a central line, if not a large peripheral vein Do not increase dose if high level AV block develops at any particular dose Monitor EKG, heart rate, blood pressure and respiratory rate Not recommended in asthma as can cause severe bronchoconstriction Reduce initial dose by 75% if on concomitant dipyridamole
Alprostadil (prostaglandin E1)	Maintain patent ductus arteriosus	IV infusion	Initial rate: 50–100 nanograms/ kg/min adjusted to lowest effective dose Maintenance rate: 10–400 nanograms/ kg/min	N/A	N/A	**Prostaglandin E1** Monitor heart rate, respiratory rate, temperature, blood pressure, and oxygen saturations (pO₂) Can cause apnea, fever, flushing, hypotension; and may be associated with NEC **Facilities for intubation and ventilation must be available**
Amiloride hydrochloride	For potassium conservation with loop and thiazide diuretics	Oral	100–200 µg/kg (max 10 mg) BD		5–10 mg BD	**Potassium-sparing diuretic** Risk of hyperkalemia with ACE inhibitors; and in renal impairment and diabetes Monitor potassium

(*Continued*)

Drug	Indication	Route	Dose			Comments
			Neonates <1 month	Child 1 month – 12 years	Child >12 years	
Amiodarone	Supraventricular and ventricular arrhythmias	IV **Loading**	25 µg/kg/min for 4h **or** 5–10 mg/kg over 1–2h			**Class III antiarrhythmic** Adjust dose according to clinical response, EKG, blood pressure, and heart rate.
		IV **Maintenance**	5–15 µg/kg/min (max 1.2g over 24h)			Administer via central line if possible
		Oral **Loading**	5–10 mg/kg (max 200 mg) BD for 7–10 days **or** until desired response **or** adverse effects occur		200 mg TDS for 7 days then 200 mg BD for 7 days	**Facilities for cardiac monitoring and defibrillation must be available**
		Oral **Maintenance**	5–10 mg/kg (max 200 mg) OD **or** lowest effective dose possible		200 mg OD **or** lowest effective dose possible	Monitor thyroid function tests, liver function tests, and CXR at baseline and then 6 monthly Ophthalmic exams should be carried out at baseline and then yearly, and also if visual changes occur Reduce dose of flecainide and digoxin by 50% if on concomitant amiodarone May increase INR if on warfarin Can cause photosensitivity, advise avoid exposure to the sun and use sun block where necessary
Amlodipine	Hypertension	Oral	100 µg/kg (max 5 mg) OD increased if necessary up to 400 µg/kg (max 10 mg) OD		5–10 mg OD	**Calcium channel blocker** Adjust dose according to blood pressure

Drug	Indication	Route	Dose	Notes
Aspirin	Antiplatelet	Oral	3–5 mg/kg (max 75 mg) OD	**Non-steroidal anti-inflammatory drug** Administer with or after food Temporarily discontinue in the presence of fever and/or viral illness (particularly influenza or chicken pox) and use paracetamol (acetaminophen). Consider replacing with dipyridimole for duration of intercurrent illness
	Kawasaki disease	Oral	25 mg/kg QDS for 14 days until inflammatory markers settle **or** until afebrile for 2–3 days **then** 3–5 mg/kg (max 75 mg) OD for 6–8 weeks until echocardiogram normal	
Atenolol	Hypertension, arrhythmias	Oral	0.5–2 mg/kg (max 100 mg) OD	50–100 mg OD	**Cardioselective beta-blocker** Adjust dose according to clinical response, blood pressure, and heart rate Dose may be given in two divided doses if necessary Use in asthma with extreme caution and under specialist supervision only when there is no alternative available
Bendroflumethiazide	Diuresis, hypertension	Oral	50–100 µg/kg (max 10 mg) OD	2.5–10 mg OD	**Thiazide diuretic** Doses up to 400 µg/kg OD may be needed initially then reduced to maintenance dose as dictated by clinical response, urine output, blood pressure, and fluid balance Monitor potassium

(Continued)

Drug	Indication	Route	Dose			Comments
			Neonates <1 month	Child 1 month – 12 years	Child >12 years	
Captopril	Congestive heart failure, hypertension	Oral	Initial dose: 50 µg/kg (10 µg/kg if <37/40 weeks) Usual maintenance dose: 100–500 µg/kg TDS (max 2 mg/kg/day)	Initial dose: 100 µg/kg (max 6.25 mg) Usual maintenance dose: 100–500 µg/kg TDS (max 6 mg/kg/day)	Initial dose: 6.25 mg Maintenance: 12.5–50 mg BD–TDS	**Angiotensin converting enzyme inhibitor** Adjust dose to clinical response and blood pressure Following initial dose observe every 15 min for 2 h for effect of severe hypotension Concomitant diuretics may need to be reduced or not administered concurrently to avoid severe hypotension Contraindicated in severe bilateral renal artery stenosis May elevate potassium levels; monitor potassium
L-Carnitine	Cardiomyopathy in the presence of primary or secondary carnitine deficiency	IV/ oral	25–50 mg/kg BD (max 3 g/day)			**Amino acid derivative (essential co-factor of fatty acid metabolism)**
Carvedilol	Congestive heart failure with left ventricular dysfunction	Oral	Initial dose: 50 µg/kg (max 3.125 mg) BD Double dose every 2 weeks as tolerated to a maximum dose of 400 µg/kg (max 25 mg) BD			**Non-selective beta-blocker with α_1-receptor blocking effects** Adjust dose according to clinical response, blood pressure and heart rate Contraindicated in hepatic impairment Administer with food May reduce the clearance of digoxin. Check digoxin levels 7–14 days after initiation of carvedilol

Drug	Indication	Route	Dose			Notes
Chlorothiazide	Diuresis and hypertension	Oral	10–20 mg/kg (max 500 mg) BD		125–500 mg BD	**Thiazide diuretic** Synergy with loop diuretics, administer at same time if on concomitant therapy Monitor potassium
Digoxin	Supraventricular arrhythmias	Oral **Loading**	Preterm: 25–30 µg/kg Term: 45 µg/kg	1 month – 2 years: 45 µg/kg 2–5 years: 35 µg/kg 5–10 years: 25 µg/kg >10 years: see >12 years	750 µg – 1.5 mg	**Cardiac glycoside** **Loading is only necessary in urgent situations**. Give 50% of load immediately, then 25% at 6 h and the remaining 25% at 12 h. Check EKG and clinical response after each dose to assess toxicity Reduce loading dose if patient has received digoxin in the previous 2 weeks Reduce loading dose by 50% in mild/ moderate renal failure and by 75% in severe renal impairment. Monitor levels
		IV **Loading** (over 10 min)	Preterm: 20–30 µg/kg Term: 35 µg/kg	1 month – 2 years: 35 µg/kg 2–5 years: 35 µg/kg 5–10 years: 25 µg/kg >10 years: see >12 years	500 µg – 1 mg	

(Continued)

Drug	Indication	Route	Dose			Comments
			Neonates <1 month	Child 1 month – 12 years	Child >12 years	
Digoxin (continued)	Supraventricular arrhythmias	Oral/IV **Maintenance**	Preterm: 2–3 µg/kg BD Term: 5 µg/kg BD	1 month – 5 years: 5 µg/kg BD 5–10 years: 3 µg/kg (max 125 µg) BD >10 years: see >12 years	62.5–500 µg OD	Start maintenance dose 12 h after loading ends Reduce maintenance dose by 50% in mild/moderate renal failure and by 75% in severe renal impairment. Monitor levels Levels taken at least 6 h post dose (time to steady state 5–10 days). Aim 0.8–2 µg/L Halve maintenance dose if given with amiodarone/ propafenone If converting from IV to oral administration, dose should be increased by 20% if taking liquid or by 30% if tablets to account for bioavailability Avoid hypokalemia as predisposes to digoxin toxicity Contraindicated in Wolff–Parkinson– White syndrome
Dinoprostone (prostaglandin E2)	Maintain patency ductus arteriosis	IV infusion	Initial rate: 5 nanograms/kg/min adjusted by 5 nanogram increments until effective clinical response or side effects occur Maintenance rate: 5–20 nanograms/kg/ min	N/A	N/A	**Prostaglandin E2** Monitor heart rate, respiratory rate, temperature, blood pressure, and oxygen saturations Can cause apnea, fever, flushing, hypotension; and may be associated with necrotizing enterocolitis **Facilities for intubation and ventilation must be available**

Drug	Indication	Route	Dose	Notes
Disopyramide	Supraventricular tachycardia	Oral	<1 year: 10–30 mg/kg/day in four divided doses 1–4 years: 10–20 mg/kg/day in four divided doses 4–12 years: 10–15 mg/kg/day in four divided doses 12–18 years: 6–15 mg/kg/day in four divided doses	**Class 1a antiarrhythmic** Adjust dose according to clinical response, EKG, and blood pressure Reduce dose to maximum TDS in mild renal impairment, BD in moderate impairment, and OD in severe impairment May need to reduce dose in hepatic impairment Drug levels may be monitored but not routine
Dobutamine	Low cardiac output, e.g. post cardiac surgery, cardiomyopathy	IV infusion	1–10 μg/kg/min (max 20 μg/kg/min)	**Inotrope** Stimulates mainly β₁-receptors (cardiac output) Tachycardia may be a problem Titrate to clinical and hemodynamic response
Dopamine	Low cardiac output with hypotension	IV infusion	1–10 μg/kg/min (max 20 μg/kg/min)	**Inotrope** Effects vary according to dose. Low doses <5 μg/kg/min cause vasodilation but there is little evidence that this is clinically beneficial. Between 5 and 10 μg/kg/min β effects (cardiac output) predominate and >10 μg/kg/min α effects predominate (vasoconstriction) Titrate to clinical and hemodynamic response

(Continued)

Drug	Indication	Route	Dose			Comments
			Neonates <1 month	Child 1 month – 12 years	Child >12 years	
Enalapril	Congestive heart failure, hypertension	Oral	Initial dose: 100 μg/kg (max 2.5 mg) OD (10 μg/kg in neonates) Usual maintenance dose: 300–500 μg/kg OD (max 1 mg/kg/day)		Initial dose: 2.5 mg OD Maintenance dose: 10–20 mg OD (max 40 mg)	**Angiotensin converting enzyme inhibitor** Adjust dose to clinical response and blood pressure Following initial dose observe every 15 min for 2 h for effects of severe hypotension Concomitant diuretics may need to be reduced or not administered concurrently to avoid severe hypotension Dose may be given in two divided doses if necessary 1 mg enalapril may substitute for 7.5 mg captopril Contraindicated in severe bilateral renal artery stenosis May elevate potassium levels: monitor potassium
Enoximone	Congestive cardiac failure	Oral		1 mg/kg (max 50 mg) TDS		**Phosphodiesterase inhibitor** Injection may be given orally but mix with milk feeds or orange juice immediately before taking Monitor blood pressure
Epinephrine (adrenaline)	Low cardiac output with hypotension	IV infusion	0.01–0.5 μg/kg/min (max 1.5 μg/kg/min)	0.01–0.5 μg/kg/min (max 1.5 μg/kg/min)	0.01–0.5 μg/kg/min (max 1.5 μg/kg/min)	**Inotrope (catecholamine)** Effects on β_1-, β_2- and α-receptors vary according to dose. Mainly β effects (cardiac output) at low doses and α effects (vasoconstriction) at high doses Titrate to clinical and hemodynamic response

Drug	Indication	Route	Dose		Notes
Flecainide	Supraventricular and ventricular arrhythmias	Oral	Initial dose: 2 mg/kg BD–TDS Adjust dose according to clinical response (blood pressure and EKG) and levels. Max 8 mg/kg/day or 300 mg/day	Initial dose: 50 mg BD Adjust dose according to clinical response (blood pressure and EKG) and levels to maximum 300 mg/day or 400 mg/day for ventricular arrhythmias in heavily built children	**Class 1c antiarrhythmic** Contraindicated in abnormal left ventricular function; haemodynamically significant valvular heart disease Reduce dose in severe liver impairment Reduce dose by 50% if creatinine clearance is <35 mL/min/1.73 m² and monitor levels Trough levels taken around sixth dose: 200 µg – 1 mg/L Reduce dose by 50% if on concomitant amiodarone
Furosemide	Diuresis and hypertension	IV infusion IV injection	0.1–0.3 mg/kg/h Dose up to 2 mg/kg/h can be used 0.5–1 mg/kg BD–QDS over 5–10 min (max 4 mg/min) Max single dose 4 mg/kg	10–40 mg BD–QDS	**Loop diuretic** Adjust dose to clinical response, urine output, blood pressure, fluid balance
		Oral	0.5–2 mg/kg BD–QDS	10–40 mg BD–QDS	Monitor potassium Usually administered with potassium-sparing diuretics to conserve potassium Bioavailability of oral preparations is variable, typically 60% of IV

(Continued)

Drug	Indication	Route	Dose			Comments
			Neonates <1 month	Child 1 month – 12 years	Child >12 years	
Ibuprofen	Closure of ductus arteriosus	IV infusion over 15 mins	As ibuprofen base, every 24 h: Day 1: 10 mg/kg Day 2: 5 mg/kg Day 3: 5 mg/kg	N/A	N/A	**Non-steroidal anti-inflammatory drug** Contraindicated if life-threatening infection, coagulopathies, necrotizing enterocolitis, pulmonary hypertension, marked unconjugated hyperbilirubinemia Monitor renal function: avoid in moderate to severe Inhibits platelet aggregation: monitor for bleeding If ductus reopens, a second course of three injections may be given 48 h after first course
Indomethacin	Closure of ductus arteriosus	IV infusion over 20 min	Doses given at 12-h intervals if urine output is >1 mL/kg/h after first dose. If urine output is <1 mL/kg/h but >0.6 mL/kg/h, use 24-h interval. Withhold doses if urine output is <0.6 mL/kg/h Initial dose: 0.2 mg/kg Then two doses dependent on **postnatal age at time of first dose:** <48 h: 0.1 mg/kg 2–7 days: 0.2 mg/kg >7 days: 0.25 mg/kg	N/A	N/A	**Non-steroidal anti-inflammatory drug** Contraindicated if life-threatening infection, coagulopathies, necrotizing enterocolitis, pulmonary hypertension, marked unconjugated hyperbilirubinemia Monitor renal function: avoid in moderate to severe Inhibits platelet aggregation: monitor for bleeding If ductus reopens, a second course of three injections may be given 48 h after first course

Drug	Indication	Route	Dose	Adult dose	Notes
Lisinopril	Congestive heart failure, hypertension	Oral	Initial dose: 100 µg/kg (max 2.5 mg) OD Maintenance dose: 200–600 µg/kg (max 40 mg) OD	Initial dose: 2.5–5 mg OD Maintenance dose: 10–40 mg OD	**Angiotensin converting enzyme inhibitor** Adjust dose to clinical response and blood pressure Following initial dose observe every 15 min for 2 h for effects of severe hypotension Concomitant diuretics may need to be reduced or not administered concurrently to avoid severe hypotension 1 mg may substitute for 5 mg captopril Contraindicated in severe bilateral renal artery stenosis May elevate potassium levels: monitor potassium
Metoprolol	Hypertension	Oral	Initial dose: 1 mg/kg BD Maintenance dose: Up to 8 mg/kg/day	Initial dose: 50–100 mg/day Maintenance dose: Up to 400 mg/day	**Cardioselective beta-blocker** Adjust dose to clinical response, blood pressure, and heart rate <12 years may be given in four divided doses, >12 years may be given in two divided doses if necessary
Metolazone	Diuresis	Oral	100–200 µg/kg OD–BD	5–10 mg OD–BD	**Thiazide diuretic** Synergy with loop diuretics, administer at same time if on concomitant therapy Monitor potassium Useful if resistant to loop diuretics

(Continued)

Drug	Indication	Route	Dose			Comments
			Neonates <1 month	Child 1 month – 12 years	Child >12 years	
Milrinone	Congestive heart failure, low cardiac output states post cardiac surgery, prophylaxis in patients at high risk of developing low cardiac output syndrome post cardiac surgery, patients refractory to escalating doses of catecholamines	IV infusion	Loading dose*: 75 µg/kg over 60 min Maintenance dose: 0.25–0.75 µg/kg/min			**Inodilator (phosphodiesterase enzyme 3 inhibitor)** *Reduce or omit loading dose if patient at risk of hypotension. Milrinone can cause a reduction in blood pressure of 10–15% Reduce dose in renal impairment Titrate maintenance dose to clinical and hemodynamic response
Nifedipine	Hypertensive crisis	Oral/ sublingual		250–500 µg/kg (max 10 mg) stat May be repeated every 4–6 h	5–10 mg stat May be repeated every 4–6 h	**Calcium channel blocker** May cause profound hypotension For rapid effect, bite the capsule, releasing the contents into the mouth and then swallow For smaller doses use liquid preparation or, liquid may be withdrawn from liquid-filled capsules. Contact individual manufacturer for further details
	Hypertrophic cardiomyopathy/ hypertension	Oral (standard release preparation)		200–300 µg/kg TDS (max 3 mg/kg/day)	5–20 mg TDS (max 90 mg/day)	
Norepinephrine (noradrenaline)	Septic shock, refractory hypotension with low vascular resistance	IV Infusion	0.01–0.5 µg/kg/min (max 1 µg/kg/min)	0.01–0.5 µg/kg/min (max 1 µg/kg/min)	0.01–0.5 µg/kg/min (max 1 µg/kg/min)	**Inotrope (catecholamine)** Used primarily as a vasopressor (α effects). Often used with other inotropes, e.g. dobutamine, epinephrine to maintain adequate perfusion. Titrate to clinical and hemodynamic response

Drug	Indication	Route	Dose		Notes
Palivizumab	Prophylaxis of respiratory syncytial virus (RSV) in children with serious congenital cardiac disease	IM Injection	<2 years: 15 mg/kg once a month during the RSV season	N/A	**RSV monoclonal antibody** Where possible, administer first dose prior to start of RSV season
Propafenone	Supraventricular and ventricular arrhythmias, junctional ectopic tachycardia	Oral	Initial dose: 5 mg/kg (max 150 mg) BD Maintenance dose: 5–10 mg/kg BD	<70 kg; see <12 years >70 kg; Initial dose: 150 mg TDS Maintenance dose: up to 300 mg TDS	**Class 1c antiarrhythmic** Adjust dose according to clinical response, EKG, and blood pressure May be given in three divided doses if necessary Reduce dose in liver impairment by 70–80%
Propranolol	Tetralogy of Fallot	Oral Slow IV	250 micrograms/kg – 1 mg/kg BD - QDS Initial dose: 15–20 µg/kg Can increase to 100 µg/kg under EKG control, given up to QDS	N/A N/A	**Non-selective beta-blocker** Adjust dose according to clinical response, blood pressure and heart rate
	Hypertension	Oral	250–500 µg/kg TDS (max 2 mg/kg/dose) 250 µg/kg – 1 mg/kg TDS (max 5 mg/kg/day)	40–160 mg BD	Contraindicated in asthma
Spironolactone	For potassium conservation with loop and thiazide diuretics	Oral	0.5–1.5 mg/kg BD	25–50 mg BD	**Aldosterone antagonist** Risk of hyperkalemia with ACE inhibitors; and in renal impairment Monitor potassium

(Continued)

Drug	Indication	Route	Dose			Comments
			Neonates <1 month	Child 1 month – 12 years	Child >12 years	
Sotalol	Supraventricular and ventricular arrhythmias	Oral	1 mg/kg (max 40 mg) BD increased as necessary every 3 days to maximum 4 mg/kg (max 80 mg) BD		40 mg BD increased as necessary every 3 days to 80–160 mg BD Doses up to 640 mg daily have been used under specialist supervision for life-threatening ventricular arrhythmias	**Non-selective beta-blocker with additional class III antiarrhythmic activity** Adjust dose according to clinical response, EKG, and blood pressure Contraindicated in asthma, long QT syndrome, and Torsades de pointes
Verapamil	Hypertension, prophylaxis of supraventricular arrhythmias	Oral	N/A	1–<2 years old: 20 mg BD–TDS 2–18 years old: 40–120 mg BD–TDS		**Calcium channel blocker** IV Verapamil **should not** be given to patients recently treated with beta-blockers because of the risk of hypotension and asystole. It may also be hazardous to give verapamil and a beta-blocker together by mouth (should only be contemplated if myocardial function well preserved). Avoid grapefruit juice.
	Treatment of supraventricular arrhythmias	Slow IV (with EKG and blood pressure monitoring and under specialist advice)		1–18 years old: 100–300 μg/kg (max 5 mg) as a single dose, repeated after 30 min if necessary		

Appendix D
Endocarditis prophylaxis

Jamie Cheong

Royal Brompton Hospital, London, UK

The American Heart Association (AHA) published recommendations on antibiotic prophylaxis against infective endocarditis (IE) in 2007. The National Institute for Health and Clinical Excellence (NICE) in the UK released guidelines in 2008. Both documents provide information for adult and pediatric patients. There are many similarities between the two reports and the recommendations in both are based on the current evidence available. They conclude that repetitive routine activities, such as toothbrushing, pose more of a risk of developing infective endocarditis (IE) than a single dental procedure (e.g. tooth extraction) due to the cumulative exposure to bacteremia. Both groups define particular groups at risk of endocarditis; however, the AHA specifically list patients at highest adverse risk from IE, whereas NICE defines those who are at risk of developing IE and those who are not (Table D.1).

Both groups agree that there is no firm evidence to support the clinical effectiveness of antibiotic prophylaxis against IE for dental procedures. However, NICE also states that there is no consistent link between frequency and duration of bacteremia with the development of IE in dental and non-dental procedures involving the respiratory, gastrointestinal (GI), and genitourinary (GU) tracts. This is because antibiotic prophylaxis may reduce the frequency of bacteremia but does not eliminate it post procedure. The AHA agrees that even if prophylaxis were completely effective, then only a very small number of cases would be preventable. NICE discussed that it would not be cost-effective to give antibiotic prophylaxis for all dental procedures, and associated it with harm due to the rare possibility of anaphylaxis and the realization of increasing bacterial resistance against antibiotics.

The AHA therefore does not recommend antibiotic prophylaxis for dental and non-dental procedures; however it does stipulate exceptions (Table D.2). NICE does not advise giving antibiotic cover for any dental and non-dental procedures, unless a procedure is being performed at the GI/GU tract where there is active infection in patients who are at risk of developing endocarditis (Table D.2). No specific antibiotics are mentioned, only that the antibiotics given should cover against organisms which cause IE. Recommendations based on outcomes of prosthetic valve IE were not made, even with the awareness that this was associated with a higher mortality rate.

The antibiotic regimens recommended by the AHA are given in Table D.3. It suggests single doses between 30 and 60 min before the procedure and up to 2 h post procedure. Adult and pediatric doses are given for IV or PO routes; it is advised that IM injections are avoided in patients on anticoagulants. If the patient is already on antibiotics, then an alternative class of antibiotic is advised with the avoidance of cephalosporins. For cardiac surgery, antibiotic doses may be repeated during prolonged procedures and for up to 48 h postoperatively.

The AHA does not mention giving patient advice but NICE recommends those at risk of developing endocarditis should be offered information about prevention, including:
- Benefits and risks of antibiotic prophylaxis
- Why antibiotic prophylaxis is no longer routinely recommended
- Importance of maintaining good oral health
- Symptoms that may indicate IE and when to seek expert advice
- Risks of undergoing invasive procedures, including non-medical procedures such as body piercing or tattooing.

Pediatric Heart Disease: A Practical Guide, First Edition. Piers E. F. Daubeney, Michael L. Rigby, Koichiro Niwa, and Michael A. Gatzoulis.
© 2012 Blackwell Publishing Ltd. Published 2012 by Blackwell Publishing Ltd.

Table D.1 Patients with congenital heart disease at risk of endocarditis

AHA	NICE
Specific cardiac conditions associated with highest risk of adverse outcome from IE	Patients with structural cardiac defects at risk of developing IE
Prosthetic heart valve/material for repair	Acquired valvular heart disease with stenosis or regurgitation
	Valve replacement
Previous IE	Previous IE
Some CHD:	Structural CHD, including surgically corrected or palliated structural conditions, but **not**:
• Unrepaired cyanotic CHD, including palliative shunts and conduits	• Isolated atrial septal defect
• Completely repaired CHD with prosthetic material or device, whether placed by surgery or by catheter intervention, during the first 6 months after the procedure	• Fully repaired ventricular septal defect
	• Fully repaired patent ductus arteriosus
• Repaired CHD with residual defects at the site, or adjacent to the site, of a prosthetic patch or prosthetic device (which inhibit endothelialization)	• Closure devices that are judged to be endothelialized
Heart transplant patients with cardiac valvulopathy	Hypertrophic cardiomyopathy

CHD, congenital heart disease; IE, infective endocarditis.

Table D.2 Recommendations for antibiotic prophylaxis

Antibiotic prophylaxis	AHA	NICE
Dental procedures	Not for all patients with an underlying condition that increases the lifetime risk of acquiring endocarditis	Not recommended, including the use of chlorhexidine mouthwash as this does not significantly reduce the level of bacteremia after dental procedures
	Should be given to those at highest risk of adverse outcome from IE for manipulation of gingival tissue/periapical region of teeth/perforation of oral mucosa	Treat infection promptly
Respiratory tract procedures	Not for bronchoscopy unless there is an incision	Not recommended, including ENT procedures and bronchoscopy
	Should be given to those at highest risk of adverse outcome from IE if invasive, e.g. incision or biopsy – tonsillectomy and adenoidectomy	Treat infection promptly
	Give if infection at site of procedure.	
GI/GU tract procedures	Not for endoscopy or colonoscopy	Not recommended, including gynecologic, obstetric procedures, and childbirth
	Give if there is active GI/GU infection	Treat infection promptly
		Give if undergoing procedures at infected GI or GU tract
Skin, skin structure, musculoskeletal procedures	Give if there is surgery of infected tissues	Not mentioned

GI, gastrointestinal; GU, genitourinary; IE, infective endocarditis.

Table D.3 Antibiotic regimens suggested by the AHA

Procedure	Bacterial cover against	Antibiotics
Dental	Viridans group streptococci	Amoxicillin, ampicillin, cefazolin, ceftriaxone, cephalexin, clindamycin, azithromycin, clarithromycin
Respiratory tract	Viridans group streptococci or staphylococci	As above or anti-staphylococcal penicillin, cephalosporin (MSSA) or vancomycin (MRSA)
GI/GU tract	Enterococci	Amoxicillin, ampicillin, vancomycin, piperacillin (if active infection)
Skin, skin structure, musculoskeletal	Staphylococci and β-hemolytic streptococci	Anti-staphylococcal penicillin, cephalosporin, vancomycin, clindamycin
Cardiac surgery	Staphylococci	First-generation cephalosporin, vancomycin

GI, gastrointestinal; GU, genitourinary.

Further reading

NICE. Short Clinical Guidelines Technical Team. Clinical guideline 64. Prophylaxis against infective endocarditis: antimicrobial prophylaxis against infective endocarditis in adults and children undergoing interventional procedures. London: National Institute for Health and Clinical Excellence, 2008.

Wilson W, Taubert KA, Gewitz M, *et al*. Prevention of infective endocarditis: Guidelines from the American Heart Association. *Circulation* 2007;116:1736–1754.

Appendix E
Anticoagulation guidelines

Sian Bentley and Alan G. Magee
Royal Brompton Hospital, London, UK

These are the anticoagulation guidelines in use at the Royal Brompton Hospital. Recommended drug doses vary around the world and from institution to institution. Clinicians should seek local advice before prescribing from these recommendations.

Prevention of thrombosis

Cardiac catheterization
During procedure (ACCP Guidelines 2012):
• **Arterial access:** Heparin IV 50–75 Units/kg (max 5000 Units) once arterial access obtained. Check activated clotting time (ACT) if procedure time is prolonged (>60 min) and consider further 25 Units/kg.
• **ASD closure:** Heparin IV 75–100 Units/kg (max 5000 Units) once venous access obtained.
• **VSD closure:** Heparin IV 75–100 Units/kg (max 5000 Units) once venous and arterial access obtained.
• **Endovascular stents:** Heparin IV 75 Units/kg (max 5000 Units) once arterial access obtained. Check ACT if procedure time is prolonged (> 60 min) and consider further 25 Units/kg.
• **Other indications (e.g. balloon atrial septostomy, venous catheterization in the newborn):** Consider use of heparin IV 50–75 Units/kg (max 5000 Units) once vascular access obtained, dependent on the procedure and clinical circumstances of the patient.
Post procedure:
• **Endovascular stents (ACCP Guidelines 2012, Andrew & DeVeber 999), ASD/VSD transcatheter occlusion, and radiofrequency ablation:**

○ Aspirin 3–5 mg/kg (max 75 mg in the UK, 81 mg in the USA) PO for 3 months (6 weeks for radiofrequency ablation)
○ This allows time for the device to become endothelialized. It is not necessary after device closure of the arterial duct

Post cardiac surgery:
• **Blalock–Taussig (BT) shunts (ACCP Guidelines 2012, Andrew & DeVeber 999):**
○ Immediate postoperative phase*: Heparin IV infusion to maintain activated partial thromboplastin time (APTT) between 60 and 100 s. Heparin loading dose **not** required
○ When feeds tolerated: Heparin stopped and aspirin (3–5 mg/kg, max 75 mg in the UK, 81 mg in the USA) started to continue indefinitely or until shunt taken down
• **Bidirectional cavopulmonary connection (Glenn):**
○ Immediate postoperative phase*: Heparin IV infusion to maintain APTT between 60–100 seconds. Heparin loading dose **not** required.
○ Confirm with cardiologist/surgeon whether continued anticoagulation required postoperatively. **If required:** When feeds tolerated, heparin stopped and aspirin (3–5 mg/kg, max 75 mg in the UK, 81 mg in the US) started, to continue indefinitely

---

*Heparin therapy is initiated when early postoperative blood loss has ceased, usually 2–4 hours after returning from the operating theater; or, where bleeding continues beyond this, any coagulopathies have been corrected accordingly.

Pediatric Heart Disease: A Practical Guide, First Edition. Piers E. F. Daubeney, Michael L. Rigby, Koichiro Niwa, and Michael A. Gatzoulis.
© 2012 Blackwell Publishing Ltd. Published 2012 by Blackwell Publishing Ltd.

- **Total cavopulmonary connection (TCPC/Fontan) (ACCP Guidelines 2012, Andrew & DeVeber 999):**
  - Immediate postoperative phase*: Heparin IV infusion to maintain APTT between 60 and 100 s. Heparin loading dose **not** required
  - When feeds tolerated: Warfarin (Coumadin) started and titrated to maintain an international normalized ratio (INR) of 2–4. Heparin discontinued when INR within therapeutic range for 2 consecutive days. Aspirin (3–5 mg/kg, max 75 mg in the UK, 81 mg in the US) ± clopidogrel (0.2 mg/kg) may be considered as an alternative where the therapeutic effect of warfarin is difficult to monitor, e.g. frequent blood tests in a small and/ or very uncooperative child
  - Other indications: Aspirin may be considered for other indications where use is not routine. This should be an attending pediatrician/consultant decision
- **Bioprosthetic valves (ACCP Guidelines 2008):**
  - In the **mitral position:**
    Immediate postoperative phase*: Heparin IV infusion to maintain APTT between 60 and 100 s
    When feeds tolerated: Warfarin started and titrated to maintain an INR of 2–4. Heparin discontinued when INR within therapeutic range for 2 consecutive days
    Warfarin given for 3 months then aspirin (3–5 mg/kg, max 75 mg in the UK, 81 mg in the US) to continue indefinitely
  - In the **aortic position:**
   When feeds tolerated: Aspirin (3–5 mg/kg, max 75 mg in the UK, 81 mg in the US) started, to continue indefinitely
- **Mechanical valves (ACCP Guidelines 2008):**
  - Immediate postoperative phase*: Heparin IV infusion to maintain APTT between 60 and 100 s
  - When feeds tolerated: Warfarin started and titrated to INR of 3–4 (mitral), 2–4 (aortic). Heparin discontinued when INR within therapeutic range for 2 consecutive days
- **Extracorporeal membrane oxygenation (ECMO)**
  - See ECMO local protocols

Other indications
- **Dilated cardiomyopathy:**
  - If severe cardiac dysfunction, heparin on presentation
  - Once patient stable and feeds tolerated: Aspirin (3–5 mg/kg, max 75 mg in the UK, 81 mg in the US) PO to continue until cardiac dysfunction recovers or indefinitely

  - Warfarin should be used when ongoing cardiac dysfunction is very severe
- **Kawasaki disease (ACCP Guidelines 2012):**
  - On presentation "high-dose aspirin"
  - Antiplatelet aspirin (3–5 mg/kg, max 75 mg in the UK, 81 mg in the US) PO once the anti-inflammatory markers have settled
  - Avoid concomitant use of non-steroidal anti-inflammatory drugs (NSAIDs), e.g. ibuprofen and diclofenac during aspirin therapy
  - Where giant coronary aneurysms are present, consider adding warfarin PO (aim for an INR of 2–4) to aspirin PO
- **Patients hypersensitive or intolerant of aspirin:**
  - Dipyridamole PO or clopidogrel PO may be used as alternative antiplatelet agents

Stopping antithrombotic medications prior to surgery

- **Aspirin (Drugs in the Peri-operative period 1999):** Should be stopped at least 5, (preferably 7 days) prior to the day of surgery
- **Clopidogrel (Summary of Product Characteristics 2009):** As for aspirin
- **Warfarin (Drugs in the Peri-operative period 1999):**
  - High risk of thrombosis, e.g. mechanical valves;
    Discontinue warfarin 4–5 days prior to surgery
    Admit 24 h prior to surgery and initiate heparin therapy if INR falls below therapeutic range
    Discontinue heparin 6 h prior to surgery and check that preoperative prothrombin time (PT) and APTT are within normal limits and INR is <1.5
  - Low risk of thrombosis:
    Discontinue warfarin 4–5 days prior to surgery
    Check that preoperative INR is <1.5
- **Dipyridamole:** Should be discontinued 24 h prior to surgery
- **Heparin (Drugs in the Peri-operative period 1999):** Should be discontinued 6 h prior to surgery
- **Dalteparin (low molecular weight heparin):**
  - Prophylaxis dose: Omit morning dose on day of surgery
  - Treatment dose: Discontinue 24 h prior to surgery and initiate heparin therapy

Treatment of femoral artery thrombosis

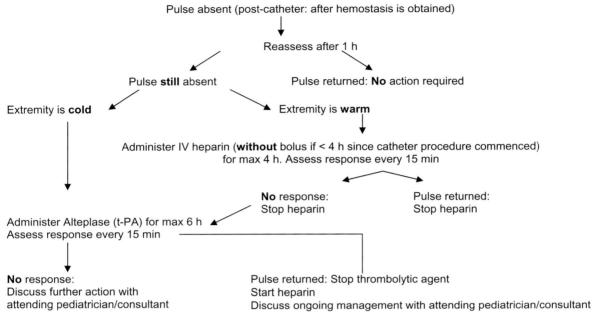

Note: Children <6 months with arterial thrombosis following cardiac catheterization: use heparin IV for a minimum of 24 h before considering thrombolytic therapy **unless** viability of the limb or organ is in doubt.

Treatment of venous thrombosis (ACCP Guidelines 2012)

<1 month old

• Heparin IV infusion to maintain APTT between 60 and 100 s **or** dalteparin (low molecular weight heparin) SC to achieve an anti-Factor Xa level of 0.5–1.0 Units/mL for 6 weeks to 3 months (the longer duration is dependent on the location and extent of thrombus)

• If associated with a central venous line, remove line, if possible, after 3–5 days of anticoagulation. If line is still in place on discontinuation of therapeutic anticoagulation (as above), use prophylactic dose dalteparin (low molecular weight heparin) SC until line removed

• Thrombolytic therapy recommended **only** if major vessel occlusion is causing critical compromise of organs or limbs. Use **alteplase (t-PA)** IV infusion and supplement with plasminogen (FFP) prior to therapy

>1 month old

• Initially heparin IV infusion to maintain APTT between 60 and 100 s or dalteparin (low molecular weight heparin) SC to achieve an anti-Factor Xa level of 0.5–1.0 Units/mL for **5–10 days**. Then warfarin PO titrated to maintain an INR of 2–4 (heparin discontinued when INR within therapeutic range for 2 consecutive days) **or** dalteparin (low molecular weight heparin) SC to achieve an anti-Factor Xa level of 0.5–1.0 Units/mL

• This should be continued for at least **3 months** for children with secondary thrombosis where the risk factor has now resolved, and at least **6 months** in idiopathic thrombosis. Where the risk factor has not resolved, anticoagulation should be continued until it has resolved (minimum 3 months)

• If associated with a central venous line, remove line, if possible, after 3–5 days of anticoagulation. If line still in place on discontinuation of therapeutic anticoagulation, use prophylactic dose dalteparin (low molecular weight heparin) SC until line removed

• Routine use of thrombolytic therapy is not recommended. Consider for patients at high risk, i.e. patients with massive hemodynamically significant pulmonary emboli; extensive venous thromboemboli with threat of venous gangrene; isolated significant inferior vena cava thrombus; pulmonary emboli not responding to standard heparin therapy

Editor's note on aspirin

Soluble aspirin is normally provided in 75 mg tablets (81 mg in the US) and this is the typical dose used for an adult. With this in mind it is easy to overdose in children. An alternative drug dose schedule that is easier for patents to administer at home can be considered:

3–5 kg	15 mg (one-fifth 75 mg/ 81 mg tablet)
5–15 kg	25 mg (one-third 75 mg/ 81 mg tablet)
15–30 kg	37.5 mg (half 75 mg/ 81 mg tablet)
>30 kg	75 mg/ 81 mg

If excessive bruising occurs, change to dose for the lower weight range.

Further reading

Andrew M, DeVeber G. *Pediatric Thromboembolism and Stroke Protocols 1999*. BC Decker Inc.

Drugs in the peri-operative period: 4 – Cardiovascular Drugs. *Drug Ther Bull* 1999;37:89–92.

Monagle, P, et al. Antithrombotic Therapy in Neonates and Children: American College of Chest Physicians Evidence-Based Clinical Practice Guidelines (9th Edition). *Chest* 2012;141:e737S–e801S.

Salem DN, O'Gara PT, Madias C, Pauker SG; American College of Chest Physicians. Valvular and structural heart disease: American College of Chest Physicians Evidence-Based Clinical Practice Guidelines (8th Edition). *Chest* 2008; 133:593–629.

Summary of Product Characteristics. Plavix (Sanofi Aventis). Last updated 21st April 2009.

Index

Page numbers in *italics* denote figures, those in **bold** denote tables.

Pediatric Heart Disease: A Practical Guide, First Edition. Piers E. F. Daubeney, Michael L. Rigby, Koichiro Niwa, and Michael A. Gatzoulis.
© 2012 Blackwell Publishing Ltd. Published 2012 by Blackwell Publishing Ltd.